When Doctors
Become Patients

When Doctors Become Patients

Robert Klitzman

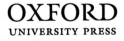

2008

OXFORD
UNIVERSITY PRESS

Oxford University Press, Inc., publishes works that further
Oxford University's objective of excellence
in research, scholarship, and education.

Oxford   New York
Auckland   Cape Town   Dar es Salaam   Hong Kong   Karachi
Kuala Lumpur   Madrid   Melbourne   Mexico City   Nairobi
New Delhi   Shanghai   Taipei   Toronto

With offices in
Argentina   Austria   Brazil   Chile   Czech Republic   France   Greece
Guatemala   Hungary   Italy   Japan   Poland   Portugal   Singapore
South Korea   Switzerland   Thailand   Turkey   Ukraine   Vietnam

Copyright © 2008 by Oxford University Press, Inc.

Published by Oxford University Press, Inc.
198 Madison Avenue, New York, New York 10016
www.oup.com

Oxford is a registered trademark of Oxford University Press

Several portions of this material appeared in different forms and contexts in
*Social Science and Medicine, Academic Medicine, Patient Education and Counseling,
Perspectives in Medicine and Biology,* and the *New York Times.*

Library of Congress Cataloging-in-Publication Data
Klitzman, Robert.
   When doctors become patients / Robert Klitzman.
       p. ; cm.
   Includes bibliographical references and index.
   ISBN 978-0-19-532767-0
   1. Physicians—Miscellanea.   2. Physician and patient—Miscellanea.
3. Physicians—Anecdotes.   I. Title.
   [DNLM: 1. Physicians—psychology—Personal Narratives.   2. Attitude of Health
Personnel—Personal Narratives.   3. Attitude to Health—Personal Narratives.
4. Physician Impairment—psychology—Personal Narratives.   5. Physician's
Role—psychology—Personal Narratives.   6. Physician-Patient
Relations—Personal Narratives. W 21 K68w 2007]
   R727.3.K575 2007
   610—dc22   2007005289

Printed in the United States of America
on acid-free paper

To the doctors who opened up their lives to me for this project,
and to Charlie

Acknowledgments

I am deeply indebted to several individuals and institutions without whom this work could not have been done. First and foremost, I am grateful to the physicians who shared their stories and lives. Their courage and candor stunned, inspired, and humbled me. Several funders assisted invaluably with various aspects of this project: the Arthur Vining Davis Foundations; Karen Davis, John Craig, David Sandman, and Robin Osborne at the Commonwealth Fund, from which I received support initially as a Picker/Commonwealth Scholar; the National Institute of Mental Health, through a Career Development Award; the Russell Sage Foundation; the Rockefeller Foundation; and Yaddo. I am very grateful to Peter Ohlin at Oxford University Press for his support and encouragement, and to Colleen McCue and Brian Desmond. For assistance transcribing and analyzing these interviews, and working on the manuscript, I am devoted to Antonius Wiriadjaja, James Zvokel, Cydney Halpin, Frank Griggs, Mary DuVernay, Davin Skalinder, Joseph Siragusa, Daniel Fishman, Shaira Daya, Jennifer Hersh, and Jonathan Weiss. Renée Fox provided additional input in the analysis of this material; and Melanie Thernstrom and Stewart Adelson provided valuable comments on the manuscript. For their support in various capacities, I also want to thank Jonathan Howe, Anne O'Keefe, Willo Pequegnat, Kristine Dahl, Anke Ehrhardt, and Masud Rahman.

Expose thyself to feel what wretches feel,
...And show the heavens more just.
William Shakespeare, *King Lear*

Contents

When Doctors Become Patients

Introduction

At 8:30 A.M. on September 11, 2001, from her office on the 105th floor of the World Trade Center, my sister Karen called her best friend. No one ever heard from Karen again.

Over the next few weeks, I helped organize a memorial service and a fellowship in her name, signed a death certificate, and packed up all of her belongings. Then my body gave out. For three months, I could not sleep. As a result, I had a flu that would not leave me. I could not get out of bed, and was no longer interested in reading books, seeing movies, or listening to music. Yet I was surprised when friends told me they thought I was depressed.

"No, I'm just sick," I said, resisting the idea. I was a psychiatrist, but suddenly, for the first time in my life, had physical symptoms of depression, and was amazed at the experience—how much it was more bodily than emotional. My body had just given way beneath me.

For the first time, I fully appreciated what my patients had to undergo, and how hard it is to put the experience of depression into words.

It was also hard to accept that I had a mental illness. I felt weak and ashamed, and began to appreciate, too, the embarrassment and stigma my patients felt.

I went to psychotherapy, memorial events, my temple and, for the first time, a Buddhist service, and a psychic who claimed to communicate with Karen—though as a physician, I was wary. I sat in Central Park in the middle of the day, for the first time in my life doing nothing for hours.

I thought my training as a psychiatrist would help, but it was quite the opposite. The experience forced me to cross the border from provider to patient, and taught me how much I did not know.

I realized that I, as a doctor, would never be the same, or look in the same way at the problems that patients and their families faced concerning depression or grief. The difficulties were far more complicated and long-lasting than I had ever imagined; closure was far more elusive. I wondered, too, how the experience of becoming a patient affected other physicians.

The psychoanalyst Carl Jung described a paradigm of the "wounded healer," who, through awareness of his or her own injuries, is able to heal others (1). Through personal suffering alone, he or she acquires deep wisdom. Observed by Jung in psychoanalysis, this phenomenon has since been delineated in pastoral care, Alcoholics Anonymous, and other forms of psychotherapy. Jung traced this concept back to the ancient Greeks. They believed that Asclepius had founded the sanctuary for healing in Epidaurus, based on self-treatment of his wounds. In various cultures, shamans have been said to undergo such transformations, drawing on their own pain to benefit others. But Jung was keenly aware of the potential dangers here as well—a healer may overidentify with patients, feeling their wounds too acutely, reawakening his or her own.

Do these processes operate among physicians today, and if so, how?

Doctors who get sick have uniquely been on both sides of the stethoscope, and possess unique *double lenses*. Their dual, contrasting sets of experiences as both physicians and patients can provide rare insiders' perspectives on the increasingly complicated contemporary medical system, but also can pose problems for these physicians as they try to treat others.

To understand these issues, I set out to interview doctors who became sick with serious disease. Through this journey, I soon saw how as patients, they drew on their knowledge as doctors; and as doctors, many came to incorporate the often painful lessons they had learned from being on "the other side" as patients. They observed how their own doctors treated them, assessing this treatment with more knowledge and higher standards of comparison than do other patients. Hence, they could be more critical. They learned to speak two different languages, talk both tongues, and could thus translate from one to the other. In doing so they offered insights and epiphanies that could help both other patients and providers.

Doctoring Today

"What do you do?"

In the United States, strangers commonly ask each other this question when initially meeting—on a plane, or at a dinner party. Often posed within seconds of the introduction, this query offends many Europeans, but suggests an essential element of American identity and culture. In many ways, *Americans define themselves by their work*. We are a "can do" nation. Here, success, "working one's way up from the bottom" and "pulling oneself up by one's bootstraps," motivate many as vital ideals. Yet in an age of corporate downsizing and outsourcing, changing and unstable economies, what does it mean to acquire and maintain a professional identity for an extended period of one's life—to put it on at the dawn of one's career and of each day—and then to be forced to remove it? Concepts of professional identity have profound implications for understanding *who we are;* how we find meaning, satisfaction, and support; and how we cope.

At the end of my medical training, I was surprised to see how much the experience had molded me: my allegiances, and cognitive and emotional responses to patients and everyday life. I wrote two books—*A Year Long Night: Tales of a Medical Internship* (2) and *In a House of Dreams and Glass: Becoming a Psychiatrist* (3)—exploring how other students and I became doctors and psychiatrists, respectively, acquiring "special knowledge." But I began to wonder what happened later on in doctors' careers, especially when they, too, got sick.

Increasingly, millions of viewers watch TV programs such as *ER*, *Scrubs*, *Grey's Anatomy*, and *House* that depict physicians in dramas, soap operas, sitcoms, and so-called reality shows. But what are doctors' inner lives and struggles really like today? Many key questions remain about how they view themselves, their work, their patients, and their power, and how they integrate their professional selves with other aspects of their lives.

Since Hippocrates in antiquity, various writers have probed the complex and unique roles and lives of physicians. Part artist, part scientist, a healer possesses special scientific understanding as well as patients' deep secrets. Every culture has "medicine men" and treatments that operate through what we in the West term "placebo effects." In the West, the Hippocratic Oath guides how physicians should behave—their roles and responsibilities toward their teachers, the healing arts, and their patients. Yet over time, doctor-patient relationships have shifted, shaped by a range of social, economic, medical, and scientific factors. In the 1950s, sociologists further advanced understandings of the roles and relationships of doctors and patients. The sociologist Talcott Parsons described the "sick role," in theoretical terms, as entailing rights and responsibilities, exemptions from certain duties, and obligations to get well, and as involving a power differential between physician and patient (4, 5). Parsons explored, too, the "situation of the physician"—to "do everything possible" for the patient's recovery, which requires probing patients' bodies and "private affairs" (4). To achieve these goals, many physicians find it easiest to maintain a paternalistic stance and rigid boundaries between the roles of doctor and patient. Long years of grueling training and professional socialization help enforce an ethos of authoritarianism. The French postmodern critic Michel Foucault has argued that physicians and medical institutions reinforce power differentials in ways that mold patients' experiences of illness (6).

But doctors also face difficulties and tensions of their own. They fear not being able to save all their patients (5). Though illness may exempt doctors from responsibilities, I soon found that when they got sick, doctors faced troubling conflicts. The New Testament admonishes, "Physician, heal thyself" (Luke 4:23), and many of these doctors felt they *should* not get sick—a situation creating dilemmas for them when they did (7).

Though the early stages of doctors' careers have been examined—how they transition from the lay world to that of medicine (2, 6)—much less attention has been given to the later stages of medical careers and the exact boundaries of the "doctor role." Little is known about how they travel back to the lay world from that of being a doctor, what stages comprise their journeys, and whether their two roles change, blur, or conflict, and if so, how.

Medical Metamorphoses

"I always thought I was Ms. Compassionate and listened," Jennifer, one of the first physicians I interviewed about these issues, sighed. She glanced down sadly as she reflected on her illness. "It was just so very different to go from one role to the other. I was really much more cavalier and uncaring than I ever would have thought! *My eyes were completely opened.*"

Though many people quip that doctors make the worst patients, these physicians can offer vital lessons, based on their multiple personal, professional, medical, and existential transformations. Forced not only to doff their white coats, but now to strip bare in examining rooms, they faced disease and the threat of death, confronting and reevaluating their views and understandings of themselves, their roles, and their interactions with patients and colleagues. *Hierarchies now turned upside down.*

Ordinarily, human beings have just one main point of view, but these doctor-patients had *two*, and elucidated how these can be held, each at times shaping, or combining with, the other. These doctors had privileged and uncommon knowledge of "the Other." Narratives, along with novels and films, can convey to us another person's point of view. Many of these doctors shuttled back and forth between these dual roles, as if between two parts of the brain; and over time, each position affected the other.

In their shuttling, these doctors illuminated the refractions between their dual roles of physician and patient—the width, depth, subdivisions, and substance of the chasm between these two poles. From Ovid to Dostoyevsky, such doublings have drawn artists and writers. The inner conflicts of the doctors here do not match the fictionalized extremes of Dr. Jekyll and Mr. Hyde (though it is interesting to note that to depict such radical discontinuity, Robert Louis Stevenson chose a physician). Nonetheless, these individuals balanced or reconciled dual aspects of their identities. All ended up somewhere different from where they began. Managed care, evidence-based medicine, consumerism, and demands for more "caring" providers pressured and embattled these doctors both personally and professionally.

They often came to see how, in their efforts to fight disease in others, and now themselves, professional institutions can help but also hinder. Institutions and colleagues pushed them to occupy just one role—as doctor or patient—not a combination of both. Through all of these processes, ill physicians became more sensitive to both sets of perspectives in unparalleled ways.

Ill Physicians Helping Patients and Others

The lessons these doctors gained can help patients and families, current and future physicians, other health care professionals, and medical administrators and policymakers. Confrontation with their own mortality

prompted these physicians to reflect on how they had distanced themselves from patients, and to learn and unlearn much. Many subsequently
tried to equalize the power differential with their patients, but faced challenges in doing so.

This book explores these individuals' complex odysseys and worlds:
how they traveled from the land of healing to that of disease. These
narratives offer patients and family members practical advice: how to
be "better" patients, and what realistically to expect as a patient with a
serious illness, having to communicate with providers. These doctors
often attained wisdom that they later tried to convey to their patients
and students. Patients feel disempowered in the system. Here, when sick,
even doctors experienced certain barriers and problems. Knowing how a
physician handles these same obstacles as a patient (what works and
doesn't) can be useful—how best to choose and interact with professionals and institutions, and what difficulties and assistance to anticipate.
These doctors probed the meanings of work and professional identity
today. In so doing, they provide a vivid cross-section chronicling American medicine today.

More broadly, for general readers and social scientists as well, these
tales of struggles with pain and displays of courage in the face of disease
are fundamentally human, touching primal issues of life and death, and
thus illuminating vital domains. These interviewees opened up their inner lives with deep and moving authenticity, providing key insights on
how men and women in general respond to crises and reconstruct their
lives. They revealed how they coped with uncertainty, anxiety, and de-
spair, and found hope. In *Man's Search for Meaning* (8), Victor Frankl
drew on his experiences in Auschwitz to describe how all humans seek
meaning in their lives. Similarly, the psychiatrist Robert Jay Lifton, based
on his studies of survivors of Hiroshima and Nagasaki over half a century
ago, explored how humans pursue "connections" to ultimate sources of
meaning through different modes: spirituality, work, family, nature, and
"experiential transcendence" (9). These doctors limned the existential
crises they faced today, the ways they struggled within the confines of
their lives—used what they had and knew—piecing together their own
particular education and experience to assist them in reconstructing a
life. For many doctors, work provided meaning. Once ill, they now battled to find renewed purpose and sustenance. As their work threatened
to slip away, many strove to clutch on to, or replace, it.

Through their struggles, these physicians illustrated much about power and magic in medicine. Chiseled over the main hospital entrance at the medical center where I work rise the biblical words "For of the most high cometh healing." In ancient Greece, healing came from, and was intricately entwined with, the gods. As the Hippocratic Oath states, healing is a gift from the gods. The healers here grappled with fears that they had now lost their power, both magical and psychological. The anthropologist Bronislaw Malinowski described how magic supplies confidence in facing uncertain and dangerous situations (10). Parsons elaborated on this notion, describing in modern medicine an "optimistic bias" that fosters beliefs that interventions and procedures will succeed. The profession "ritualizes" optimism (4), but treatments can fail, leading to conflicts between hopes and realities. Broad historical contexts shape scientific thinking (10), but how do microsocial and psychological contexts—the hourly encounters of doctors and patients—mold views and approaches to science, pseudoscience, and magic? Do ill doctors change how they view and approach scientific data, and if so, how?

These men and women wrestled, too, with tensions between science and faith. Controversies over evolution versus intelligent design rage, among the most intense of our time. Of the physicians here, some became religious; others mixed and matched various beliefs about spirituality or, in part because they were scientists, couldn't bring themselves to believe, though they longed to.

They elucidated, too, a closed world, and the workings of a profession and institutions more broadly. In ever-evolving and, arguably, ever-expanding ways, large institutions shape our daily lives. For these doctors, scientific dictates, institutional pressures, and personal needs and desires now clashed. These men and women faced difficult trade-offs. Aspects of their roles competed with, or reinforced, each other.

As a result, these physicians did not always practice what they preached, or seek the best care. What previously helped them as doctors (e.g., beliefs about their own invulnerability to disease) could now impede them. Frequently, they pursued VIP treatment—which celebrity lay patients do as well. Yet no prior studies have been done of how VIPs themselves look at the treatment they receive.

These doctors' experiences shed light, too, on several recent theories about improving health. Health behaviors—from dieting and smoking cessation to taking medications for high cholesterol—may be shaped by an individual's perceptions of the costs and benefits of the action (11). As they move toward adopting a particular change in health behavior, individuals may pass through several consecutive stages, from precontemplation to action (12, 13). But what happens when serious disease threatens a *whole life*, and all aspects of it must shift? Periodically, we all engage in unhealthy behaviors, but these doctors have spent years training, pushing patients to alter activities. The physicians here now observed themselves behaving like their patients. In addition, they self-diagnosed and self-treated, and saw themselves doing so—at times as if they were a third party. Rarely can or do people who experience such split identities talk about the experience. Many came to weigh risks and benefits and end-of-life decisions differently, and now deviated from professional norms, pursuing novel approaches. In politics, where one sits, affects where one stands. I soon saw the degree to which this phenomenon worked in medicine, too.

Their stories also say much about how people construct their identities more generally, in an ever more complex and fluid world: the stages and strands of our lives. For millennia, artists, poets, and philosophers have explored the phenomena of personal transformations. Ovid's *Metamorphoses* all concern mythic figures changing: Narcissus transforms from a man to a flower; Pygmalion's statue changes from stone to flesh. In Kafka's *Metamorphosis*, a man wakes up to find he has become a cockroach, and sees the world as an insect.

Yet major debates persist about notions and natures of selfhood. Emerson and American ego psychologists such as Heinz Hartmann have urged individuals to find their "true selves" (14). Yet Proust writes of characters who are a composite of *many* selves. His hero Marcel has a self that tries to enter high society, a self that interacts with his mother, one that prides itself on possessing a lover, and one that mourns a lost love. Postmodernists such as Jacques Lacan and Foucault further question essentialist notions of "the self" as a single entity, arguing that identities are multiple, fluid, and socially constructed in different settings (15, 16, 17, 18). What does it mean to "be" Indian or African, male or female, Western-educated or not, gay or straight, a doctor or a lawyer, healthy or sick, or an amalgam of several of these categories? Such identities can be shifting and flexible, rather than rigid and fixed.

Most of us usually alter our lives only gradually, but serious disease transformed these doctors more dramatically—into patients.

Generally, patients with serious medical problems have to manage stigma. The sociologist Erving Goffman described how individuals learn to conceptualize and manage "spoiled" aspects of their social or personal identities (19). Those with a particular stigma often alter their conception of self, resulting in a "moral career," sometimes attempting to conceal its symbols and to "pass." Others become fully involved in groups of similarly stigmatized individuals and become "professionals." Gaps may widen between their pre- and post-stigma acquaintances. Sick doctors face dilemmas: whether they should try to "pass" (i.e., as healthy) or are morally obligated to disclose their illness to patients and colleagues. Sissela Bok and Immanuel Kant have argued that individuals should rarely, if ever, lie or deceive (20, 21). But how, then, should ill physicians navigate between these poles of honesty and professional transparency on the one hand, and secrecy and silence on the other? Indeed, in his earlier work, *The Presentation of Self in Everyday Life*, Goffman described how all individuals in fact act as if they strut upon a stage, trying to manage how others see them (22).

I wondered how these doctors negotiated these difficult transformations—what, exactly, changed versus stayed the same, and why. As we shall see, some resisted such change, grasping onto the status quo—and demonstrating what I term a "will to wholeness." Others proved far more protean. These doctors drew differently upon their own experiences with disease, from profoundly metamorphosing to modifying only smaller or subtler aspects of their outward behaviors with patients. Not all wounds affect one equally; and no particular wound moves all individuals in the same way.

Postmodern critical theories of Foucault and others focus on broad categories of gender, race, and class. Yet individuals of the same gender, race, or social class may vary significantly. But in what ways do they? These doctors can help elucidate how critical theory intersects with individual psychological responses, with differences between individuals within only one broad social category.

Making Better Doctors

Increasingly, these topics have become important, as both health care providers and their patients face mounting challenges. The health care system continues to grow as a portion of the U.S. economy and to alter rapidly. In one way or another, we are all patients: growing up seeing doctors, stripping before them, divulging our secrets and souls. Yet as biotechnologies quickly advance, geneticists further crack the human genome, and baby boomers age and face more disease, the medical system is becoming ever more complex and frustrating. Managed care continues to spread and evolve, and debates about national health insurance boil without clear resolution. Patients are becoming more educated consumers, while the health care system becomes ever less user-friendly. Some critics fear that trust in physicians is eroding, that doctors and patients feel themselves to be antagonists, and that doctoring is becoming less of a noble and respected profession, and more of a mere job.

Recent studies have highlighted several specific problems: for example, how doctors and patients fail to communicate. Physicians disagree with patients 50 percent of the time about the latter's main problem (23), and have difficulty discussing sensitive but important topics such as end-of-life care (24). Providers may raise the topic, but often too vaguely. Physicians miss important emotional cues (25) and have trouble talking about sexual issues (26). Doctors and patients even disagree about the importance of effective communication (27). Yet good physician-patient communication can improve health outcomes (28) and patient satisfaction (29, 30), and decrease how often patients switch doctors (31). Jerome Groopman has vividly explored how doctors miss diagnoses (32), and he offers many important cautions and suggestions. But the individuals here illuminate how they miss as well many key aspects of patients' experiences with illness. Often, only the experience of becoming seriously ill finally compels them to change their thinking, and see themselves and their work more broadly, and from a different vantage point—to realize how their prior professional view is just one of several possible perspectives.

Attempts have been made to foster more compassion in physicians (33, 34), yet many uncertainties persist as to whether empathy can in fact be systematically taught, and if so, how and with what effectiveness (35). Disagreement exists even as to whether empathy is a skill or an attitude (36). Medical students learn values from senior doctors implicitly, by modeling, rather than explicitly (37, 38, 39), yet through their training, medical students generally become more cynical and less compassionate (40), and medical schools are teaching growing amounts of other, scientific information. Medical education leads doctors to distance themselves, build defenses, and feel immune from death and suffering around them. But if physicians adopted more "rational" views, they might easily feel more threatened by the surrounding illness and death. Further obstacles to compassion exist, since physicians face multiple stresses, confronting sickness and death, and working long hours. Doctors avoid admitting psychological difficulties (41, 42), yet such problems can potentially affect patients adversely (43).

Educational efforts to help improve physician communication have been attempted, but many physicians still clearly have trouble inter-acting with their patients (44). Recent efforts to increase students' em-pathy through reading and discussing literature (45) to improve commu-nication skills may help in the short term, though results have not been entirely consistent (46, 47) and the long-term impacts remain underassessed. Questions of how doctors and patients can best interact are of rising consequence.

For their colleagues, these doctors' experiences can be more poignant and compelling than those of lay patients. They can help other trainees and practitioners in medicine, nursing, psychology, social work, and other health fields to see more clearly how patients perceive them. These stories of sick physicians can encourage fellow providers to be more open and sensitive to problems in communication, and to see what specifically needs to be improved. Frequently, physicians dismiss patients' criticisms: "Oh, it's just the patient complaining." But these sick doctors can say, "No, I am one of you, and these are legitimate gripes that I, as a patient, know." Other providers may come to recognize more fully that they, too, will one day be patients, that the boundary between physicians and patients is, in the end, nonexistent.

Prior Writings About Ill Physicians

Physicians such as Oliver Sacks, Fitzhugh Mullan, and Jody Heymann have described their own personal experiences with particular disorders (48, 49, 50). *The Doctor*, a film starring William Hurt, depicted one ex-treme case: a cold, chauvinistic surgeon whose illness made him more humane (51). Two books, by Pinner and Miller in 1952, and by Mandell and Spiro in 1987, compiled single accounts by physicians, each describing his or her particular experience with an illness (52, 53). But these two compilations of individual stories, while valuable, were not organized the-matically, to analyze issues systematically, investigating the same set of concerns and questions with each physician to detect and examine pat-terns, similarities and differences, and areas (e.g., death and dying) about which individual physicians may be reluctant to comment, or do not mention at all. These two books organized individual doctors' reports by disorders, like a medical textbook, with each report standing by itself.

Many insights are scattered through them, but these accounts tend to enumerate medical events one after the other, shaped by these physicians' experiences gathering medical histories. The focus of these books was not to identify or explore commonalities and differences (e.g., between diseases). It is also not clear how these individual contributors were chosen.

Hence, I have integrated here such doctors' stories to present cross-cutting issues, analyze underlying concerns, and provide a sense of the full scope and range of the challenges faced.

Moreover, though these earlier individual and compiled narratives represent self-reports, I have tried to shed light on aspects of experiences that such physicians have trouble discussing as well. For example, of the fifty doctors in Mandell and Spiro's book, over 80 percent come out publicly about their illness, a fact that in itself may shape what they say or feel comfortable admitting. To avoid embarrassment, they may frame their experiences in particular ways. Yet at times, choked by emotions, the doctors who spoke with me couldn't fully express themselves as they wished: halting, and unable to complete sentences about difficult events. Spontaneous speech differs from written text that physicians in these other works have revised calmly over time. Such editing can conceal the role of unconscious processes such as denial.

Nonetheless, these relatively few prior single, anecdotal cases have highlighted certain aspects of ill physicians' experiences with illness. Doctors often undergo a difficult transition, denying their illness (54) and seeking treatment late, because of attitudinal and organizational barriers, including stigma and peer pressure (55, 56). They may hesitate to relinquish the role of the physician, and instead diagnose and treat themselves, entering the dual roles of observing their symptoms and being observed. Personal illness is additionally stressful because physicians frequently define themselves by their work (53). Other physicians may be unsupportive of ill colleagues (57), and can be silent, judgmental, or avoidant, based on embarrassment and anxiety. Some ill physicians become more aware of how they had previously depersonalized patients, made them into "cases," and approached the doctor-patient relationship with paternalism and domination (58). Physicians with cancer tend to self-doctor in some form, approaching their own care along a continuum between typical physician and patient roles (59). Yet, within very broad categories of being more like a doctor, or more like a patient, critical subdivisions and distinctions may occur that have to yet to be explored. Several strategies for treating ill physicians and negotiating the relationship have also been recommended, given that ill doctors are similar to, yet different from, other patients (60). Some systematic research has been done on managing physicians with substance abuse (61), but not on physicians with serious, life-threatening medical problems per se.

In short, many crucial questions have received little, if any, attention. It is not clear how ill doctors treat their own patients differently, view health care communication, and deal with stigma, disclosure of illness, spirituality, retirement, or multiple other topics. How thick or thin are the white coats that doctors wear—the armor that protects them from disease? Prior work also tends to view self-doctoring as a single entity, focusing on self-prescribing rather than distinguishing between types of self-doctoring (e.g., self-prognosing). Prognostication of other patients has recently received discussion (62), but *self*-prognostication—gauging one's own future—has received little, if any, attention.

Are Doctors Different from Everyone Else?

My own experiences as a doctor and as a patient, and what I learned from prior research and the interviews presented here, indicated to me how doctors, in confronting illness, differed from, and in some ways resembled, lay patients. In *Being Positive: The Lives of Men and Women with HIV* and *Mortal Secrets* (63), I examined the experiences of patients wrestling with one of the great crises of our age, HIV. *The Trembling Mountain: A Personal Account of Kuru, Cannibalism, and Mad Cow Disease* drew on fieldwork I conducted while living with the Stone Age Fore group in Papua New Guinea, studying the kuru epidemic (spread by a prion similar to that responsible for bovine spongiform encephalopathy ["mad cow disease"]). This book explored fears of patients and providers in confronting one of the great unknowns of science today, prion diseases (64). Recently, I have been examining, too, the experiences of patients facing genetically-associated diseases, from breast cancer to Huntington's disease (65, 66, 67).

When sick, both doctors and patients fear bad outcomes and engage in denial. But only physicians can order themselves medications, and have trained for years to approach and treat disease in others, probing all parts of strangers' bodies. Doctors possess unique knowledge, rights, responsibilities, moral commitments, and placebo effects. I saw how patients taught and inspired them. Many physicians felt they did not have the right to give up the profession, to let people suffer. Even when they became ill, some continued to place their patients' health above their own. Doctors can access care more knowingly and effectively than lay patients, but do not always do so when facing life-threatening disease.

Methods

To address these questions, I interviewed seventy individuals in depth. I first conducted twenty sets of pilot interviews to focus the range of topics, and then conducted the remainder of the interviews for the full study, doing so in two phases. I initially studied HIV-infected doctors—who raise many of these issues in bold relief—and then, in order to broaden understandings of these issues, expanded the study to include physicians with other kinds of medical problems. I recruited participants through the Internet, through e-mailed announcements and Web sites (e.g., "Are you or do you know a physician with a serious illness?"), word of mouth, and ads in newsletters. For the full study, I was contacted by 48 doctors, a medical student, and a dentist. These individuals (referred to below as "doctors") had HIV, cancer, heart disease, hepatitis C, Huntington's disease (HD), infection, bipolar disorder, and other diagnoses. They ranged from twenty-five to eighty-seven in age; one was Latino, the rest were Caucasian. They lived in several cities; and included surgeons, internists, pediatricians, radiologists, neonatologists, endocrinologists, infectious diseases specialists, anesthesiologists, neurologists, psychiatrists, and trainees. Many had observed and treated other ill colleagues, and had family members (parents, siblings, spouses and children) who were physicians who had been sick as well. These participants observed and commented on these others, too.

I could have summarized these participants' stories and spoken for them, but that would fail to capture the power and poignancy of their own words. Their voices best convey the struggles and conflicting identities, poetry and pain they described. Sick, contemplating the ends of their lives, they divulged things they had sometimes told no one else—at points embarrassed, but searching. Through suffering, many found sagacity about doctors, patients, death, and life.

One of my former teachers, the late anthropologist Clifford Geertz, and others have advocated understanding social phenomena from the experiences of those in a particular situation to provide a "thick description," rather than imposing explanatory frameworks from outside (68).

"Illness narratives" can shed light on approaches toward, and ways of coping with, disease (69). Studs Terkel and others have shown the value of oral histories in conveying the grit and detail of individuals' lives (70, 71). Here, for example, stories can communicate not just the fact that discrimination or denial exists, but also how individuals experience it—how even well-meaning colleagues discriminate, and well-adjusted doctors deny their problems, unaware.

Due to space limitations, I cannot present all their stories. To illustrate key points, in the pages that follow, some individuals appear more than others, and in the background or foreground. The pilot interviews very much informed the project, and at times I have drawn on these as well.

To give an overview and help orient the reader, these individuals' names (all pseudonyms) and brief descriptors are given on the next page. To further protect confidentiality, I have changed certain identifying details.

I conducted all the interviews myself at the subjects' offices or homes or in my office—whatever was most convenient for them. The Columbia University Department of Psychiatry Institutional Review Board approved the study; and all of the interviewees provided informed consent.

All informants spoke to me twice, for two hours each time, about their experiences as patients and as providers, and about other aspects of their lives. As I was a fellow doctor, they opened up to me. Many felt that these interviews—having a trained psychiatrist listen to them—were therapeutic. Though the interviews clearly did not constitute psychotherapy, many of their stories were wrenching, and they found the opportunity of reviewing, organizing, and synthesizing what they had learned to be helpful. They also valued entrusting me with their stories to convey to others. By nature, a few were not very introspective. But almost all were forthcoming, and some called me later to follow up, a few of them shortly before they died. Their openness enriched these interviews, elucidating many issues that the literature on doctoring has wholly or largely ignored.

I audiotaped, transcribed, and content-analyzed the interviews, informed by grounded theory (72), developing hypotheses during the process of conducting the interviews. An assistant and I examined all the narratives to assess factors that shaped experiences, identifying categories of recurrent themes and issues. I drew on my past ethnographic experience, and consulted with an eminent senior sociologist.

The experience of becoming patients prompted these doctors to reflect on numerous aspects of their lives at the most fundamental levels. Invariably, these interviewees discussed, too, the illness experiences of

Name	Brief Description
Albert	Internist who had a myocardial infarction (MI) while driving on the highway
Alex	Dentist with HIV
Anne	Swiss internist with metastasized cancer
Bill	Southern radiologist with HIV
Bradley	Internist who became depressed for the first time after an MI
Brian	Pediatrician with hepatitis
Charles	An internist with HIV who became an "underground researcher"
Dan	Oncologist with chest metastases
David	Psychiatrist with HIV
Deborah	Psychiatrist with metastatic breast cancer
Eleanor	California health care professional whose physician-husband had diabetes and cancer
Ernie	Midwest internist with Huntington's disease
Frank	Surgeon who had an MI in the operating room (OR)
George	Internist with HIV; also a government committee member
Harry	Internist with heart disease; also a World War II refugee
Herb	Neonatologist with MI
Jacob	Religious Chicago radiologist with skin cancer
Jeff	Adolescent medicine specialist with HIV
Jennifer	Internist HIV-infected by a needle stick
Jerry	Philadelphia surgeon-lawyer with HIV
Jessica	Pediatrician with Hodgkin's lymphoma
Jim	Drug company researcher with leukemia
John	Public health official with HIV
Juan	Retired Latino internist with HIV
Kurt	HIV-infected internist who had used crack
Larry	Anesthesiology resident with HIV
Lou	Physician with cancer; had an award on his office wall
Mark	Internist with HIV; interviewed in a diner
Mathilde	Pennsylvania physician whose husband died of AIDS
Nancy	Endocrinologist with metastatic breast cancer
Neil	Neurologist with HIV
Pascal	Lebanese internist with HIV
Paul	Internist with HIV who lost a job offer
Peter	Medical student with HIV
Rochelle	Surgeon with breast cancer
Roger	Surgeon with HIV

(*continued*)

Name	Brief Description
Ronald	Suburban Connecticut radiologist with AIDS
Roxanne	Gastroenterologist with abdominal cancer
Sally	Internist with cancer who brought her laptop to the ICU
Scott	Internist with an infected foot
Simon	Radiologist who refused to be audiotaped
Steven	Suburban endocrinologist with HIV
Stuart	Retired internist with HIV; now teaching
Suzanne	Psychiatrist with bipolar disorder
Tim	Dermatologist with leukemia
Tina	HIV-positive pulmonologist
Tom	Physician whose lover died of AIDS
Walter	Politically active internist with lymphoma
Wilma	Elderly physician with a severe GI infection

medical colleagues and family members—many of whom were also health care professionals.

I have organized thematically the experiences these interviewees discussed. Many of the themes they raised are closely related; for instance, they encounter particular problems (e.g., depression) and also have trouble communicating about these problems with their physicians. Clearly, such distinctions are in some ways artificial—one can only with difficulty separate the form from the content of poor communication, but doing so allows for more precise analysis of each set of subthemes and problems. The phenomena here have diverse implications. For instance, views that physicians are immune to disease can both diminish preventive health behaviors and prompt doctors to continue to work long hours, even in the face of disease. Moreover, a story can make more than one point at a time. I beg the reader's indulgence in my making such distinctions in order to provide a sense of the whole. At points, I have added italics to highlight certain key phrases and points.

Yet overall, for these diseases, the similarities far outweighed the differences. These doctors shared key experiences, desires, obstacles, self-treatments, fears of discrimination, forms of denial and coping, and decisions on how much to follow preventive health behaviors, and how to confront fundamental issues of meaning, identity, work, worsening disease, mortality, and hope.

I have pointed out where contrasts emerge, but I was most struck by the similar problems, crises, and types of insights. Doctors with HIV shared much in common with those who faced cancer and other kinds of serious medical problems: dilemmas of whether and how to tell colleagues, treat their own patients differently, be more spiritual, and continue to work, or retire and lose their career. Uncertainties loomed as to how long the benefits of treatments would last before disease reasserted itself. At times, experiences with HIV presented many of these issues writ large, yet physicians with cancer also often confronted risky and invasive treatments (e.g., toxic chemotherapies and radical surgeries), and uncertain prognoses—given the possibility of disease recurrence and increased risk of other types of primary cancers. Opportunistic infections arise among both immunocompromised doctors on chemotherapy and those infected with HIV. Doctors with HIV who had retired on disability, and now felt better on new medications, faced dilemmas of whether and how to restructure their professional and personal lives. Physicians recovering from cancer also encountered the possibility of recurrence, and hence the same issue, even if at times less starkly. Many ill doctors now came to identify more with their patients (e.g., getting results to patients faster); gay doctors with HIV who treated members of the gay community often encountered this issue with added urgency. Some doctors with HIV confronted particular stigma or discrimination due to fears that they might infect patients, and to aspects of a physician's background, such as sexual orientation. Gay men—the group most affected among doctors—may face added stigma. Yet fundamental issues of stigma and discrimination arose for other physicians, too. Whatever these doctors who courageously talked to me experienced, others whom I did not interview surely feel, too.

I have tried to illustrate these themes and the variations within them, rather than merely presenting a sequential series of isolated doctors speaking one after another. The material itself strongly dictated that I not simply offer a series of short, distinct tales of each physician's life. Therefore, to highlight commonalities as well as differences, I have chosen to present a group portrait, a montage, a collage, similar to a documentary, in which interviews with different people are intercut, with each person commenting on a specific issue in turn, and then reappearing. I have tried to present these areas in the order and arc through which they occur in these physicians' lives. Granted, film documentaries have an advantage over written text—the viewer can *see* the person speaking, and does not have to be reminded each time that Mr. X is a spry, gray-haired, elderly man wearing thick black glasses, or that Mrs. Y is a shy, young Latina with dangling silver earrings. I refer to each person by providing not a photo of each, but their descriptions of their inner and outer worlds. Invariably, any such attempt to break up an individual's narrative into discrete topics risks doing some disservice to the "whole." In the end, such distinctions are both real and artificial, since these categories interrelate. At times, similar underlying themes emerge in different guises. For example, denial manifests itself in many aspects of individuals' lives, from how they treat themselves to how they interact with colleagues and friends. I have tried to organize these types of implications, to present them coherently rather than diffusely. In the end, I think the reader will gain a sense of both the common themes and these doctors as individuals, grasping both the breadth and the depth of these extraordinary lives.

Below, I first lay out the ranges of problems that these individuals confronted—as patients, and as doctors treating others—and then the ways that they addressed and often solved these. Through their journeys, these doctors questioned many areas. Part of my intention here is to present the full scope of the issues in these individuals' lives, and the fissures, cracks, and successes of contemporary medicine. Eradicating the problems that these physicians identify will require further efforts. But to recognize them is itself a vital first step toward cure.

Part I

BECOMING A PATIENT

2

"Magic White Coats"

Forms of Denial and Other Internal Obstacles to Becoming a Patient

"We doctors wear magic white coats," Dan said. A middle-aged oncologist, he had metastases (spread of cancer from one place in the body to another) in his chest. "We destroy disease all the time," he explained. "How could it ever attack us?" His comment amazed me, but was hardly unique.

When confronting disease, the physicians I interviewed faced a wide variety of *both internal and external challenges:* medical, logistical, social, psychological, and existential. Physicianhood proved to be a double-edged sword, both aiding and impeding response to disease.

Repeatedly, I was struck by the levels of denial these doctors evidenced when they were facing the horror of illness—how their fears as patients overcame their objective knowledge as physicians. The profession abetted this psychological response to diagnoses.

MD as ID

"Who are you, compared with what you do?" one doctor asked me. In becoming patients, these physicians felt threatened in their roles and identities as doctors, and reflected on what their profession had meant to them, and why they had entered it in the first place. Their past relationships with the profession molded their current views. They described trajectories through which they had passed, integrating their professional roles into their lives before becoming ill. They had become physicians for a variety of reasons that in turn shaped how they viewed medicine, what they expected, and how they now reacted to their condition.

Regardless of why they entered the field, these individuals had soon come to define themselves by their professional identity. Juan, an internist, struggled to become a physician in part to overcome affronts to his self-esteem that he had felt as a sickly gay Latino child. "A doctor's a doctor's a doctor," he said. Nothing, he felt, could take away what his sweat had earned him. Similarly, after being diagnosed with AIDS, Jerry, a Pennsylvania surgeon, went on disability and attended law school, but his identity remained that of a surgeon, not a lawyer. Having lost his surgical practice, he tried to keep busy. Yet for a long time, he did not know what to say to people who asked him what he did.

> The first thing people always ask you is "What do you do?" That defines 90 percent of who you are, it seems. I get tired of telling people, "I'm retired." Their next line is "You're so lucky!" Sometimes I say, "It's not quite like that," and I'll tell them the story. I have to stay very active. I got a law degree, but it didn't give me the sense of identity I had as a practicing physician.

Such identification with one's job is particularly strong in medicine, but as we shall see, it can reinforce a rigid hierarchy and authority.

For many, medicine offered enormous personal gratification beyond financial rewards, providing the major, or main, *sense of purpose* in life. Roxanne, a gastroenterologist, was diagnosed with abdominal cancer. Even before that, she derived deep *moral* meaning from her work. After her diagnosis, she continued to see patients because she liked to, and because being a physician was a "calling" that sustained her. "An MD degree is a privilege. You use all that knowledge to help others." As we will see, for her, her work carried a sense of religious vocation.

The medical profession also provided structure that organized and directed lives. Mathilde, a Pennsylvania physician, talked about her husband—a fellow doctor who had recently died of AIDS that he had acquired from a blood transfusion. She felt that their daily work with patients provided connection and fulfillment. "I enjoy my job, and *love* my patients and they love me. That helps a lot." Indeed, physicians can develop deep relationships with the field as a whole. About her husband, Mathilde said:

> The most stressful thing for him was that he was in love with medicine, and it had failed him. He could deal with tragedy and adversity, but not with losing his love.

Becoming Patients

Ill physicians faced not only loss of their role, but also burdens in entering a new one, that of the patient. *The difficulties of this new identity surprised them all, especially since they had assumed beforehand that they knew what to expect.* Their prior and present senses of self now began to separate radically.

They struggled to articulate and describe this profound disruption in their self-conceptions and sense of the future. Lou, an elderly pediatrician in remission from cancer, said, "I can *taste* these things about being a patient differently now," grasping for a metaphor. "I knew them before. But it is very *different* now."

Many of these doctors said they knew intellectually what patienthood would be like, but still hadn't always "believed" it. Even when they were aware of this discrepancy, and tried to prepare themselves for it, the reality still shocked and overwhelmed them. Jim, a physician who worked as a drug company researcher, developed leukemia. "You can't be completely prepared for it," he said. "Even though people told me, 'You're not going to feel well for thirty-six months, or feel like yourself, or want to go back.' Still, I was surprised." He strove to keep working. While he was in the hospital for the first time, he bought a laptop. He was disappointed that he could not bring himself to open it.

Firsthand knowledge of illness differed from book knowledge in several significant ways. Epistemologically, these physicians gained deeper personal comprehension that led them to perceive their work differently. Heretofore, they had education about *treating disease*, but not about *being sick*. The philosopher John Dewey wrote of different forms of learning, and of the importance and benefits of active and experiential, not simply passive, education (1). These doctors revealed the limitations of their prior education, only now becoming aware of former barriers to heightened sensitivity to patients.

"Post-residency" Disease: Denials of Disease

In "post-residency disease," which I am here defining, these physicians, established in their professions, often minimized symptoms that in fact were present. "Medical student's disease" has been described (2, 3) as referring to trainees who fear that they have symptoms of the diseases about which they are learning. Students then overdiagnose themselves when they are in fact completely healthy. In contrast, post-residency disease involves worries about legitimate physiological disorders, and can in fact lead to decreases in care sought, or to various forms of self-doctoring. Hence, the consequences can be more serious. Medical student's disease, after all, is a response to *nonexistent* medical symptoms, while post-residency disease refers to symptoms and diagnoses that could threaten to terminate one's life and career. After medical school, physicians can still suffer from hypochondriasis. But here, "post-residency disease" proved far more prevalent and involved denial—not worrying too much, but *too little*, about medical problems. Health professionals appeared to cross the divide between "medical student's disease" and "post-residency disease" after they had extensively treated patients' diseases, and now had a real disease themselves that needed treatment, evoking fears of mortality and triggering psychological defenses.

Self-diagnosing

The initial stage of these physicians' passage into patienthood was *diagnosis*. This stage proved far more intricate and challenging than they had anticipated. Many diagnosed themselves, assessing their own prognoses and treatments.

Yet errors clouded these judgments. Some physicians minimized or failed to recognize the significance of their initial symptoms, and didn't use their medical thinking—they failed to think of themselves as patients or to look at themselves as a doctor would. Jim, the pharmaceutical company researcher with leukemia, didn't view his early symptoms as he would if they had been those of another patient.

> For about a week, I had been sick, and thought it was the flu. But it got worse. So I saw my physician and was diagnosed with leukemia. I was surprised. I had been thinking about what else this could be *besides* a flu. I was even doing some reading, *but I just never used the kind of medical thinking that I might have with somebody else*, and said, "Let's go through everything: Is it infectious? Autoimmune? Malignant?" I could have picked up on other clues, but didn't: I cut myself shaving, and it took a while to stop bleeding.

Even after the disease was identified, Jim still doubted it. He continued:

I questioned the diagnosis—it probably could be something else: just a very high blood count. But my docs were pretty clear that the diagnosis was not in doubt. My primary care doc drove me right to the hospital himself!

Even after the diagnosis was made, based on objective data, ill doctors often had trouble believing it.

Many sick physicians were surprised at the degree to which they misinterpreted early symptoms and failed to conceptualize these correctly. Roxanne, the gastroenterologist with abdominal cancer, first felt pain one night while preparing slides for a lecture. She examined herself, but then kept working for hours on her lecture, and did not look at herself with a clinical gaze, as she would another patient. Only in retrospect did she put the events together.

I wanted to do a good job, but the lecture would not gel. It was 2 A.M. and it still wouldn't click. I had the slides laid out on the floor, and I was watching TV. As I bent over, I felt something, a mass.

Nonetheless, Roxanne struggled with her talk for several more hours. Even though she had had other significant symptoms, including the loss of menstrual periods, she still hadn't linked all her symptoms and signs. The social role of a doctor and its accompanying perceptual framework can take a long time to change.

For six months, my periods ceased. I thought I was too young for menopause. Four weeks before, I woke up in the middle of the night with epigastric pain. But there was no pain on my liver when I palpated, and there was no pain in the back. I'm a gastroenterologist. I examined myself. I thought it was irritable bowel syndrome, and I was surprised how painful, how *terrible* it could be! I had bloods drawn on my own. I picked up the results, and the only thing abnormal were platelets less than normal. But I still didn't put the whole thing together. A week after that, I was going to the symphony, and in the taxi, the pain came again, and lasted two hours. In retrospect, that was the expansion of the spleen. But I didn't know it at the time.

Roxanne had not yet accepted the disease or the role of patient, suggesting the width of the chasm that separates doctors from patients, established through years of rigorous professional training, and compounded by psychological defenses of denial. Revealingly, Roxanne referred to "the spleen" rather than "*my* spleen," as if it were someone else's. She illustrated, too, the vast gap between knowledge of pain and experience of it. Though she had treated many patients with abdominal pain, she was astonished at just *how horrible* it could be.

Such resistance to switching roles led to many physicians continuing to work full-time, despite their early symptoms. For example, Frank, a surgeon, developed a heart attack while rushing a patient into the operating room (OR). He continued to operate even though he began to experience chest pain.

Minimizations can continue not just in making a diagnosis, but afterward. Lou, in remission from cancer, hung on his wall a plaque awarded to him by a professional organization. The plaque included a framed photo of him taken when he was receiving intensive chemotherapy. The picture showed him bald, emaciated, and weak. He debated whether to keep the plaque on the wall—the award gratified his ego, but the photo reminded him of how bad his disease had been. The cancer could return at any time. "Every bone in my body told me I should not meet with you today," he immediately said as I entered his office. He did not want to reopen psychic wounds by discussing his disease. Several times he pointed to the plaque on the wall.

> They put this award with the picture in a frame and gave it to me—it just happened that the photo was in it. It doesn't bother me. *It doesn't bother me at all!* Yet it *is* a reminder. Somebody else would say, "Who needs it?" But they wanted to give it to me. If the illness was depressing me, I might take it down.

Lou's repeated protestations of *not* being troubled about the illness seemed to belie underlying conflict about it, and the insult to him that the disease represented. In part, he and others felt that to adopt a new role, as a patient, would necessitate giving up the other, as a doctor—*as if individuals had a zero-sum identity.*

Rationalizations and magical thinking could foster denial, too. Mathilde and her husband danced around the possibility of his being HIV-infected. They both employed magical thinking: because he was exercising, he must be fine. In addition, she believed, irrationally, that because they continued to have unsafe sex, he must be uninfected.

Doctors rejected the patient role in particular when the disorder was psychiatric, suggesting that acceptance of the sick role can vary widely, based on the nature of the disease. Accepting potential threats to one's mental functioning was extremely hard. Suzanne, a psychiatric trainee, said about being diagnosed with bipolar disorder:

> I am a highly functional person, and had to admit that I had some paranoid ideation. It was really hard to accept needing an anti-psychotic. I was entering *a new category*.

Resistance arose to transitioning not only from healthy to sick, but also from minor to serious illness. Brian, a young pediatrician, acquired hepatitis C from a patient. He felt that he crossed a critical boundary when he moved from merely being infected into the *"land of more advanced disease."* Hence, within the broad category of the "sick role," key subcategories of various "symptom roles" emerged that affected these individuals' lives.

Resistance to adopting the role and identity of patient can extend to numerous realms of one's life. Lou, the pediatrician with the award on his wall, tried to stay active, determined that nothing in his life would change. He saw his response as "denial," and defended it.

> I passed an internal law: if I fatigued early, I would exercise more. If my stomach hurt, I would eat more. I swam and ran more. Rest is not useful! If you're not using the brain, it atrophies. Nothing changed...except I lost my hair.

Lou dealt with his illness by acting as if it did not exist. "I had an unreality about it: I was not sick! I dealt with it by *denial, essentially ignoring it.*"

Yet such rejection of illness could extend to the point of impeding health. For example, at times, doctors, though suspecting and fearing a disease, resisted diagnostic testing. Many delayed the initial steps required to get a full or official diagnosis. Paul, a young internist, later lost a job offer because of being HIV-positive. Earlier, he had postponed HIV testing, suspecting that he was infected, just as he was embarking on his post-medical school training.

> It took me a year to get tested, because I was starting residency, and didn't really want to know I was positive, and have that hanging

over my head. The second month of residency, I finally got tested, and found out I was positive. That was really hard. Here I was at the beginning of my residency, concerned about whether I could even finish.

Not until the symptoms or evidence became *irrefutable* did many of the physicians I interviewed begin to accept their illness. Eleanor's husband, a physician, had hypertension and diabetes, but never sought medical assistance. He minimized his cancer and stroke until forced to confront his own X-rays depicting metastases. Eleanor said:

He was diabetic, but never sought care. He managed his own case. Then, he was diagnosed with cancer, had two strokes, and was forced to leave medical practice. He was diagnosed with metastatic cancer, and had a third stroke.... He had hospitalizations. *But his response to all of his illnesses was to deny them. For years, he still didn't go for checkups!*

Such minimization could take substantial effort. Some physicians constructed their world, citing or ignoring evidence to support their beliefs. Denial could verge, too, on magical thinking. Eleanor, a fellow health care professional, observed about her husband:

He just did not see himself as a patient. There was an element of magical thinking: If he didn't stick to his diet, he wasn't diabetic. If he didn't have a biopsy, he didn't have cancer. If he didn't ac- knowledge the cardiac arrhythmia, there was no cardiac problem. If he didn't acknowledge the aphasia, there was no stroke. There were two separate compartments: the magical thinking ("this can't possibly happen to me") and the physician-scientist, trained ob- server and diagnostician. There wasn't any connection between the two. Only when he got really backed up against the wall—when he saw the bone scan, and when I called ambulances to take him to the ER—did he feel sheer terror.

He had his second stroke at work and then drove home. I took him back to the ER. He said, "I just need to rest." For the first stroke, we were headed out to the movies and he had problems zipping his jacket and getting his seat belt on. He said he just wanted to go home, because he needed to rest, and was fine. He tried unlocking the house with his *car* key. I grabbed his hand, and said, "Look at what you're doing!"

There came a point when I was managing all of his medications, because it was so complicated. More and more, he just abdicated responsibility to me. That was as close as he got to acknowledging he was sick.

Yet even when Eleanor's husband admitted his illness, it was only in a dissociated and cursory manner.

In the end, he was informed of having metastatic bone disease by having his bone scan put up on an X-ray box. He took one look, turned to me, and said, "Yup, I'm a dead man."

Even after that point, he could allude to dying only indirectly.

When he finally decided to retire on disability, I bought him a pair of dogs to keep him company. One of his big concerns was whether I was going to keep the dogs after he died. *That was the only acknowledgment of dying he could make.*

Doctors as Invulnerable

Through their professional training and socialization, these doctors frequently had come to see physicianhood as protective against illness—as immunity and defense. They believed that doctors were magically invulnerable to disease. Their professional roles shaped their thinking.

Charles, an internist with HIV who later became an "underground" researcher, experimenting with new treatments, had earlier felt that because of their white coats, doctors simply did not get sick.

As medical students, we were once wearing white coats, walking through the medical center, and a sign said "No One Permitted— Sanitary Area." I remember a mother telling her son not to go in there. He pointed to the group of us, and he said, "But *they're* going in." She said, "Yes, but *they're doctors.*" People think you can't be diseased because you're the one who *cures* disease. I used to wonder how doctors could die, except by accident. I had so much confidence in medicine. Surely anything that might go wrong with a doctor physically, he would pick up early, and prevent.

This belief in invulnerability can easily border on magical thinking. Indeed, many doctors felt they donned a *"magic white cloak"* giving them authority and protecting them against strangers' bodies and disease. Such authority and belief can reinforce one another. Charles added:

> We have the right to give drugs and do things that no other human being has. I can put a needle into your spine and thread a wire up it. I have this tremendous power over people, and therefore maybe over myself. Maybe I can keep anything bad from happening to *me*, because I know that if I'm diligent, I can keep anything bad from happening to *patients*. If something bad *does* happen to a patient, I think, "How could it have happened? I was perfect."

Charles suggested here, too, the lack of self-reflectiveness that physicians may often have toward their work.

Some thought that morally, physicians in fact somehow *should not* get sick—that they implicitly had a contractual and *moral* imperative not to. David, a practicing psychiatrist with HIV, said:

> I tell myself, "You have to hold onto your end of the bargain. You said you were going to take care of a patient and now you can't." People say, "Patients would understand." But I know they wouldn't. They got screwed.

Intuitively, David felt that illness was not part of the agreement that doctors make with patients. This attitude, instilled through years of training, marks the thickness of the psychic armor that doctors don—the belief that, for various reasons, physicians simply do not get ill.

These beliefs assume the status of myth, inculcated through training and reinforced throughout the culture of medicine. Deborah, a psychiatrist-in-training with breast cancer, said:

> It's arrogance: "I'm a doctor, I'm protected." It's a myth: "I know how to take care of myself and diagnose my problems." Doctors think it will never happen to them. But that is such a mistake. Because it can and probably will happen.

Medical students identify first with patients, and only later with fellow physicians. Medical training radically challenges these trainees, taking them apart psychologically, *wounding them*. They must then put themselves back together, and end up identifying with fellow doctors.

Yet given these defenses, carefully built over years, the eventual loss of this sense of invincibility can prove devastating, undermining prior rationalizations. Now sick, they strongly resist giving up their role as doctor. Jacob, a devout Jewish radiologist with skin cancer, said:

A dent in the armor of invulnerability was a surprise, a startling change. I wasn't expecting it. It changed the whole focus of my life. I always assumed I would live longer than anybody else—because my pulse is low, my blood pressure is low, I don't get upset....

Jacob sought varying reasons to bolster his belief in his immunity.

These myths can be ingrained in doctors to such a degree that confronting disease can precipitate deep depression. Dan, the middle-aged oncologist with chest metastases (or "mets"), had been very assertive throughout his life. He had a busy and successful practice in a major hospital. Yet now he had changed. "Knowing I have a disease that could kill me produced a mild depression which I did not have before. We're not invulnerable, immortal, perfect."

Other physicians did not sufficiently plan for the possibility of disease or death in their lives, not yet writing or sufficiently updating wills. Mark, an internist, was very open about being HIV-positive, suggesting that I interview him over lunch at a diner near his office. As will be discussed later, as a result of being a patient himself, he felt that he had improved at dealing with end-of-life decisions for patients. But, surprisingly, he had not been able to bring himself to write a will. "I don't think it means anything Freudian. Maybe it does. I really should do a will—that's my intention." Yet he still could not bring himself to do so.

These physicians' surprise was itself surprising, indicating the extent to which they had previously been socialized to feel otherwise. These beliefs persisted to such a degree that physicians may not only distance themselves from patients, but also look down at, and stigmatize, them. Some doctors thought that being a patient was "the worst possible thing" that could happen to them. Eleanor, whose physician-husband had recently died from complications of diabetes, said about him:

He thought that the world was divided into two groups—us and them—*us* being the physicians, and *them* being the patients. If you have an illness, you become one of *them*. Doctors think, *"We're not patients."*

These doctors revealed the degree of stigmatization of patients that can exist within the medical profession. Charles, who had become an "underground" researcher, said, *"To be a patient is suddenly a step down."* His diagnosis led him to voice this sense that others felt as well. This stigma reflects ostracism of the sick more broadly in society, and is of concern in and of itself, impeding physician readiness to enter this new role of patient.

Only now did some physicians become more fully aware of the extent of human fragility. Deborah, the psychiatrist, said, "When I became a patient, I realized how vulnerable we all are and that you can get sick." Though she had treated patients for many years in various capacities, it took her own illness to bring her more completely to this realization.

In sum, as their disease marched on, these physicians engaged in resistance and denial at multiple points, starting with the initial recognition and integration of symptoms and diagnosis as they struggled to cope. As we shall see, they came to rely on many tools that they had long used with others.

3

"The Medical Self"

Self-doctoring and Choosing Doctors

"When am I a doctor, and when am I a patient?" Stuart asked. He and others grappled with this question.

As their disease progressed, these physicians were finally forced to acknowledge their illness in some way, but had to decide exactly *how* and *to what degree* to do so. After all, they could treat themselves, order and interpret their own lab tests, and prescribe medications—choosing drugs, doses, and lengths of treatment. These capabilities could all help. Yet such self-doctoring had limitations.

They also self-doctored in the contexts of dynamic doctor-patient and doctor-colleague relationships that can shape these self-treatment decisions. These ill physicians had to choose and interact with their own doctors, but faced obstacles in doing so.

I found that most of these doctor-patients wrestled with questions of whether they *should* self-prescribe, and if so, to what extent. They also faced dilemmas in selecting doctors to treat them. Generally, they tried to balance treating themselves and being treated by others, but wondered how to establish such boundaries. In these matters, many thought they were not wholly objective.

Several physicians described going within a few minutes from seeing patients in a clinic to being seen *as* a patient. The physical contexts of clinics and their own doctors' offices also structured and shaped their roles, informing how they behaved.

Letting Oneself Be a Patient

Once they were sick, a few readily acknowledged their diagnosis and chose to "let themselves be patients"—to adopt and embrace that role and let another provider heal them. Usually they did so if their disease lay outside their area of expertise. Thus, pediatricians and psychiatrists with cancer accepted their doctors' treatments almost fully, while internists with diabetes, such as Eleanor's husband, felt they could and should handle their illness themselves. Some suggested that if they *did* have more expertise in their own illnesses, they might self-doctor more. Jacob, the radiologist with skin cancer, for example, accepted his physician's advice, and adopted a submissive role as a patient. He did not check the medical literature concerning his cancer; his wife did so for him. He adopted a relatively passive stance because his illness lay outside his area of specialization as a radiologist, and he had ready access to colleagues with proper expertise.

> I don't know anything about my melanoma, because I'm not clinical. *I'm the picture reader, not a symptom finder.* I don't know how I would react if I were more adept at dealing with symptoms—how easy it would be to write prescriptions and self-diagnose.

Jacob doesn't mention here that his wife researches his disease for him.

Other physicians tended to "let themselves be patients" if, when first diagnosed, they were young, or early in their careers. Suzanne, the psychiatrist-in-training who was on lithium, for example, said, "I'm perfectly comfortable being a patient because I've been seeing psychiatrists and therapists since I was nineteen!"

At least initially, passivity as patients could arise, too, from familial models. Ronald, the WASP radiologist in his thirties who lived in Connecticut and was HIV-positive, said:

> My family was very passive when it came to the doctor-patient relationship, and that's what I also fell into: "I better not bother the doctor and ask too many questions, because he'll get offended."

Yet even those who more readily accepted patienthood tended to judge their doctors' decisions carefully. For example, David, the psychiatrist with HIV, said, "I'm not 'the aggressive patient' in terms of dictating my care. My internist is good and caring—that's what I want.

I can tell she knows what's going on. I know *enough* that this is a competent person." He still relied on his own medical knowledge in accepting that of his doctor. As he implied, increased trust of one's physician can diminish impulses to self-doctor.

Worsening of symptoms could also prompt heightened acceptance of the patient role. Jim, the drug company researcher with leukemia, said, "There was no way to maintain any denial at all. I was sick—sicker than most people I had ever known."

After treating patients for years, a few ill doctors were glad to have another physician assume the responsibility and burdens of being in charge. Bill, a Southern radiologist with HIV, said, "I play doctor all day long. Part of me wants to be a patient who can trust the doctor to make the decisions." It should be noted that HIV treatment lay outside his specialization.

Other physicians did not self-doctor, but for potentially less healthy reasons. For instance, they sought to avoid accepting and acknowledging that they were even sick. Neil, a neurologist with HIV, tried not to treat himself, but did not want to hear about certain aspects of his medical condition, either.

> I cannot stand hearing lab results. I just told my doctor, "Tell me if
> I'm doing ok. But nothing else." *I know that sounds crazy, and I'd*
> *never recommend it for my patients, but I didn't want to deal with being*
> *sick.* I didn't feel sick, and didn't want the numbers to make me sick.

Ironically, it could take denial to halt self-doctoring. Neil engaged in a behavior (denial) that he would never suggest for his patients, but that he pursued nonetheless, highlighting a disconnection that will be explored further below. As we shall see later as well, other physicians neither self-doctored nor consulted other physicians. Rather, they resisted the role of patient altogether.

But adopting a passive stance as a patient had potential pitfalls: placing one's self and well-being wholly in another's hands, despite potential medical errors that might ensue. Jacob, the religious radiologist with skin cancer, accepted the word of his doctor; somewhat analogously, he accepted that of God, too. He acknowledged that his approach with doctors might make him vulnerable to medical mishaps.

> I don't ask a lot of questions. Just tell me what I'm supposed to do
> next. I select a doctor, and that's it. If the doctor makes a mistake,
> tough luck. Doctors are supposed to make mistakes.

Jacob saw respect for authority as a virtue. At one point, however, he prescribed a bone scan for himself, intimating that he may have engaged in more self-doctoring than he perceived himself as doing.

Others varied over time in how they balanced their roles as doctor and patient, and the degree to which they adopted the stance of patient. Jacob added, "I went that patient route a little *too far*, and now am trying to get more involved in my health care."

"Insider Status" and "Remaining in Control": Self-doctoring

In contrast to those who "became patients" more fully, others strove desperately to remain "doctors" and "in control," in order to avoid yielding power to a colleague. Their acts of self-doctoring ranged widely in degree, from "being proactive" and using their insider status within the complicated bureaucracy of managed care, to prescribing for and diagnosing themselves.

In some way, most ill physicians drew on their own health resources, which were unavailable to ordinary patients. Their greater access to the medical system allowed them to "manage" the system. Jeff, an adolescent medicine specialist with HIV, said, "I know how to get great care and deal with the system." As a physician, he had learned skills that he now used for himself as a patient—for example, calling physicians a second time when phone messages weren't returned. Since he had heightened access to medical information, he thought he received better care. "The system responds to me. If I were just playing patient, I would be more frustrated. I wouldn't be privy to all the information, or understand the system."

Jeff suggested that, at least in part, one *plays roles* of patient and doctor—parts one performs.

Many of these physicians were tempted to use their status as insiders simply because they could. For example, Jeff possessed the hospital directory, which provided him with direct phone numbers.

> I don't go through public phone lines—the receptionists, the barriers. I have the direct line to the doctor or nurse—the directory. I know the nurses personally. I've developed connections and friendships over years of working there. Everybody does it at their companies.

This privileged status helped in procuring referrals to the "best" physicians and getting appointments as soon as possible. Many of these physicians had access that permitted them to consult frequently with doctors, and obtain second, third, and fourth opinions. Jacob said, "I was two phone calls away from getting the best person in the business." Daily physical proximity to experts facilitated such access.

These physician-patients were aware of the marked contrast with "how it works *on the 'outside.'*" Here, the distinction between "inside" and "outside" referred to both geographic and social space—working inside or outside of the hospital or the profession. These two types of distinctions were also interrelated, strengthening the walls between these two "locales." Roxanne, the gastroenterologist, said:

> I can call up whomever I want and solicit expert advice: "Who knows about this? I want to be involved in certain trials." Yet even for me, sometimes it's hard to get information, and I *know* whom to ask. So *I can't imagine what it's like for some patients "out there."*

Given the health care system, even for these physicians, accessing optimal care was often still difficult.

The advent of managed care and changes in the health care system exacerbated these self-doctoring behaviors. As the system itself has become more cumbersome and bureaucratic, proactive stances get further rewarded. In the past, physicians had a relationship of professional courtesy, treating each other for free or for whatever fee insurance companies provided. But managed care eroded this custom. Many of these physicians bemoaned the loss, which in turn furthered self-doctoring.

The desire to remain as a doctor resulted, too, from desires to avoid dependency on others. To accept illness is to relinquish control. For example, Deborah, the psychiatrist with metastatic breast cancer, primed (set up) her chemo herself. She made sure the staff didn't have to do anything, as she did not want to rely on others. Her actions, however, violated hospital procedures.

> When I do chemo, I prep all the solutions. So when the nurses come in, everything's ready. The only thing they have to do is stick me. I also used to pull the IV out when I was done. But they got very concerned: "We can be cited. *Because you are a patient, you can't behave like a doctor.*"

Deborah did not oppose getting the treatment, but being given it by others, which represented dependency. These physicians found it hard to accept help in part because both the profession of medicine and the prevailing American cultural ethos encourage rugged independence.

Deborah resisted entering the sick role in other small but symbolic ways as well. As a result, her oncologist admonished her to "be a patient":

> My oncologist says, "Why don't you put a gown on and be a patient for a while?" I don't change into the gown every time.
> She does a physical exam, and I don't change until we talk. She gets upset and says, "*You should really be a patient!*" But I don't want to.

Similarly, as a patient in the hospital, Dan, the oncologist with chest mets, who had been assertive throughout his life, insisted on wearing surgical scrubs rather than patient pajamas.

> The hospital staff have seen me over the years and know who I am. But *it's very strange to sit there in a hospital gown with my butt hanging out.* When I go for my scans, I bring along a pair of scrubs, and change into scrubs, rather than into one of their sets of patient pajamas which, because of my girth, don't fit me.

Additionally, many doctors are controlling by nature; and self-select to enter the profession. Premed courses and medical school encourage and reward obsessive traits, weeding out individuals with more casual attitudes. Harry, an elderly internist and World War II refugee who had a myocardial infarction (or MI), said:

> It's the great failing of most physicians: they are controlling people. But to be a *good* patient, and get the best care, you have to say, "I'm the doormat. You can do what you want," and not second-guess.

Medicine may attract individuals who also seek mastery over disease and death. When they were young, several of these doctors observed disease in a family member or in themselves, and vowed to try to conquer it.

Self-doctoring could result, too, from more overt denial. To enable doctors to perform their job, a degree of denial may be necessary to allow physicians to be physically close to patients, despite potential fears of contagion. But patienthood can exacerbate this denial, which can prove maladaptive and interfere with treatment.

Self-treatment created potential difficulties, too, since, as mentioned earlier with regard to self-diagnosis, problems could be overlooked and decision-making authority could be unclear. Jeff, the adolescent specialist, took the lead in his own care. But as a result, his physicians may not have followed up with him or taken full responsibility as much as they would have otherwise. Physicians-of-record may relinquish some of their control to these physician-patients. Jeff said:

I take the lead *a lot*. Sometimes maybe when I shouldn't. But my primary doctor's already let me have it, so she drops it. My counts dropped a couple of weeks ago. My primary doctor got the lab results, but hasn't called me. It might have come across her desk. But I take over, and *who's running the show?* When it works, it works really well. It saves her time and makes it easier for me. But when it doesn't work, things could get missed. I'll go fill out my own lab slip. But if I don't do it, they're not going to miss it. *They assume that I'm doing it because they know I can.*

Yet receiving optimal care may require surrendering a degree of self-reliance and control. This need to yield and cooperate undermines notions, too, of patient self-empowerment. Harry, the internist and war refugee with an MI, drew analogies, describing how being hospitalized in many regards resembled being in the military.

I was in the army, which in some ways is similar to being a patient—an outside "force" controls you. In basic training, I tried to maneuver my fate. I went to the personnel office. I was being a smart-ass. It got me nowhere. When I let the army do what they wanted, in their own seemingly illogical way, things seemed to work out. In the hospital, you can try to modify the system as much as you can within limits—knowing the system—a little bit, so that you can wear more comfortable slippers that won't drop off your feet. But in the end, if I'm relaxed, instead of fuming things will work out better.

Some physicians felt torn or even "guilty" about exercising aspects of self-doctoring, aware of professional propriety. "I felt guilty because I was in medicine, and wasn't being a scientist about it." Still, many self-doctored anyway, given competing needs. The fact that some felt "guilty" about self-doctoring suggested the degree to which the profession implicitly questioned this behavior.

Varieties of Self-testing

As indicated above, self-doctoring can include several stages: self-diagnosing, self-testing, self-prescribing, and self-interpreting of tests. Some physicians ordered diagnostic tests because, they argued, getting other doctors to do so was hard or inconvenient. Scott, an internist with a foot infection, chose his own diagnostic tests, even arranging to grow the infectious agent that caused his cellulitis. "I cultured the stuff: collected it in a sterile tube. None of the trainees wanted to culture the stupid thing. Even the surgeon didn't want to!"

Self-doctoring can also involve researching one's illness, including providing information to one's physicians—"filling in the gaps," performing tasks that otherwise might not get done. Sally, an internist with cancer, loved her work, calling it her "therapy." When hospitalized in the intensive care unit (ICU), she brought along her own laptop and conducted Internet searches on aspects of treatment about which her physician said he could not find any articles.

> In the ICU, I did my literature search. The attendings couldn't find the literature on my condition and low calcium. It took me about five seconds. They didn't really look. I went to Medline and typed "hypocalcaemia with pneumocystis." Out came five wimpy articles. But these doctors said they couldn't find *anything*!

Ill physicians arranged not only to access certain procedures, but also to avoid others that they deemed unnecessary. Herb, a neonatologist in his sixties with an MI, for instance, was able to eschew invasive procedures that he felt were not fully warranted: "A cardiologist friend said I could pull my IV out, call a cab, and go home, and my prognosis would be identical."

Self-prescribing

Among self-doctoring behaviors, the most controversial and potentially dangerous was self-prescribing. Commonly, these doctors ordered medications for themselves, determining types, amounts, and lengths of drug treatment. Yet self-prescribed drugs can range from the innocuous to the risky. Implicitly or explicitly, self-prescribers had to face questions of whether these behaviors were inappropriate, and where, if at all, to draw the line. Moreover, only these doctors themselves—not their physicians-of-record—assessed, monitored, and limited these behaviors. Self-prescribers approached these tensions in a variety of ways. Scott, who had an infected foot, treated his own hypertension, since, he claimed, he couldn't get his MD to do so.

> I've been treating myself because I can't get a doctor to. My doctor takes my blood pressure every once in a while, and it's pretty normal. But I can take my blood pressure *all the time*. So I'll futz with my doses—add this, that, adjust, etc.—and I've gotten the readings I like.

When undergoing surgery, Scott even *brought his own addictive opiates as pain meds with him to the hospital* "because the nurses made dosing errors."

Other doctors drew limits on how much self-dosing they permitted themselves. After all, not all self-prescription was equally dangerous or worrisome. Yet explanations they offered could at times constitute rationalizations. Dan, the oncologist with chest mets, said about his operation:

> I'm playing my own doctor, which is probably not the most brilliant thing. But as long as I'm playing my own doctor, being *conservative* rather than radical, I tend not to be concerned.

Even these doctors had difficulty revealing their self-doctoring to their physicians—not always disclosing fully. Scott, who self-prescribed experimentally, did not tell his doctor until afterward. Some *never* divulged their self-prescribing to anyone. For example, Jessica, a pediatrician with Hodgkin's, secretly gave herself antidepressants.

> From time to time I have medicated myself with Paxil. But I stop because of fear of long-term side effects. I don't go see a psychiatrist, for multiple reasons: time and money, and I would probably find it difficult to talk about very private, intimate things. My nature is to be very private. So I medicate. I can write prescriptions for myself. I usually use low doses. My sister was taking Paxil, and it helped her, so I said, "I'll try *that*." I never really wanted to be on it, but I needed it. I stopped after a while, but then needed to start it again. Obviously, it's altering my brain chemistry, and nobody really knows how in the long term. So it makes me a little nervous.

Still, Jessica never told her doctor, even though variations in her symptoms implied that consistent treatment by a professional might benefit her. Even when asked, she maintained secrecy. "The oncologist asks, 'Are you taking any medication?' I'm not going to admit to taking the Paxil! I don't want them to know about it." She feared discrimination, and felt shame.

A range of rationalizations arose for self-prescribing—from convenience to beliefs about innocuousness. Deborah rationalized that she was taking only a *small* dose. Kurt, an HIV-infected internist who had once used crack, now self-prescribed Prozac. He said he did not like the psychiatrist he had been consulting, so now he saw none.

> Maybe I still have a little residual depression. I have not seen the psychiatrist, and have been self-prescribing the same medicine. I stopped seeing the psychiatrist because I think he was using drugs.

Alternatively, Kurt could have found another psychiatrist, yet he felt ashamed about his problems coping.

Some physicians self-prescribed because they felt they knew more than their doctors did. Ill physicians may in fact have more experience than their treating physicians—particularly if the latter are interns or residents. Yet such perceptions may not always be correct. Dan, who had chest mets, said:

> The intern said, "We don't think you need your patient-controlled anesthetic. We're going to put you on oral medication." I said, "I still get severe pain." She said, "It's going to be very difficult to transition when you go home." I said, "I'll tell you how we could do it very easily." She said, "In my experience I think we ought to take you off." I said, "Come on—you've been a doctor for a month. *I've been a doctor more years than you've been alive! This is my expertise." I yelled and screamed and got what I wanted.*

Still, perceptions of having more knowledge than one's colleagues may be only impressionistic and ego-gratifying. Pascal, a Lebanese internist with HIV, treated himself, feeling he knew more than any other doctor in his town. He didn't want to consult "and pretend I'm the patient. Because I feel I know more than any of them." He laughed, hinting at a degree of embarrassment and discomfort about his claims of superior skill, but continued self-prescribing.

Self-prescription can lead to problems, as these individuals may disagree with their own physicians' recommendations, and may not maintain objectivity.

Many physicians self-doctored without thinking of themselves as doing so. Harry, the elderly internist and war refugee, felt that he had been able to relinquish control. He said, "I'm a patient-physician"—as opposed to a "physician-patient"—emphasizing one role over the other. He added, "I'm a very controlling person, basically. But under these circumstances, I think I have the attitude 'Do what you think is best.' They say, 'What do you think?' and I say, 'Do what you think is best.'" Nonetheless, Harry started treatment with an experimental medication on his own:

> I initiated it. I called it to the attention of my physician, looked it up, and asked my doctor for permission to do it. I almost always order medications for my wife and myself. It's much simpler that way.

Thus, his self-perceptions and actual practices of self-doctoring clashed.

Some physicians set up standards and boundaries concerning self-prescribing, but did not always follow these either. Herb stated:

> I would never write prescriptions—well, that's not true. I will write them. The second tick bite I had, knowing that there is a lot of Lyme disease around, I decided to treat myself.

Herb implies a distinction based in part on the severity of the medical problem. He self-prescribes for what he considers minor, but not major, problems. But others might question where he draws the boundaries.

Many of these doctors treated other ill physicians, and had to deal with the latter's self-prescribing, observing these issues from triple perspectives. Observations of colleagues treating themselves poorly could prompt one to set rules and vow to be a "good patient" oneself. Stuart, an internist who retired due to HIV and was now teaching at a local university, reflected:

> Sick doctors who treated themselves or didn't come in for follow-ups annoyed me. I had to keep the ground rules straight: you should adopt the role of the patient here, because you'll get good care. If you muck it up, I can't be responsible. So I came to my doctor with that sense of "I'll behave."

Yet when treating ill doctors, such ground rules can be hard to follow. Tensions and deceptions marked such negotiations. Herb continued:

> I'd say, "I'd rather you don't write your own scripts." But a couple of patients got a little demented and frightened, and broke down. It became a real push-and-pull.

Because of such self-doctoring efforts, lay patients may be more straightforward to treat than doctor-patients. Herb added:

> It was easier for nondoctors to see my role as I saw it, and understand: "Come into the office. Let me treat you like a patient." Docs would say, "I'm busy; I can't do it this week." Other patients would say, too: "I'm busy at work." But I can pull rank on them. With the docs, it was hard to put my foot down. Some talked back.

Herb did not feel strong enough in his beliefs about appropriate standards to argue.

Practicing "Research-Level Medicine": Aggressive Treatment

Many ill physicians not only self-doctored, but approached treatment decisions *more aggressively* than they standardly would for their patients. Some practiced "research-level medicine"—using less proven, experimental treatments that were "off-protocol," not yet approved for the particular use in question. These behaviors offered insights for lay patients as to what else patients might do if they had the knowledge and professional connections of physicians.

For centuries, doctors have self-experimented. But here, this tendency appeared as part of a larger trend: of physicians approaching risks and benefits *differently* for themselves than for their patients, accepting different standards and levels of safety. For example, Charles, the underground researcher with HIV, continually tried experimental drugs on himself, "leaving no stone unturned."

Roxanne, the gastroenterologist with abdominal cancer, flew to the West Coast for a treatment that had been used in only one other patient.

> There's no cure. But an expert on the West Coast was using a new medicine. It was not yet approved. Still, I wanted it right away. My doctor said, "You shouldn't take medication unless you have to. Wait until the right time to treat."

Roxanne flew to the West Coast anyway, and took the medication.

Many physicians were more aggressive in part because they *could* be, possessing better access to the health care system. Their position let them learn more readily about, and obtain, experimental treatments—including those not yet regularly available. Jeff, the adolescent specialist, for example, distinguished his care from that of "a *regular* patient." He spoke to me as use of new HIV medications was beginning to spread.

No one is aggressive in my care, telling me about studies. I want my doctor to say, "We think maybe you should do this." But they're not looking at my case, knowing what I've been through. I initiate the conversation. I don't know what my physicians would have done if I were just a *regular* patient.

Such aggressiveness enabled physicians to avoid periods that otherwise often occur of "waiting to see what happens." Waiting produces anxiety, feelings of helplessness, and pain of inactivity. Dan, the oncologist with chest metastases, for example, said, "I want to be more aggressive. But my doctor will say, 'Let's get another study; let's wait a month.'" Assertive throughout his life, Dan now sought to remain so.

Frequently, having observed and employed aggressive treatment with others, physicians were now less afraid of it themselves. Nancy, an endocrinologist with breast cancer, said, "I had this feeling: these are bad cells, I want them off of me—which a lot of doctors with breast cancer do. They choose a mastectomy over lumpectomy" (removal of an entire breast rather than just a lump) "even though supposedly they're sort of the same" (i.e., in terms of long-term outcomes).

Dan knew the high risks of his treatment, but tried to minimize these by getting the "best possible" doctors to perform the procedure. He took advantage of the fact that known risks of a procedure reflect aggregated statistical data that fail to account for differences between practitioners.

Though a doctor's job was to "protect" patients from danger, the calculus changed if the patient was oneself. The responsibility to safeguard potentially vulnerable patients from harm outweighed the desire to undertake such risks on behalf of others. Yet no such duty existed to protect oneself from dangers one knowingly chose to confront oneself.

I'm willing to take more chances with myself than I am with other people, because it's *me*. A physician is a *protector*: protecting the patient from himself, and from others who would be more aggressive.

Such aggressive treatment stemmed in part from doctors' sense that they better understood, assessed, and could accept risks. Indeed, these views and approaches toward risk were often deeply ingrained. Harry, the internist and war refugee, said, "I can be *more realistic* and hopefully less emotional. The amount of risk I'm willing to take is *part of my personality.*"

Jacob's wife asked whether doctors were "morally obligated" to volunteer for experimental treatments in order to help other sufferers of a disease. She argued:

> A Jew is supposed to want to preserve life. So if a patient has lung cancer, and is told, "We have this treatment, a potential cure," then, as an observant Jew, are you required to do it? To go for every single thing offered?

Often, these doctors were grateful for the ability to be aggressive, as this approach succeeded. Dan commented, "Very few surgeons have experience *taking out* a sternum. If I wasn't aggressive, my sternum would still be there with tumor."

But such experimental treatment can be difficult to procure. Walter, a politically active internist with lymphoma, tried research treatments to which other patients did not have access. But he found even these interventions difficult to arrange.

> I tried this experimental use of interferon, because a cancer researcher I consulted thought it may help me. My oncologist said, "I don't agree, but if you want to, it's ok with me. I'll write the prescription." But weeks went by, and I could not get him to give me the prescription. As a doctor, I was asking another doctor—but couldn't make it happen. When I stopped being really sick, I dropped down *a lot* on his list of priorities.

These differences in degree of aggressiveness raised questions about how physicians treated patients generally. Doctors must triage, but a patient sees his or her own serious illness as critically important. With their own patients, these physicians also tended to be more conservative; only gingerly suggesting, but not "pushing," less conventional and more research-level treatments. Dan said:

> *I am much more aggressive for myself than I would be for my patients.* I would offer these options to my patients—sort of *hint* that these were possibilities—but wouldn't push them. For myself, I have really pushed: I've had over *double* the usual doses of radioiodine, to be as aggressive as possible: research-level medicine.

I'm saying, "Let's do it off-protocol. I know enough to give in-formed consent."

With patients, doctors ordinarily try to find the appropriate balance between erring a little on the side of too much versus too little treatment, and most tend to be cautious. Harry, the internist and war refugee, said:

Compulsive overdoers order every test in the book. Maybe they are insecure. But it costs somebody a lot of money and blood. Occasionally, they find something that they didn't suspect. But you hope to do the *proper* amount of tests. You want to be in the middle. Which is worse—overdoing it a little or underdoing it a little? I overdo it a little—I hate to stand there with egg on my face. But I always attempt to have some justification.

These differences also underlay the questions patients commonly ask their providers: "What would you do if you were me, doctor?" or "What would you do if your mother were the patient?"

As a result of being a patient, a few doctors occasionally did become more vigorous in treating their patients. For example, some tried to provide test results more rapidly. A few tried to order treatments more aggressively, too, but this alteration was rare. Pascal, for example, said that if he were not HIV-infected himself, he wouldn't push as much for his patients as he did now.

I am much more aggressive in finding other ways of doing things. I don't think I'd be as aggressive, or come up with novel ways of treating patients when I've run out of options, exploring things that you can only get through compassionate use, or combining multiple medications—things a "straight" doc wouldn't do. He'd think, "Well, this drug doesn't work...you're dead anyway."

Other ill physicians wanted to be more assertive with patients, but refrained for various reasons, in part legal liability. Harry, the war refugee, explained, "Malpractice is somewhere in the back of my mind. We physicians are more aware of the consequences, and can deal with the side effects" (i.e., when treating themselves).

But these doctors suggest that perhaps norms should change—patients should be offered riskier treatments when no other therapy is available, providing these patients can understand the risks and benefits involved—which they frequently can.

Practicing What They Preach: Health Behaviors

"I tell patients to do a lot of things that I don't do myself," Deborah
sighed. Despite aggressiveness in their own medical treatment once they
became seriously ill, many had previously found it hard to practice what
they preached concerning preventive health behaviors. Many failed to
engage in health prevention: not seeing a doctor for decades until becoming seriously ill, not extending their roles as doctors to their own care.
These physicians were "only human." These discrepancies in behavior
illuminated the divides between treatment of present illness and prevention of future ailments; treatment of self versus of others; and *one's
medical self versus one's patient self*. The pursuit of future health proved less
motivating than the elimination of present symptoms.

Many physicians were aware that they didn't follow the recommendations that they gave others, but they remained unable to alleviate this
discrepancy. Deborah said, "I give advice, and think: Why don't you give
that advice to *yourself?*"

Repeatedly, gaps arose between doctors' advice and practice concerning, for example, *diet*. Many doctors consumed high fat diets, despite
having high cholesterol, and advising patients to do otherwise. Jessica, the
pediatrician with Hodgkin's lymphoma, ate unwholesomely, and avoided
accessing medical treatment for fear that doctors would reprimand her.
She rationalized that she would die young anyway.

> I have very bad eating habits. My diet is unhealthy and my
> cholesterol is high. I preach about it all the time to my patients,
> then go eat at Burger King. I don't have a lot of willpower. I
> say to myself, I'll deal with it when I get something really life-
> threatening—my first heart attack. After I turned forty, I put on
> a lot of weight, as many people do—but a *lot*. My oncologist
> always yells at me. I don't exercise. I say, "I've had cancer, I'm
> going to die early anyway"—which is kind of crazy—or "I'm going
> to die from some other cancer." It makes me see doctors less.
> I know I'm fooling myself.

Jessica recognized that she was rationalizing, but still found it hard to
change. She resisted because of countervailing reasons—enjoying life and
gaining pleasure now trumped logical concerns about future harms. It was
hard even for these doctors to imagine their feelings in the future, high-

lighting again how doctoring does not overcome certain preexisting human traits, but gets grafted onto them.

Unhealthy behaviors continued even in the face of pressures from colleagues. Coworkers may remind doctors of dietary restrictions, but to no avail. Herb, the neonatologist with an MI, found, for instance, that nurses with whom he worked reprimanded him for eating junk food when they saw him doing so in the staff lounge, warning him of "the evil temptation of pizza." He suggested that we live in a new era of morality, employing moral terms of "good" and "evil," focused on diet and health. Albert, a white-haired internist in his mid-sixties, looked like a small town doctor from an earlier era. He had had an MI while driving on a highway, and said that afterward, he suddenly became "religious" about his diet, alluding to the high sense of obligation entailed—as if such health behaviors were special, sacred, and subject to laws.

> I had never cared how much fat was in my diet. As soon as I became aware of it, I realized that everybody in the room but me would know the fat content of a bag of potato chips. Then, for a while, I could quote the fat content of every food I ate. I got a certain amount of satisfaction from being religious about that.

Individuals may try to act on medical findings in their everyday lives, yet doing so requires vigilance and energy. It took his own unexpected illness to prompt Albert to alter his outlook and activity.

Many doctors failed to practice what they preached with regard not only to diet, but also to safer sex, which may affect others as well. For example, David, the psychiatrist with HIV, had unprotected sex though he knew he shouldn't: "I had unsafe sex after I knew better...with a guy at a gay physicians conference, even as we were sitting there talking about this stuff." Physicians are not alone in engaging in risky behavior despite knowledge that they shouldn't, but they are unique in simultaneously urging patients to engage only in healthy behaviors.

At times, magical thinking—that MDs were somehow invulnerable to disease—abetted unhealthy behaviors. David felt that his unprotected sex was somehow safe.

> One of my dead boyfriends was a doctor. I rationalized that because he was a doctor, his unsafe sexual practices were somehow safe. Because he was a doctor, he *couldn't* be positive. It made no sense. I was just avoiding the subject.

Here again, recognition of avoidant behavior was not sufficient to eliminate it.

Substance abuse also emerged—including the use of recreational drugs that were perceived as unhealthy, particularly for those with impaired immune systems. Physician stress can compound substance abuse. Indeed, doctors may have higher rates of abuse of certain substances than do nonphysicians (1).

As a result of beliefs in invulnerability, doctors often protect themselves less than they should against disease. They may self-protect less than nurses, who generally do not follow as "macho" an ethic. Stuart observed, "The doctors are the last ones to wear protective gloves. The nurses are much more likely to do so."

Even more dangerous, several doctors who had lowered immunity, making them acutely vulnerable to disease, nonetheless still treated infectious patients. This behavior suggested both commitment and denial. Lou, who debated removing the award from his wall, in retrospect perceived such actions as having been unwise. "Maybe that wasn't so smart, because my white blood cells went down to zero. But the Good Lord smiled down on me."

As indicated, a variety of rationalizations could arise. For years, Sally, the internist with cancer who brought her laptop to the ICU, had avoided seeing a doctor, using the excuse of "never having enough time."

> I was "too busy." I got basic blood testing done, and figured if that was ok, I was ok. Then, I had a high white count. So I asked a colleague to look at me. This colleague is still beating herself because she didn't feel the enlarged spleen tip.

Jessica rationalized that many other professionals had personal problems, too. Hence, she didn't need to consult a mental health professional for her depression.

> I think: why is it that most psychiatrists and psychologists are crazy? Or family counselors are divorced and are not speaking to their relatives? The flesh is weak.

Perceptions of laypeople's shortcomings justified these doctors' own, and eased guilt. Kurt sought to justify unsafe behavior as not being unusual: "A lot of people I know take some risk: get drunk, do drugs, throw caution to the wind."

Yet Kurt had gone further than many by using crack, which is highly addictive.

Others rationalized that preventive medicine generally was not very effective anyway. Albert, who had an MI on the highway, believed that overall, routine physical exams, for example, were not very useful, since physicians-of-record are increasingly lax about preventive health efforts.

The arduous work hours to which physicians become inured through their training can further impede preventive health behavior. Jeff said:

> Part of the training is an endurance test—irregular meals, poor sleep habits, and, unless you consider running up and down stairs exercise, irregular exercise—no balance in your life. *Fried bologna at midnight for supper!* The whole system is geared toward not paying attention to what a healthy lifestyle is for yourself. This is "for the patients." Patients come first. We are only rewarded for cures. If patients need a great deal of education, we refer them to a nurse practitioner or a nutritionist. If they need behavior modification, they go to the psychologist. *Since these things are devalued by the profession, they become unimportant to do for yourself.*

Some doctors recognized the disparity between what they preached and what they practiced, but did not seem able to reconcile the two—either to advise their patients more sensitively and effectively, or to engage in healthier behavior themselves. Neil, the neurologist with HIV, said:

> I don't truly believe what I tell my patients about the need for adherence. I take medications anyway, because I have seen that my immune status and skin have improved, and I believe that I'll be around for a long time—until the next round of medications comes around. But I tell them that the medications should be like *breathing,* or like the necessities: you eat not to starve to death, or drink water in order not to become dehydrated to death. It has to be integrated as a major part of your life because it is necessary to live, and that's how you have to look at it—*which is a great way for them.* For *me,* it's drudgery.

Hence, Neil realized the limitations of the medical recommendations he gave others, but still did not feel compelled to alter his spiel to patients. He uttered the words, but did not act on them himself.

Tensions between what they practiced and what they preached existed even despite beliefs that doctors should, if anything, abide by a higher standard. In the past, Kurt, who had used crack, had not disclosed his HIV infection to sexual partners when using condoms. But he now wanted to set a moral example. He wondered whether doctors had different moral obligations than did nondoctors, and if so, how, and what the implications were if they did not follow their own standards.

> I like to set an example. If an HIV-positive person fucked with a condom and didn't tell his or her partner, that would be ok. But I don't feel it's ok for *me*: it's a slippery slope. I want to hold myself to a high ideal, so I don't deviate from it.

However, Kurt felt guilty because he had gone further, and had even had sex with a former patient.

> I've been so "off" in the past. I ran into people who were patients. A former patient—I had been fired—had sex with my boyfriend, and I had sex with someone else in the same bathhouse room. This patient had a problem with crystal meth, and was whacked out of his mind. So was I. I felt really awful—*because I was his doctor*, and was getting fucked by some other guy without a condom, and he was fucking my boyfriend without a condom. *I should be setting an example!*

Yet moral standards may not always be clear. If an MD should adhere to the highest possible standard, what was it? Kurt wondered, for example, whether he was obliged to disclose to partners if he engaged with them in oral sex.

> If I'm in a park or a bathhouse, I'm not sure: Do I have to tell them I have HIV? Am I morally obligated? Ideally, especially since I'm a physician, I should tell everyone. I like to hold myself to that standard. So when I don't do that, I start questioning it. If the condom breaks, do I tell them *then?* What is ok, and what isn't?

He remained unsure.

The fact that these doctors deviated from their preaching illustrated the degree to which knowledge alone was insufficient to alter health behavior. Perhaps with patients in general, incentives can help. For example, insurance companies can request that patients engage in preventive care, or pay higher premiums. Such approaches may or may not work, but these doctors' experiences clearly raise the need at least to consider such possibilities, given the deep psychological obstacles that exist.

In addition, physicians appeared to "put on" the role of doctor without always fully integrating it into their lives and deepest senses of self. These doctors saw illness as residing in the patient. Hence, since it was in the patient, it could not also reside in these doctors themselves. Thus, they did not feel sick or at risk for disease. These implicit attitudes indicated a significant degree of distancing or projection. Though generalizing about psychodynamic defenses among a large group is difficult, these patterns of responses appeared common.

The Medical Self: Self-prognosticating

Many physicians looked at the worst possible outcome—the prospect of death—as if they were observing another patient rather than themselves. In essence, many saw themselves as if they were a *third person*. Physicians, when they became ill, often faced prognoses as physicians rather than as patients. For example, Nancy, the endocrinologist, stated matter-of-factly, "I have metastases in my head." Her cancer had now spread to her brain, and hence was beyond treatment. She reported:

> My physician said, "We'll just keep doing drugs. Eventually they will stop working and that will be it." I've stopped thinking about the future as much as I can. It's a weird feeling not to have any idea if I'm going to be living next year. When I discovered that I had brain mets, I spent this very funny weekend, thinking, *"This is the last weekend with my brain."*

Nancy's comments indicated a wide distancing from oneself—a surreal otherworldliness evoking profound, existential quandaries. After all, it is not clear what it means to have one's "last weekend" with one's brain; what happens the following weekend; whether one is then no longer "with one's brain," and if so, what it means to be one without one's brain—who and what the "one" is in each case; and what one's identity is without one's brain. Nancy suggested she would encounter mental deficits, but she raised questions as to whether and at what point one was no longer oneself. Is one still one if one has one's body, but not one's mind? In some ways, the answer may be "yes." These questions, which have plagued philosophers for millennia, plumbing the very depths of philosophical inquiry, now confronted many of these doctors daily.

Walter, the political activist with lymphoma, looked from a great distance at himself as a patient. His medical conceptualizations helped him cope, providing him a framework through which to view his illness and telling him he could survive, based on the statistics.

> My *medical self* said, "A lot of people survive Hodgkin's. You can
> get through that." But when I was told I had a very *malignant*
> non-Hodgkin's lymphoma, *that* was a shock. My sense of mortality
> and vulnerability—that I could really die from this—was much
> more heightened.

Walter felt he had a "medical self" observing himself. This self responded to medical facts, and was separate and distinct from other, emotional aspects of himself: his fears and worries. The contrast between his *physician-self* and *patient-self* astonished him. Heretofore, he and others had not recognized or appreciated the depth of this divide.

This prognostication of one's own death, leading to discontinuity in one's identity and sense of self, was so threatening that at times it revealed itself only in flipness or "gallows humor." For example, Eleanor's husband's curt comment on seeing his X-rays ("Yup, I'm a dead man") suggested irony, resignation, and distance all at the same time.

A few physicians recognized this discontinuity and self-distancing, even if still perplexed about it. Stuart, now teaching at the university, for example, felt he spoke about his illness as if it affected "a third person"— not himself.

> It's easy to talk about now—almost as a *third person*. Before, I was
> not connecting much of the emotional—the darkness that was
> definitely there. That came to me later. When you say "hurt,"
> there's almost a certain amount of nonchalance, as I proceeded to
> say this happened and that happened.

In talking about himself, Stuart switched here back and forth from the first person to the third person to the second person, hinting at this separation from part of himself.

Some physicians viewed themselves as though they were "a case," barely a full person. Sally, who brought her laptop to the ICU, went so far as to consider writing up her own case for publication in a medical journal. The fact that her physician raised this possibility with her did not wholly surprise her.

The head of the medical ICU wanted to write it up, so they invited me to join them. I said, no, that's fine. I gave them the references, after they basically couldn't find any. Why should I write up my own medical case? There are some cases in literature, though this is a better one. It may be helpful to others.

Sally pondered the decision, still intrigued by the possibility, recognizing the value of the endeavor. She based her decision on the fact that other articles already existed, not the oddness of the situation. Similarly, Mathilde's husband was asked to present his own case at his departmental rounds.

The degree to which one saw oneself as "the other" varied over time, as ailments progressed. With initial symptoms, some looked up their symptoms in textbooks to help diagnose themselves. Albert, who had an MI on the highway, checked a reference to learn that his symptoms were consistent with an MI.

I was driving and started to feel a little indigestion. I started to take some back roads, and thought maybe I'd stop and grab a glass of milk somewhere. But the prospects of getting on and off the highway argued against that. So I just hung tough, and got home, and the pain, which was mostly mid-upper gastric, changed its nature, and got a little more intense. It was not relieved by milk at home. The subscapular region started to bother me. An idea that I might have some skipping heartbeat problems popped into my mind, and I was curious because the pain was in my back and scapula region. It didn't make sense from what I remembered. So I pulled up my old medical textbook, and sure enough, cardiac pain can be there.

His thinking process remained that of a scientifically trained clinician weighing the evidence pro and con. Albert checked references, but resisted the notion that he was experiencing a heart attack—which he had treated in many patients. He thus delayed responding to it medically as quickly as possible.

In deciding how to integrate these dual identities, ill physicians confronted concrete questions of whether to check their own lab results, which might indicate disease progression. Some did so, interpreting their own lab results and facing their own worst fears unbuffered by the "framing" or objectivity that their physicians could provide. Anne, a Swiss doctor with breast cancer that had metastasized to her spine, found that picking up and reading results herself could be an error. She obtained her pathology results herself, and wept.

> I said to my internist, "I'm really scared of going to the pathology department to get my slides. Can you get them?" He said, "Yes," but he didn't do it. So I had to go to the pathology department myself. I had my slides in my hand, and saw that the inside was full of cancer. The surgeon said he had taken everything out. But all the perimeter was full of cancer. "Shit!" I tried to find him, but he was on vacation. I was absolutely climbing the walls! I was in the hospital, and went to the breast clinic, because I couldn't find any other doctors. I arrived there crying, totally hysterical.

Over time, others struggled, varying in how much they assessed or interpreted potentially devastating prognostic tests. Nancy, the endocrinologist with breast cancer metastases, shed light on the strains involved in maintaining these conflicting roles of both observer and observed, object and subject—and the discontinuities between these.

> I had a very aggressive doctor who liked to follow CEA [carcinoembryonic antigen], a controversial tumor marker. She doesn't do scans. But there was a very hard period of about two and a half years when I was fine, but would come in every three months and get the CEA checked. It's literally going to tell you if you will live or die. I struggled with how to do this: I can go to my office and get on the computer and check it myself. At first, that's what I did. But then, it was just too weird and scary to be sitting there thinking, "Ok, I'm going to check now...." Still, if I waited for my doctor to call me, I'd have to sit by the phone, and I'd get hysterical waiting. So finally, I figured out her office hours, and would check that morning. If it was bad, I would run to her office.

Thus, in myriad unanticipated ways, these doctors had to decide exactly how involved and aggressive to be in their own care. Self-doctoring included a range of behaviors, and the reasons to adopt or eschew these approaches varied. Fear and denial led some to avoid getting diagnosed or, once diagnosed, visiting a physician. Many factors contributed to degrees of self-doctoring—from lack of expertise about one's diagnosis, to psychological needs to maintain control of one's body and life. As we shall see, these tensions mirrored and anticipated others as well.

Doctors Choosing Doctors

The individuals I interviewed had to select physicians to treat them. Whether they acted fully or only partially as patients, these ill doctors had to decide the qualities they themselves sought in health care providers. In so doing, they had to balance a range of personal values and technical, interpersonal, and emotional factors, engaging in highly subjective processes. They made these decisions in the contexts of complicated relationships with family members and caretakers, physicians-of-record, and colleagues. Yet their relatively informed decision-making processes offered many lessons and insights from which lay patients and others might learn.

Therapeutic Tastes and Styles

In selecting their own physicians, most of these interviewees used "inside knowledge"—usually their own, but sometimes that of others. Several of the doctors made use of the fact that they could find "the best" physician in a field, and relished their privileged status as cognoscenti. In their assessments of, and search for, appropriate specialists, some were highly elitist, wanting only "the best." Wilma, a physician in her eighties with a severe GI infection, said:

> I discovered there were only four people in this city who could
> be considered for doing my surgery. Similarly, I went to a lab—
> probably the only one east of the Mississippi that does a proper
> job—and got a proper tropical disease examination, and discovered
> I had an intestinal parasite.

Wilma, wary of the quality of many physicians, felt her standards were justified.

These doctors often looked to particular colleagues, specialists, or friends for information, and cited *subjective* characteristics—aspects of styles and tastes. The *ability* to choose a good doctor may itself vary. Sally, who brought her laptop to the ICU, described a colleague who judged such distinctions well.

> She's very fussy about the doctors she picks, and has always been
> my main source of information. *She has very good taste in doctors*:
> They have to be competent technically, but also able to listen.

Still, within these broad parameters, Sally does not wholly specify what, exactly, constitutes "good taste." The specific criteria may be somewhat intuitive and elusive. Such an assessment may be made in part by observing a physician's work over years. For example, Albert, who had an MI on the highway, ended up in a local hospital, not his own. To choose a doctor, he realized he should ask the head nurse for the name of the best physician.

> They asked me, "What cardiologist would you like?" Of course I knew no one. They would not refer by name easily. And they didn't have a roster. So I excused everybody from the room except the head nurse, and said, "Who would *you* call?" So I got a name. She called him, and he came.

Nurses, after all, have observed physicians' comparative abilities and characteristics closely. Albert's insight—to ask an experienced nurse who has seen a range of doctors, and their successes and failures—can potentially help lay patients as well.

Many spoke of finding physicians with similar practice *styles*—whether "therapeutic nihilists" or "minimalists," on the one hand (who believe that much disease will resolve on its own, and are concerned that physician aggressiveness can at times cause more harm than good), or aggressive "therapeutic enthusiasts" or "overdoers" on the other. Larry, a young anesthesiology resident with HIV, thought he should not yet start medications. Early in his career, he neither wanted to use his insurance for them, nor could afford them on his own. He chose and liked his internist because they were similar: both therapeutic nihilists. "I've read the papers, he's read the papers, and we sort of bounce back and forth. So far we've been on the same wavelength. Everything's been okay, because he's not that med-crazy."

Similarly, Albert, who had an MI on the highway, described himself as "*conservative*" in his medical style. "My doctors didn't feel I had to do anything. I thought that was good. I'm basically conservative about that. You can get into trouble with one of those vessels blown open." Here again, the term "you" referred to his doctors, himself, and other patients, his roles as patient and physician melding.

Preferences for minimalism frequently arose. This approach suggested wariness of the potential dangers of excessive interventionism, with its possible concomitant iatrogenic (treatment-induced) problems. In the end, many doctors felt that Nature ineluctably eludes and overpowers them. As a result, physicians' abilities are inherently limited. Mathilde thought that "Nature has a way of getting back at us. We have defeated streptococcus, staphylococcus, and maybe TB. But Nature comes up with something else."

Ultimately, the inevitability of aging and death curbed physicians' powers. Harry, the war refugee, perceived this limitation starkly.

> I used to tell my patients that they could cheat on their wives or their income tax, and lie to their children, but not change the forces of nature, which are immutable. We are subject to forces of nature—aging, disease, mental processes. We struggle as hard as we can against these forces, and modify and subjugate them if we can. But everybody struggles.

Harry's strong awareness of relative powerlessness grew, in part, from his personal experiences. As a child, he fled Nazi Germany as a refugee. "I'm acutely aware that other forces play a major part in our lives—having to leave the country in which I was born."

Some felt that, in fact, doctors had the ability to reverse the course of only very few diseases, that the profession's perceived powers are over-emphasized. Herb, the neonatologist with an MI, said:

> Eighty-five percent of disease is completely self-limited, and 10 to 12 percent is progressive in the face of all treatment, which leaves only 3 percent in which you could maneuver. When do you ever give a medication that you immediately see results for? In few situations can you do something, and be present for the results.

He distinguishes between the occurrence and the observation of cures, but sees the low rates of both as supporting his point.

Yet such therapeutic nihilism can facilitate self-doctoring. Ill physicians often chose a doctor with a similar practice style who would make treatment decisions similar to these patients' own—achieving results similar to self-doctoring, but not self-doctoring per se. Alternatively, awareness of doctors' ultimate limitations can prompt aggressive stances, to ensure that everything that *can* be done *is* in fact done.

With different styles and approaches toward these issues, doctors may implicitly *choose* their patients as well. Harry said, "Every physician has a practice that reflects his or her personality. After several visits, things sort themselves out. One tries to find a doctor whose skill, worldview, human characteristics, and sentiment reflect yours, and with whom you're confident." Consequently, doctors and patients may each, to a degree, self-select.

Doctors may also assess and take into account these differing styles in deciding to whom to *refer* patients for treatment. As Harry put it:

> There is this wonderful business: if you refer a patient for chemotherapy, you have a choice of sending them to a therapeutic nihilist or a therapeutic enthusiast, or anything in between. You know who's doing what before you send the patient to them—what they're going to do. You determine to some extent the patient's therapy. Should you tell that to the patient? That's the issue I present to students. I did and didn't tell, depending on the patient.

Yet conversely, barriers can arise to finding and being able to choose a doctor who matches one's own ideal approach. Insurance plans can limit choices of physician. Harry described himself as being at one point a "prisoner of a minimalist."

Good Bedside Manner versus Technical Skill

Technical skill, and the balance between it and "bedside manner," also shaped choices of the interviewed physicians. Among these ill doctors, a minority emphasized that for particular types of medical problems and treatments, empathy alone was insufficient. Harry, the war refugee, said, "I know a son of a bitch who's a wonderful surgeon."

The appropriate balance between humanism and scientific ability could depend on the medical problem faced. To a friend requiring surgery, Harry therefore recommended technical skill over "niceness."

> A good friend was diagnosed with carcinoma of the uterus, and went to the cancer hospital's surgeons, who always just cut everything out. There are untoward side effects, but the cancer hospital doesn't care about that. They just want to eradicate Cancer, with a capital C. She had only a little bump in her myometrial wall. So I said, "Go to Dr. X. He's a wonderful surgeon, but not only doesn't talk much to his patients—he's nasty." She interviewed him, and he just insulted her. He said, "We'll get in there, do a biopsy first, and see what needs doing." He did a fine job. It turns out she had only this little localized cancer. But in the

hospital, he came to see her only once. She wanted to ask him a question. He said, "I've been with you all my time in the OR. Good-bye." He's a mean son of a bitch. But if you can tolerate that kind of idiocy, that's what you should do.

In this instance, Harry recommended acceptance of this surgeon's extreme style because of a specific medical treatment.

Most of the doctors prioritized a combination of technical and emotional strengths, and marginally more interpersonal skill over marginally more scientific know-how alone. Thoroughness and provision of necessary time were important. For example, Lou, with the award on his wall, described the category of a "classical" doctor—a "doctor's doctor"—and how he chose one.

I didn't go to 400 doctors, getting opinions. I found the person I trusted—a superb internist, a *classical* physician. He practices holistic medicine, though he wouldn't call it that. He gets a detailed history and is empathetic. He practices medicine the way it's supposed to be practiced. You don't see it that much. He is a "doctor's doctor," thoughtful and listening. He understands things and knows the literature. In law, they have a "counselor of the law." We should have a "counselor of medicine."

These ill physicians thus drew fine, often implicit distinctions among their colleagues.

Others spoke more explicitly of valuing the psychological comforts they received from their providers. Many appreciated their physicians' ability to ameliorate anxiety. Roxanne, the gastroenterologist, liked her doctor in part because he soothed her psychologically. "He was the best because he was experienced: he calmed me down." She valued, too, not being abandoned as a patient. "He was always there, saying, 'You are not alone.'" Even Lou, the physician with the award on his wall, wanted more reassurance than he received. His doctor was "civil," but not encouraging—providing facts but not interpreting them.

He wasn't a cold fish, but was not warm. He wouldn't say, "The outlook is good," but "The CT is negative." The chances of cure were pretty good, but he wouldn't say that.

This doctor would merely provide "the facts" without their emotional implications.

This preference for more bedside manner over more technical expertise matched that of many patients. Indeed, slight gradations of technical expertise, as well as broader distinctions in reputation, were difficult to assess. Bradley, an elderly but athletic internist who first felt symptoms of an MI while playing tennis, and afterward became depressed for the first time, said:

> The major input to people's sense of the hospital experience was
> the personal contact, not the size of their incision or the fact
> that they had no postoperative infections. Consumers aren't that
> good at evaluating the quality of medical care anyway—even re
> ferring physicians aren't that good. What does it mean when
> the newspaper lists "the best doctors"? They run a hundred-yard
> dash faster to the operating room? How do you know?

Confrontation with illness and mortality provoked rare professional candidness on assessments of the quality of colleagues. Bradley added,

> Two or three guys were significantly above the rest of us in terms of
> their ability to make patients well. But that's rare. Most of us
> have good days and bad days. Sometimes we miss something, or
> astound the world by picking up something subtle. But basically,
> the level of performance is pretty standard. There's no correlation
> between my role in making people better and the feedback I get
> from them. The feedback is proportionate to how much time
> I spend with the patient. The average patient would choose a
> sympathetic, soft, and gentle hospital experience that had a slightly
> greater risk of poor outcome, over a sterile, stark, unfriendly ex
> perience that had a slightly higher chance of a successful outcome.

Bradley felt that physicians' attention to personal and psychological issues was not only preferred, but medically important.

These doctors came to realize—often painfully—that reputation alone was insufficient in choosing a doctor. Sally, the internist with cancer who brought her laptop to the ICU, chose an internationally renowned expert for whom an important procedure was named. But his poor bedside manner appalled her, illustrating the gap between skills as a researcher (that may build a reputation) and those of a clinician.

> A colleague recommended his mentor, who was very smart but
> quite dishonest, and not at all encouraging of anybody else's
> opinion. He wrote a note in my chart when he didn't even see me!

I said to him later, "We did a good job." He said, "There's no 'we.' It's just *me*!" He has an aura of being really smart, but he's not systematic. Out of his stubbornness, he did a couple of dumb things. He put me on a drug that dropped all my counts. He didn't recognize it. He was hell-bent that he knew how to do this. I put up with him, but it became intolerable, and ultimately dangerous.

Here, as elsewhere, these doctors revealed discrepancies between colleagues' reputations and technical competencies. Department chairs, too, may have impressive reputations, but not the most up-to-date "hands-on" experience. Herb, the neonatologist with an MI, said:

My chairman said, "The chairman of cardiology is willing to treat you." I had no interest in that. I wanted a "bread and butter" doctor who has more day-to-day experience. When was the last time the chairman handled a basic MI? Probably a long time ago.

These ill doctors became more aware of the difficulties and limitations involved in assessing colleagues' abilities. Harry, the internist and war refugee, said:

You don't know how good a doctor is—whether from hearsay or reputation. You have to be their patient to find out—in terms of caring, empathy, and understanding. None of these qualities are described by the conventional measures of excellence: faculty position, number of referrals, size of practice. Well-reputed people, when I was their patient, were technically fine, but that was it. They had very little interest in emotional, psychological, empathic, or relationship factors. I thought I knew an internship mate of mine well. I'd seen him work. I went to him, and he was willing to treat me over the phone or in the hallway! That's where you make your biggest mistakes.

This gap between reputation and performance can be shocking. Harry continued, pointing out the importance not only of personal and technical skills, but of integrity as well, and reflecting on the underlying causes of these discrepancies.

I was startled by my own discovery that I didn't really know who they were. Everybody says they're wonderful, so they must be wonderful. But what is that based on? Presumably manner, kind voice, apparent interest, and enough time to listen and respond.

But how does one get a reputation? Presumably he or she is honest and honorable—knowing his/her limits, admitting errors. But those are surface phenomena that don't make a good doctor.

Questions therefore emerged as to the nature and notion of "reputation" itself. These physicians realized more than before the limitations of assumptions about such assessments. Moreover, if *they* encountered difficulties judging a colleague's shortcomings, lay patients must invariably face even greater barriers. Nonphysician patients may be unable to judge their doctors' competence or limitations adequately.

> The patient doesn't know whether technically docs are any good.
> So "the good doctor" is to some extent a myth. We don't do
> outcome studies. The state is beginning to, but mostly in surgery:
> a gallbladder operation is more or less a gallbladder operation.
> You can compare them. But in medicine, everything's mixed up.

Getting Treatment Elsewhere

These ill doctors had to decide, too, whether to find a physician and receive treatment within their own hospital, or elsewhere. Some obtained their care relatively far away, in other cities, states, or institutions, rather than their own, to protect privacy and avoid being seen differently. Boundary violations occurred when colleagues, chairmen, and supervisors came by to visit, read, and comment on ill physicians' medical charts, often with little sensitivity to the implicit impropriety.

Many traveled elsewhere for treatment because they feared discrimination—even by "enlightened" colleagues—whether subtle and implicit, or more drastic. Sally said:

> I didn't want my diagnosis to be anyone's business around *here*. It's
> a feeling I subsequently confirmed: no matter how enlightened
> people are, they put you in a different category.

Stigmatization may be unconscious as well as conscious.

With HIV, state reporting laws further impelled physicians to seek out-of-state treatment. George, an internist with HIV who served on government committees designing policies concerning HIV-infected physicians, said, "My state has name-reporting, so patients with money go to the next state to be tested or treated. It's unfair for people who can't afford to." Steven, the suburban endocrinologist with HIV, traveled to another city for treatment, and envied patients who could get care closer to home.

Conversely, other physicians avoided treatment elsewhere, due not to inconvenience but to desires for "VIP treatment." Outside their own institution, they might be treated as a "mere" patient. Eleanor's husband sought treatment at his own hospital so he wouldn't lose his VIP status. "When I go to my own hospital, everybody knows who I am. When I go somewhere else, I'm *just a patient!*"

Second Opinions

"When I went for a second opinion, my internist got mad," Jessica, the pediatrician with lymphoma, said. "He had a hissy-fit. As if I were his lover and had cheated on him." An aggressive stance in their own treatment led many doctor-patients to "*doctor shop*" and pursue second opinions. Yet, though officially sanctioned, second opinions were often mutually difficult, as they could be seen as questioning a colleague's expertise.

Nonetheless, many physician-patients sought second, third, fourth, and even fifth opinions, consulting experts around the country. Unfortunately, confusion could then arise over who was ultimately responsible for the patient's care. Stuart, now teaching at the university, said about treating other ill doctors:

> I saw my role as being a primary care doc; but the docs I treated as patients, especially specialists, never really respected that. They thought they needed someone with expertise. So it was difficult. I would find out only later that they were seeing docs all around town. I wondered if these patients were still my patients. That was the biggest confusion: *am I still your doctor, or are you now seeing them over there, or just talking to them?* Some didn't really want a doctor at all: they were just doing serial consultations.

Not surprisingly, many doctors-of-record disliked their patients' obtaining second opinions, implicitly challenging the first physician's authority. Some seemed to take it personally.

Many sick doctors felt that on principle they should simply choose a physician they trusted, and then abide by the latter's decisions. Jacob, the radiologist with skin cancer, felt this logic should extend not only to treatment, but to diagnosis as well—to interpreting one's own radiographic scans. "It's not a good idea for a person to read their own X-rays. I wouldn't do it *out of principle.* It's low-class to be your own lawyer. My father used to say, 'A man who is his own lawyer has a fool for a client.' "

Feelings arose as well that criticizing fellow physicians was taboo. Respecting authority fully was important. Yet, as we shall see, this taboo could potentially impede professional mandates to help patients as much as possible. At times, these physicians made nuanced decisions whether to obtain second opinions or not that were based on the magnitude of the problem, doing so only for "major things."

Yet even if an ill physician avoided pursuing a second opinion, his or her family members and friends could urge such a consult, precipitating conflict. Eleanor said about her physician-husband, "My daughter and I both tried talking him into getting a second opinion after his surgery. He refused."

Yet these doctors also had to decide whether to *provide* second opinions for friends, family members, and others. Jacob did so, though questioning the practice. Nonmedical acquaintances routinely asked him to read their radiologic images. "People in synagogue give me scans to look at. I seem like such an empathetic guy, so therefore I am the greatest MRI reader, the greatest doc." He criticized these common assumptions, yet obliged the requests. He felt that he wouldn't pursue second opinions himself, but that others had a right to do so.

Doctor-Patient—Doctor Relationships

"What is a doctor's role to a doctor?" one physician asked. How should a provider approach and treat a patient who is also a colleague? The relationships of ill physicians to their own doctors differed from those between doctors and nonphysician patients. Relationships between doctors and lay patients have been explored, largely in attempts to learn how to increase empathy and the quality of decision-making (2, 3). Yet how doctors treat fellow physicians has not been systematically examined. Boundaries can muddle with lay patients, too, but here do so at times in wider and far more complex ways.

Frequently, colleagues were not only physicians, but friends as well, thus occupying *three* roles that could conflict or shape one another. Given the increased risk of identification, ill doctors challenged their own physicians' defenses. Physicians-of-record had to decide how much leeway to give an ill physician—whether to modify standard practices, and if so, how much. Doctor-patients in turn often expected special, VIP treatment, or purposefully handpicked their physicians-of-record from among friends and colleagues in order to ensure certain types of care. Questions arose about how to proceed.

Entitlement and VIP Treatment

Awareness of the pitfalls of VIP treatment arose, but was rare. "VIP syndrome" has been described (4), in which hospitalized VIPs receive substandard care due to the reluctance of medical staff to treat the VIP as a "mere" patient. Ill doctors faced similar issues, though important differences arose, since physicians were not only VIPs, but *doctors* possessing medical knowledge. Moreover, the VIP syndrome has never been examined from the point of view of the VIPs themselves—only from that of the treating medical staff.

A few of the doctors here expressed caution about receiving "special treatment." Albert, who had an MI on the highway, felt that being treated by a generic doctor on call at his local hospital was appropriate: the system then operated as it was supposed to.

> When President Reagan was shot in Washington, the doctor was a vascular surgeon on call. Several other doctors could have been mobilized. But sometimes the system functioning according to the way it's designed is a bigger plus than the increment in quality of care you might get from somebody with a better reputation.

Hence, Albert had asked the head nurse whom she would recommend.

Nevertheless, the majority of these doctor-patients sought or received VIP treatment, often because, as suggested earlier, they were patients at institutions where they were well-known as doctors. Ill physicians who knew their provider as a colleague might trust him or her more, but decrease how much authority they ceded.

Indeed, many physicians felt they were members of a "fraternity," and hence *deserved* good care from each other. Jim, the drug company researcher with leukemia, felt he had taken care of others, and as a result he now expected special treatment in return: "I am part of this group, this profession, and have contributed to it. I've done my share of taking care of people—that may be selfish, but that's reality."

Many simply anticipated VIP or "special" treatment in some way. For example, Jacob didn't ask for favors, but just *expected* them. He became angry at having to wait weeks for biopsy results. He felt he should be treated the way *he* would treat a fellow physician.

> I had to wait two weeks for a biopsy, then ten days for a second opinion. If I were taking care of another physician, I would probably Fed Ex the slides to a pathologist I knew to get a second opinion within a couple of days. If you call someone up and say, "I really want you to look at the slides this afternoon, I'm going to Fed Ex it to you today," they'll look at it two days later. I'm the kind of guy who never *asks* for any favors. I just *assumed* my doctor would hurry the process. I waited ten days. He still didn't have the result!

Some people requested favors more than others. To get what they wanted, ill physicians often tried to manipulate the system—taking advantage of their knowledge, perhaps unfairly. Dan, who had chest mets, said:

> I know the system: If I keep pushing the bedside button often enough, the nurse will get angry, and may or may not come. But if I tell her that I'm going to spill urine all over the bed, she's going to come in a hurry, because that way she's not going to have to change the sheets.

His assertiveness could succeed, but vex his providers.

Other ill physicians used their knowledge in refusing to accept their doctors' excuses. They implicitly raised questions of whether there was a limit to how much doctors *should* manage or manipulate the system, and if so, when. Did they sometimes go too far? Presumably, they should not self-doctor at the point at which it interfered with their own or others' quality of care. But how did one know if one had reached that point? Can one know in advance, or only afterward?

This sense of entitlement and the demands to be treated as "special"— as a physician, not a patient—can stem from a variety of social or psychological factors, including poor self-esteem. Juan, the Latino internist with HIV, for example, became angry when treated simply as a patient, having been sickly for much of his earlier life. He felt ostracized as well because of being gay and Latino.

> All my life, I've been a patient for different things. Once I was a physician, I did not want to be babied anymore. What frustrated me most was getting a doctor with a paternalistic approach,

hearing me using technical language, and still going back to layman's terms, and dumb, inaccurate layman explanations. I would
correct him: "*I am a physician!* You need to be a little more precise." Some doctors got up and said, "Then find yourself another
physician." Fine. Others said, "I'm sorry. I didn't remember.
I was just going on automatic mode, and gave you the little spiel
I give everybody."

His personal history made Juan particularly sensitive to slights. His remarks underlined how much doctors had "automatic spiels" they gave
without considering patients' individual characteristics. Doctors saved
time and energy through such rote speeches, but seemed unaware of such
habits and the costs involved.

Problems with VIP Treatment

"The worst care I ever saw was for a multibillionaire's son," Harry, the
war refugee, said. In many ways, VIP treatment could be suboptimal.
Entitlement can simply be unrealistic—impractical or unproductive—
and anger health care providers. Yet to counter these ill physicians' expectations can be hard. Harry described how VIP care provided the son
of one of the richest men in the world the worst possible treatment.

This son had a cranial pharingioma, and was under the care of the
five chiefs of neurosurgery here and at the four other medical
schools around the city. Nothing got done. I was his medical
consultant. They disagreed, and the father would not relinquish
control and say, "You're the doctor: do what's right." He thought
he was doing the best for his child by having the five chiefs be
quasi-joint physicians. That was the *worst* thing you could do.

Such VIP treatment can interfere with the chain of command, paralyzing
processes of decision-making and care.
VIP treatment can also prompt demands for information that then
overload the patient. Scott, the internist with an infected foot, said,
"Doctor-patients with entitlement want you to report daily on their
baby's every bowel movement. That's just unrealistic: 'You don't really
want to know that.'" Doctors facing illness in themselves or a loved one
may believe that more information is better, but this belief may not be
entirely correct.

Colleague-Physician-Friend: Collusions and "Denial Systems"

Though they were not self-doctoring, some doctors came close by selecting physicians whom they knew well, in order to negotiate for better
treatment. Roger, a surgeon who became suicidal when diagnosed with
HIV, said he knew which physicians could work with his "boundaries"—
specifically, his abhorrence of hospitalization.

> I state my boundaries up front: you're not going to hospitalize me
> for pneumonia, and I'm not going to go on a ventilator. I left a
> physician because he wanted to put me in the ICU!

On the other hand, others chose a doctor-friend who would consult
only if they were doing well. Walter said about his physician:

> We've known each other since internship. He said that if it looked
> like I was going to die, he didn't want to be my doctor. For that,
> he wanted to be my friend.

Over time, as patients' conditions worsened, these boundary distinctions
could be hard to maintain.

Many chose good friends as physicians in order to have a "physician-
of-record," while still controlling their own care. Juan, the internist
with HIV, and a colleague/friend wrote prescriptions for each other.
Juan termed this practice "incestuous" and "not kosher," suggesting degrees and *gradations* of inappropriate or unethical behavior. Each was
physician/friend/patient to the other.

> My current "physician-of-record" is a former officemate. I used to
> be his physician. When I need something, I just call him and get
> it. If I want something checked out, most of the time I know what
> it is, and just get it confirmed. Because I know what I'm dealing
> with—what the risks are.

Juan's phrase "not kosher" suggests that these behaviors are not, strictly
speaking, unethical, but not fully appropriate either.

Over decades, Albert, who had an MI on the highway, reported that
colleagues and he "routinely signed each other's forms for yearly physi-
cals" required by some hospitals. Friends completed disability forms, too,
for each other. Albert continued, "I've had a friend who is a doctor fill out
my disability form forever as a favor. I see him every three months and

bring some labs." Heightened bureaucratic demands on physicians furthered these practices, even if the latter were problematic.

Conversely, to avoid imposing on others, some physicians vowed *never* to ask a friend to treat them. Paul, the internist with HIV who lost a job offer, said, "If I needed a physician, I would probably use a friend's new office partner. He's not a friend. I would just hate to burden a friend with having to take care of me."

Given these potential conflicts and pitfalls, others sought care from colleagues/friends, but tried to set limits. Still, the potential blending and confusion of roles could present problems. For example, some enlisted friends to provide certain aspects of care but not others. Kurt, who had used crack and now had HIV, referred to himself as the "dictator of my medical care," and picked a doctor he knew. But Kurt drew firm parameters concerning what he would and would not do.

> Occasionally, I would have my nurse draw my blood, and I would check my T-cells every six months. I did my own stuff, off the record. My doctor chose the meds I wanted. If he hadn't, I would have told him. If he wouldn't prescribe them, I would have gone to someone else. If I develop fever or night sweats, I would see him. But for my anti-viral management, I know as much as anybody. Since I know what drugs I've been on, I'm in a better position to choose them.

Yet as to "being in a better position," Kurt may be rationalizing here, since alternatively, he could tell his doctors what meds he had tried.

Based on their recognition of their own tendency to want to remain in control as patients, and sensing the potential problems, a few physicians purposefully chose physicians who would be firm and objective, and challenge any self-doctoring. Frank, the surgeon who had an MI in the OR, for example, feared he would undermine his own treatment, and hence picked a doctor who would strongly oppose such behavior: "I selected a doctor that doesn't take any nonsense, so that I could not manipulate my own position, which I would have been prone to do."

A treating physician may contribute to these boundary problems by *deferring* to his or her doctor-patients, shifting the relationship from doctor-patient to colleague-colleague: from a relationship of hierarchy to one of equal power. A few physicians deferred to their doctors—normally, as mentioned earlier with regard to entering the patient role, because their illness clearly lay outside their area of expertise. Brian, the pediatrician with hepatitis C, said his doctor felt hesitant and awkward treating him as a patient. "The first time I went to my doctor, he said, 'All right, I'm going to test your prostate. Drop your pants. That doesn't bother you, because you're a doctor, does it?' I said it would bother me if he didn't!"

Collusion commonly occurred. Eleanor said about her husband:

> Part of the problem was that colleagues were willing to be cornered in the hallway for quickie consults. Colleagues would say, "You really ought to come in and be checked." But that's where it began and ended. That facilitates more denying: if it's a quickie consult in the corridor, it's not really serious. *Both sides* were willing to do that.

Many physicians-of-record gave ill doctors more latitude, seeing them less often if these patients wanted. Scott, the internist with the infected foot, said about caring for fellow physicians:

> I yielded a lot more to docs than to other patients. If I would normally see patients at three-to-four-month intervals, I'd probably hold docs to half that. They could talk me out of it. I tried not to buckle under. If I hadn't seen them in a year, I'd say, "Am I still your doctor?" To try to avoid this confusion, I'd say, "Let's try not to let this happen again," without sounding rude. I wanted to say, "Be nice to me. Respect me!"

In a small city or town, finding a physician whom one does *not* in some way already know can be difficult. Awkwardness may be inevitable. As mentioned earlier, Pascal, the Lebanese internist with HIV, concluded he simply couldn't have a doctor in his small town. "If I were in a larger city, it'd be easier. I wouldn't know anyone."

Doctor-colleague-friends may shirk roles or functions of a physician. They may not only fail to perform full or partial physical exams, but also defer treatment decisions to these ill physicians. Jerry, the surgeon-lawyer, said, "My physicians definitely treat me differently than they do their other patients. They pretty much leave my care up to myself."

Colleagues may have trouble treating a sick peer. Paul, for example, decided he did not want to care for friends, since objectivity would be difficult and their illness would distress him. It would be hard if and when they got seriously sick.

Emotionally, it's draining. It gets to be more of a social than a medical encounter. I like my job because I'm buffered. When people are acutely ill, I do not see them. They're hospitalized. Previously, if outpatients were really acutely ill, they would be in hospice or home care, so I was able to separate from those really intense, emotion-draining times. I do not look forward to doing it with friends. I haven't taken care of any friends who got really sick.

A colleague succumbing to illness can threaten the rigid structure of doctor and patient roles, and make physicians feel vulnerable in ways that could affect the care they provide. Some colleagues couldn't fully acknowledge Eleanor's husband's illness, as they were also his friends and now his physicians.

They had tremendous difficulty accepting the fact that one of "them" had become one of "us." He was treated where he had worked. All his physicians were also his colleagues, and many were friends. That played a large part in how he was managed.

These doctor-patients may in fact be expected by their physicians to exercise a large role in treatment and follow-up, reducing the responsibility of the doctor-of-record. Sally, the internist with cancer who brought her laptop to the ICU, was in fact told to take a greater role in her own care. Her doctor expected her to self-prescribe, ostensibly because Sally was a fellow physician.

One doctor said they expected me, as a physician, to take more responsibility for my own care than I did. He assumed I would follow things more myself. He said he'd never seen pneumocystis pneumonia in patients like me because he always puts patients on bactrim to prevent it. I thought: Well, why didn't you ever tell me to do that? He assumed I'd know.

Deborah agreed. "Doctors assume that if you're a doctor, you know everything." Yet physicians' specialties vary widely. Scott, with the infected foot, said, "I'm in an altogether different field—what the hell do I know about feet?"

Though doctor-patients and their physicians may agree about treatment—whether from collusion or not—disagreements can occur, and be thorny to negotiate. At times, ill physicians openly dissented from their doctors, and then had to decide what to do: whether to speak out, and if so, how much and in what way. These two parties then fought over hierarchy and authority.

Some questioned, but did not disobey, their physicians' advice. Nancy said that despite her qualms, she tended to follow her physician's suggestions because otherwise, "I would be pulling rank and I would rather not do that." Respect for the system could then clash with feelings of entitlement. With more seniority, Lou, who had a plaque on his office wall, went further, challenging his physician. "I wouldn't sign myself out against medical advice, but I asked, 'Is there anything that we're doing here that I can't just do at home?'"

Others felt no hesitation about confronting their providers more forcefully or fully. As patients, some doctors were sometimes very demanding. Simon, a radiologist with HIV, refused to be audiotaped because he was terrified of losing his disability insurance. He said he was a "better" doctor than patient. In the first role, he had to act "professional," but in the second, he could be "bitchy." "I can be very nasty as a patient, demanding that I want something done *stat!*"(immediately).

The awkwardness of consulting physician-colleagues could lead to doctor-shopping. Some sick physicians visited multiple doctors, previously known or unknown, before finding a "good match." Jennifer, who had become infected with HIV through a needle stick while treating a patient, illustrated the lengths to which one could have to go to find a physician.

> I was a colleague of everybody in the area that treats HIV. I had become friendly with all of them on a professional basis, and we did a lot of social things. Then, I needed somebody to take care of me. It works better if the patient is anonymous. Otherwise, there is awkwardness, not really knowing who is in what role.
>
> My first doctor was the most knowledgeable. We had been friends. I went to him, but didn't get examined. It just felt wrong. Then I thought I'd really rather have a woman physician, and one who doesn't know me. I heard wonderful things about a new infectious disease woman on the other side of town. I went, but then got really sick, and she was not very accessible. I ended up at my local county hospital ER, miserable. No doctor could take care of me there. The only doctor I would even consider in my area was a good friend. He didn't think it was a good idea, but finally

said, "Ok, I'll try it." It didn't work. He never once examined
me, except doing cranial nerves. The first time I had any problem,
he just freaked, basically saying, "You could just go home now
and die." He gave me this huge prescription for Seconal—for anxiety or to kill myself. I said, "I don't need Seconal. I need a head
scan and a lumbar puncture!"

To find an appropriate provider, others, too, meandered far. Jennifer also
presented an important category here: "friendly...on a professional
basis," that is, "professional friends"—more than co-professionals but not
entirely friends. Such friendships ranged widely in strength, length, and
trust.

Questions arose of what to call such colleagues who offered some aspects of treatment, but were not formally or officially one's doctor. Pascal,
the Lebanese internist, for example, referred to "the person" that writes
his prescriptions for him—as distinguished from "his doctor." Pascal
made his own medical decisions, but did not order his own drugs.

I'm sort of my own physician. I make the decisions, and discuss
them with *the person that writes my scripts*. I haven't been to physicians for a physical exam for years.

Pascal saw problems with this arrangement, but no alternative.

I wish I had someone to go to, and be a patient. But there's no one
here. I don't feel *un*comfortable making these decisions. I think
they're good decisions, but that's probably not a good thing to do. I
don't think of it as an ethical problem, but I just would like it to be
different. I want someone to be objective.

Pascal felt awkward with this situation, but not strongly enough to prompt
him to change it.

Such collusion and denial could have several implications. Eleanor's
husband chose staff who colluded with his minimization of his illness, and
did not, for example, discuss end-of-life care much. She quoted a discussion between her husband and his doctor:

"How are you feeling?" "Fine, thank you." "Are you interested in
radiotherapy?" "No." "Do you have a living will?" "Yes." "Any
interest in hospice care?" "No." *That* was the end-of-life conversation. Everybody was very complicit with his denial, and did
not address the outstanding issues.

Other dynamics, perceived norms, and rationalizations could further perpetuate denial. Taboos against criticizing peers could impede colleagues from reproaching a physician's self-treatment. Often, colleagues could only gingerly suggest better follow-up. Eleanor added about her husband:

> Some colleagues would say, "You really ought to come in and
> be checked." But that's where it began and ended. If he didn't show
> up, nobody came down the hall after him.

Even though her husband was now also a patient, his autonomy as a physician extended to his own self-care, and went unchallenged. The fact that ill doctors had more power than other patients often led to confusion.

In part, colleagues didn't want to offend a physician by implying that he or she was *incapable* of caring for his or her own disease. Eleanor continued:

> Physicians do not want to confront their colleagues—it's the doc-
> tor's prerogative to remain in control of his or her own case. Col-
> leagues almost felt they would be offending my husband, or
> implying that he was not capable of managing his particular case.
> Friends didn't want to harass and infantilize him, and turn him into
> a patient—just as they would never want to be turned into pa-
> tients themselves. The only physician who truly confronted him was
> his diabetologist, and my husband would just not go see him. My
> husband saw his neurologist only because otherwise, he wouldn't be
> allowed to drive.

Norms of not criticizing colleagues outweighed colleagues' concerns or responsibilities regarding each other's health. This dynamic of avoidance was exacerbated by the fact that ill physicians had the status and power to eschew physicians' admonitions and recommendations. Professional hierarchies, if any, with colleague-physicians are generally less rigid and more fluid than those with lay patients. Eleanor continued: "If a patient-physician says, 'Everything is fine,' it's offensive to question his ability."

A physician-patient may either avoid friends who treat him or her as a patient, or confide only in nonphysician friends. Eleanor's husband confessed his feelings only to his sole lay friend. Eleanor said:

> All his close friends were physicians. One friend was not, and was
> the only one he spoke to about being ill. He would talk to this
> friend about the fact that he was sick. But he would not discuss that
> with his physician-friends. With this friend, he didn't need to be "a

physician"—clinical, detached, in control. He could acknowledge fear, talk about what he couldn't say to his physician-friends. To *them*, he couldn't say, "I'm tired." They'd say, "Of course! You have cancer! You understand the process. Why is that surprising?" as opposed to "Yeah, it must really be tough."

Colleagues supported him as a fellow physician, but not as a patient. For some physician-patients, only debilitating illness or cognitive decline halted this mutual denial.

Even at the end, Eleanor's husband entered the role of patient only with reluctance. To alter such a *"denial system"*—as opposed to a support system—could be difficult. A social system can support particular beliefs about a diagnosis, even if these are maladaptive. Eleanor tried to confront her husband's denial, but couldn't.

I'd say to him, "You are dying. I really need to know what you want, and don't want, done." The conversation would get turned on and off, depending on his mood. It was generally "We've discussed this before." But we really hadn't. Many times when I'd raise the subject, he would just literally turn the TV on, to head off the conversation.

In sum, in confronting diagnoses, treatments, and prognoses, these doctors had to decide whether and to what degree to let themselves be patients versus "remain in control" and self-doctor. They tended to be patients if they had comparatively less experience treating their own diagnoses. Others used their "insider status" to "manage the system" and access or forgo procedures. Controversy swirled most around self-prescribing, from the innocuous to the potentially problematic. Some rationalized the practice, while others tried to limit it. They self-doctored because they could, did not want to depend on others, were obsessive by nature, or denied or had difficulty accepting their illness.

Self-doctoring increased due to deeply ingrained professional identities and to managed care's obstacles in accessing care, but at times decreased when the disease grew more severe. Some of these individuals self-doctored without thinking of themselves as doing so. Others did not discuss their self-treatment with their physicians-of-record, though medical problems could then be overlooked. At times, sick doctors and their physicians attempted to impose ground rules or constraints on self-doctoring, but these efforts often failed.

For themselves, many doctors took more aggressive approaches than they would for their patients, leaving no stone unturned, and at times experimenting on themselves. For themselves, they accepted relatively higher risks of harm. Often, this aggressiveness succeeded, but such double standards raised disturbing questions: whether and when protecting patients interferes with accessing beneficial treatments for them. The success of such aggressive treatment challenges the cautious conservatism dictated by malpractice concerns.

Many doctors did not practice what they preached, particularly regarding diet, treatment adherence, and preventive care. Changing unhealthy behavior proved hard. These physicians tended to feel invulnerable, and the demands of medical training facilitated poor health behavior. Knowledge of preventive behaviors alone was not enough to instill them. This resistance among physicians presents challenges for interventions aimed at improving health through prevention among lay patients as well.

Prognostication, particularly of one's own demise and death, was especially difficult, and led to self-distancing, viewing one's self as a patient from the standpoint of one's "medical self" or "medical gaze."

In choosing their own doctors, these men and women revealed a wide range of "tastes" and "styles"—generally, but not always, preferring minimalists to obsessive overdoers. They also sought to balance good bedside manner with technical skill. Most favored marginally more of the former over the latter. They now witnessed, too, how much colleagues' clinical reputations could fall short. Still, particularly in certain surgical fields, a few of these physicians valued colleagues' technical prowess over obnoxious behavior. These ill physicians had to decide, too, *where* to get treatment—at one's own institution versus elsewhere—balancing privacy and potential stigma versus convenience and VIP care.

Frequently, these doctors shopped for additional opinions, though doing so rankled other physicians who felt that this behavior implied criticism of colleagues, which was taboo. Second opinions can be vital. Their rate and efficacy have been examined with regard to invasive procedures, as means of avoiding unnecessary surgery (5, 6), and obtaining additional information about breast cancer treatment (7). But many aspects of second opinions have not been explored: barriers, facilitators, norms, and attitudes among physicians and patients, and the ways first and second opinions vary. Lay patients, no doubt, also find that their doctors resist these potential critiques.

Ill physicians interacted with their doctors differently than did other patients. Self-doctoring muddled boundaries and roles. Sick physicians tended to expect and/or receive VIP treatment. As a result, roles at times clashed, and decisions emerged on whether openly to disagree, confront, or challenge their physician-of-record. Some chose close colleagues as physicians, further confusing or colluding roles, and avoiding confrontation with one's disease. Through these choices, denial assumed multiple forms.

These narratives raise key questions of how therapeutic styles function more generally in lay patients' preferences and experiences concerning treatment referrals. Therapeutic nihilism has been mentioned, usually as a strategy to be avoided. Professionals often face countervailing pressures to help severely ill patients as much as possible now, rather than waiting for the completion of definitive studies at some point in the future (8, 9). But I have not found any studies of therapeutic nihilism as an approach or principle in clinical decision-making: when and how commonly it shapes physicians' decisions in referring patients or prescribing treatments. Are colleagues' perceptions of therapeutic nihilists correct? How *consistent* are physicians in their styles? Lay patients as well no doubt perceive such differences among physicians in therapeutic tastes, styles, and nihilism, but patients' observations, preferences, and responses concerning these categories remain unknown. The role of subjective factors in clinical referrals more generally has also been neglected.

Similarly, these doctors reveal that physician reputation influences referral patterns in ways that might impede patient care. Yet little research has been done on the composition and accuracy of physicians' judgments of colleagues' reputations, which thus need to be explored.

To some degree, physicians here *chose* their patients. But it is not clear how this phenomenon operates more broadly, and how commonly, and whether lay patients experience or observe this process. Research on patient satisfaction has focused on whether patients feel they have a choice or not, rather than examining other key components of satisfaction, such as aspects of the compatibility or "match" between doctors and patients, and the ways lay patients balance trade-offs between empathy and skill, and resolve disagreements with their providers.

Prior research has viewed patterns of self-doctoring dichotomously, as either present or absent. But questions emerge here of *how* doctors decide where to be on this spectrum, and how they support, maintain, or alter their position in the face of illness, and handle tensions between the relationships they seek and those they end up having with their own physicians.

These narratives have important implications—for example, in exploring the ways that these elements of style shape trainees' decisions, and the ways medicine is an art—even more than most doctors generally like to admit. These doctors offered a key suggestion for lay patients, too: to ask a head nurse (or other nurses) for recommendations for physician referrals, as these staff members have seen many doctors' successes and failures over the years.

Lay patients who choose friends as their doctors or have been treated by a doctor for a long time may similarly face blurred roles that can cause or reflect denial by either party. In confronting these tensions in choosing physicians, and maintaining appropriate doctor-patient relationships, lay patients certainly face analogous obstacles—without the same resources.

4

"Screw-ups"

External Obstacles Faced in Becoming Patients

"I've made terrible mistakes," Harry murmured, shaking his head and glancing down. "I've *killed* people."

Medical errors occur, yet now, for the first time, many of these physicians became fully aware of, and reflected on, the *range* of problems and lapses in health care—from fatal flaws to poor communication. They faced challenges, too, in how to respond to these shortfalls, either as patients or as fellow doctors. As patients, they now faced hurdles due not only to their illness and self-doctoring, but also to deficiencies in the wider medical system. They evaluated their treatments as patients from the perspectives of fellow doctors. Lay patients need to be aware of these issues as well—to prepare for these tensions and inform their expectations, even if they do not lessen their hopes for optimal care.

Institutional Obstacles

Though most of these doctors encountered problems and disappointments with "the system," a rare few were pleased with their treatment, and had few, if any, complaints. As mentioned earlier, several received VIP care. Given well-known problems in health care, such special treatment could cause surprise, even embarrassment. Bradley first noted chest pain when he could not hit a drop shot in tennis. Well-respected at his institution, he had his operation performed the next day. "My treatment was unbelievably, embarrassingly good. I got cared for in minutes to hours. Other people have to wait longer."

Yet, far more commonly, these physician-patients encountered problems in their care.

Problems with Hospitalizations and Bureaucracies

These ill physicians now became more aware of difficulties concerning the larger social organization of health care. Their complaints ranged from the physical plant to the bureaucracy of hospitals. These institutions' vast size and complexity caused problems beyond inconvenience and aesthetics alone. At the extreme, some saw these shortcomings as symptomatic of a larger crisis: the system as a whole was "falling apart." They saw these deficiencies, too, as reflecting *institutional bias against patients*, and as communicating messages that patients "do not matter" much to the institutions designed to benefit them most. These organizational failings incurred high psychic costs, reinforcing humiliation and degradation due to disease.

The extent of problems with the physical plant astonished these physicians. Harry, the war refugee with heart disease, described the situation thus:

> I was put in a room with a broken window—a big crack, and a missing piece. It was a cold night, but they said they didn't have any other place to put me. I thought: hang a sheet or a towel over it! I had a bad night. Silly meals at silly times ... but that's the system.

Surprisingly, at times these problems constituted the most dissatisfying and disappointing aspects of medical treatment. In the current era of fiscal restraint, institutions devalued not only amenities, but even basic necessities, as priorities. Herb, the neonatologist with MI, said:

> My memories now are of the physical environment—the room was ugly, spartan, inhospitable. A roach was on the wall. The catheterization lab was crowded and cold. This medical center is erecting a big new cancer research building that is probably not going to treat a single patient. Less money proportionally goes into patient treatment.

To Herb, medical centers increasingly focus not on patients, but on fundable research.

Similarly, Nancy, the endocrinologist with breast cancer, felt that "hospitals are filthy, dirty, and the food sucks: awful, inedible." Institu-

tions supposed to promote health may thus themselves induce risk. Nancy
and others saw these aspects of patienthood as in fact declining further.

> The physical part of being a patient is going to get worse. The
> dietary people said they used to have the food made upstate, and
> even *that* is now too expensive. So they are just going to buy
> prepackaged frozen dinners!

Other hospital employees may disappoint, too—not being available,
for example, to hook up the telephone or television at night when patients get admitted. The deficiencies Nancy saw included:

> . . . having a phone, a TV, or any comforts, or things to do. There's a
> library: one lady, a volunteer, walks around with magazines and
> candy. That's it. Some transporters are unprofessional.

Nancy also complained, "There are no fresh flowers." As a result, she
now routinely bought bouquets for the clinic she ran. Policymakers may
consider these concerns to be secondary to medical care, but the physicians here argued otherwise. Aesthetics played far more of a role than
these doctors had anticipated, due to the symbolic meanings involved.
Frustration about the poor quality of the physical plant and of amenities
reinforced senses of helplessness and dependency.

Bureaucratic inefficiencies compounded these shortcomings in the
physical plant. Many of these doctors cited unwieldy management and
personnel structures. Difficulties began at the outset, during procedures
for admitting patients to the hospital. Nancy continued, "The method of
getting people into the hospital is barbaric—waiting for a bed in the ER for
hours."

These problems were so pervasive and deeply ingrained that not even
being a physician wholly eradicated them. Despite the fact that both
Walter and his wife had trained at the hospital, staff proved unrespon-
sive.

> The surgeon arranged for me to be admitted directly—not through
> the ER. But the admitting department couldn't find any docu-
> mentation. So, with intense pain and vomiting, I waited two hours
> in the admitting office. My doctor did what he was supposed to,
> and it didn't make the mechanism of the hospital function.

Only Walter's ability to "pull strings" helped. He ended up having a friend
run into the OR and grab a surgeon, who said his beeper wasn't working.

The system's inefficiencies may hamper patients not only in being admitted to the hospital, but also in getting evaluated once there. During another hospitalization, when seriously ill, Walter got a bed, but was not evaluated for hours. Finally, he was seen only after he phoned his physician, with whom he was on a first-name basis.

> I called his office, and said, "Tom, I still haven't been seen by anybody, after two hours." He called an attending, who came and saw me. In the meantime, they had drawn my blood and took a portable chest X-ray. But I had not seen a doctor. They had not assessed or treated me. Six hours after my admission, the intern and resident came. I said, "I have to tell you how upset I am with you. I say this as a doctor to another doctor. You needed to have assessed me." The intern said, "Well, I ordered all the tests." That was their perception of what was needed to assess an acutely ill cancer patient: "I was busy. A patient arrested in the X-ray suite." There was a series of "explanations," all of which really just amounted to bad medical care. But if *I* couldn't get decent-quality medical care, it says something about the difficulty lay patients have!

Increasingly, hospital bureaucracies seemed organized more for their own benefit than for that of doctors, and last, for that of patients. Hence, as both a patient and a provider, Walter felt frightened:

> Hospitals and the health system respond to their *own* needs. Doctors would be aghast at me saying this, but hospitals have been shaped around the needs of the doctors, administrators, and businesspeople who run them, rather than around the patients. The system isn't designed to meet the needs of patients—that's almost incidental. So it must be working for other reasons, though *these days it doesn't function very well for doctors, either.* If I hadn't been a doctor, I would have been frightened because I wouldn't have known what was going on. I *was* frightened *as* a doctor because I *did* know what was going on.

From ERs to childbirth centers, patients were positioned—at times both literally and figuratively—for the benefit of doctors more than patients. Part of the problem arose because of the multiple functions of teaching hospitals: to educate trainees, provide care, and stave off fiscal crisis.

But no built-in feedback existed to change the system. Patients were too sick to provide any. Walter continued, "I had to devote all my attention to myself and my own well-being and pain." Stasis persists. Nonetheless, as we shall see, some physicians tried, even in small ways, to remedy these problems with their own patients.

Insurance

Among the hardest aspects of "the system" proved to be arranging details of health insurance coverage and reimbursement. Tim, a dermatologist with a rare leukemia, reported that in being a patient, the difficulties involved with insurance coverage surprised him most. "I don't know how patients do it when they aren't also physicians, and don't know the system. It's a full-time job."

Problems arose with managed care referral systems for seeing physicians, particularly specialists. Scott, with an infected foot, felt that managed care forced physicians and patients to be antagonistic.

> Insurance companies create a system that puts patients at odds
> with physicians in a very clever and deceptive process.... My sur-
> geon said, "You need to get a new test. The insurance company will
> pay for it, but it has to be prescribed by your primary care provider
> [PCP]." My primary care doc has never heard of the test, and
> is reluctant to write a prescription for it because of the liability.
> I had a medical emergency, but couldn't get to see him. If he saw
> me, he would send me to an infectious disease person. But I can't
> get the referral because the people at my PCP's office say I need
> twenty-four hours to get a referral. "But," I said, "I've already
> arranged the appointment with the specialist. He's on my insur-
> ance. The PCP only needs to sign at the top." But his staff is
> bitching and moaning. My PCP is standing five feet away. When
> they finally hand it to him, he says, "Ok, sure."

A sense of entitlement may exacerbate Scott's frustrations with this complex bureaucracy, but many other ill physicians shared his experiences.

Concerns surfaced as well about whether insurance companies would maintain confidentiality. Physicians often feared submitting medical bills that could disclose diagnoses to insurance companies and human resources departments. Especially given computerized databanks, information might not be kept confidential, and could impair present and future employment. Those with HIV faced particular problems, and most initially paid out of pocket for their medical care rather than submit claims to third-party payers or HMOs, for which these physicians often served as providers as well. Yet the high cost of HIV medications (up to $20,000 per year) forced many infected physicians to submit insurance claims, and therefore divulge their diagnosis. The steep price of these drugs left them little choice.

Medical Errors

In their individual care, many ill physicians became more aware, too, of "screw-ups" in care. Generally, they were far more cognizant of these errors—at times potentially lethal—than lay patients would be. For example, some of these doctors were dispensed the wrong kind or dose of medications. Nancy, the endocrinologist with metastatic breast cancer, was given the incorrect amount of blood thinner.

> The nurse made a mistake and gave me a ten- or a hundred times concentrate of heparin, so I started bleeding uncontrollably. They couldn't figure out why. So I had to go back and have a procedure repeated the next day!

Their medical training made these physician-patients more conscious of medical mistakes than they might have been otherwise, and reveals the kinds of errors that can occur. Deborah reported, "When I was hospitalized, the aide wrote down my temp as 104, instead of 100.4, and a fever workup was ordered. Luckily, I realized what was going on." No harm occurred, though extra blood was drawn, and unneeded tests were run.

Many physicians also became more acutely aware of the extent of differences in the quality of care between hospitals. Some institutions may have less experience, particularly with complicated procedures. Jim, the drug company researcher with leukemia, sought to transfer from his nearby "St. Suburbia Hospital," where he received no workup, to an academic medical center in a major city.

> At my local hospital, very little was done for me. I had a fever and didn't get any X-rays. They didn't know any genetics, or do a bone marrow biopsy. Over the loudspeaker, I kept hearing requests for people to come in to donate platelets. Then they said to me, "We can't do this procedure right now because we don't have enough platelets." That clinched it! I transferred to the city.

Within forty-five minutes, they did a bone marrow biopsy, and in two hours had the results, and started antibiotics.

Seasoned staff and specialized facilities can help avoid mishaps. Jim explained:

> You have to be in a place where the nursing staff, in particular, takes care of these problems all the time. My local hospital didn't have a specialized oncology floor or leukemia service.

Over time, attitudes toward medical errors have changed. As suggested earlier, an unwritten code exists against criticizing fellow doctors that extends particularly to suing. Physicians, aware how malpractice suits have become out of hand, hesitated to engage in this same process themselves. Jacob said, "Suing doctors for malpractice is a crime—worse than a crime, a *religious* crime! Because it assumes that doctors are as good as God."

Before the era of wider malpractice suits, mistakes may have been more accepted: readily discussed and recognized as inherent in medical practice. Indeed, Harry, the war refugee with heart disease, described a yearly ritual at his hospital, designed to permit talk and laughter about mistakes.

> The hospital furnished the beer. It was a nice, amusing occasion, and you got to know your people. One doctor did a sigmodoscopy, found an obstruction, and biopsied it. It came back "normal cervix"! He thought he was in the colon, but he had gone into the vagina! Another doctor thought a woman was pregnant. He followed her, wondering why she didn't get *more* pregnant. Finally, he did an abdominal tap and got a lot of fluid. The woman wasn't pregnant. She had ascites. One doc described a patient as smelling "uriniferous." He'd forgotten that he'd examined the patient at night in the men's room. Then malpractice came, and that was the end of that.

He thought such an event had many beneficial functions.

> Doctors would tell their own stories. Dignified physicians put an Indian blanket over their heads and went in a circle, chanting and waving tomahawks. You didn't even know who was under this blanket. . . . Interns were pleased: everybody loosened up. The department was very cold. It was an opportunity to get a little closer to the attendings: relaxed, friendly, quasi-intimate.

Yet this event—an institutional ritual—was anonymous, and implied forgiveness and pardon. Unfortunately, nothing had replaced it, leaving doctors terrified of mistakes and guilt-ridden. Yet medical mishaps can, of course, be serious or even fatal, and not humorous.

Questions arose of what to do with *colleagues'* "screw-ups"—whether and how physicians should handle *others' errors*. Harry described how nurses complained to him about fellow doctors' care. Nurses could potentially serve as checks on a physician's care, but were ultimately limited in their capacity to do so or to intervene.

> I was the physician for the nurses, so I always had a special relationship with them. Sometimes they'd say to me, "Isn't there something to do about this patient? Her doctor doesn't talk to her, and she is worried sick about XYZ." Or "What can I do about Mrs. So-and-So?" There is no mechanism for the nurses to deal with that. They can't go to their supervisors. If they went, nothing would happen.

Yet in the end, physicians' abilities to influence colleagues' decisions were restricted, too. Harry continued:

> It's tough: none of my business, basically. A colleague might be *outraged* and complain about the nurses, or say, "That's the way the patient *ought* to be treated!" or "That's *my* patient. That's the way to do it." I have enough worries of my own to take on the world. If the doctor in question was a good friend, I'd chat with him. But it's hard to criticize. I'm not the world's most courageous person. I don't want a bloody nose.

Thus, informal checks may exist, but often only if the doctors are close. However, the lack of such feedback may end up hampering the quality of care. Moreover, doctors in private practice "depend on referrals" from colleagues, whom they therefore don't want to alienate. Physicians also hesitate to criticize colleagues, rationalizing that "We all do things wrong."

Still, occasionally, feedback worked. Harry added:

> One oncologist clearly mistreated patients: overtreated them, charged them excessively, and kept them too long in the hospital. Finally, his colleagues rebelled, and went to the chief. He was let go, went elsewhere, and almost lost his license. So *there*, a corrective process worked.

Yet such success appeared to be the rare exception. Though close colleagues may give each other feedback, it may be limited. Changes in the structure of health care delivery may have curtailed venues for such interactions. Harry continued:

> In my covering group, we correct each other. Somebody might say in a nice way, "Gee, now. . . ." That was wonderful about the hospital lunchroom, which doesn't exist anymore: Everybody came to lunch, and you could solve problems by talking to people. Professors would be there if you had physiological or biochemical questions. Now, there is less opportunity to have corridor con-sultations. You have to call somebody. It is difficult to see what somebody else is doing. You don't read their charts. Once in a while, there might be an opportunity to mention a patient indi-rectly, try to get a point across. But I couldn't say, "The nurses told me. . . ."

Still, in the complex system of the hospital, nurses could potentially serve a greater role as checks, providing corrections, as doctors once did for each other. Nurses have experience, observational skills, and judgment that could benefit patients, even more than at present. Yet professional boundaries can preclude optimal use of their input.

"Blowing off" Mild Symptoms

These ill doctors became more aware, too, of colleagues' lack of profes-sional appreciation of the inconvenience of seemingly minor symptoms, including medication side effects that can impair adherence to treatment. Previously, many of these doctors had merely been frustrated by patients' failures to follow treatment. They now came to appreciate the difficulties involved far more. These physicians became more acutely aware of the stress of symptoms that they had previously minimized, or even ignored as mild or nonspecific. Symptoms may not cause abnormal lab results or necessitate biopsies, but nonetheless trouble the sufferer. Before, these doctors had frequently minimized the impact of particular adverse effects that they saw as nonspecific, and hence as potentially or relatively unim-portant or even volitional. Now, they tended to identify further with pa-tients, no longer dismissing such nonspecific complaints, but taking them more seriously. Pascal, the Lebanese internist with HIV, said:

A physician that's not been affected personally may blow off mild symptoms. But I understand that mild symptoms can devastate your regular, day-to-day life, and I would probably treat them more aggressively than somebody else. I have taken one drug, and it's given me mild pancreatitis—just a 100-point increase in lipases; clinically, probably not that significant. But it's enough to nauseate me, and give me stomach discomfort and diarrhea. So when a patient tells me that, I understand. Another physician might say, "It's not high enough to stop the medication." I might say, "We'll stop it for a few days, restart on a lower dose, and I'll give you some lipase supplement, and anti-diarrheal."

His own disease thus prompted him to treat his patients differently.

Symptoms such as physical pain, too, can in fact be virtually indescribable. As suggested earlier by Roxanne, the gastroenterologist, though she had treated countless patients with abdominal pain, she had never fully appreciated the degree of difficulties they experienced. After all, pain is pre-linguistic: animals lack language, but feel pain, too. Yet health care professionals are often unaware of the impossibility of conveying such symptoms in words. "When my spleen enlarged, I could hardly eat," Roxanne said. "Appetizers would be enough for me. I'd get full. Afterward, I would feel pain, but was still hungry in my head. . . . My spleen crossed the midline. I realized *how painful* it must be for patients!"

The quality of pain differed radically from what these doctors expected. Albert, who had an MI on the highway, described difficulty communicating the experience or even the location of pain because of his fears of its implications.

When I was a medical student, we used to ask, "How far down does the pain go?" We tried to get the precision we wanted, but never really knew. My cardiac pain had a different quality than when I'm burning my finger or itching my skin. The fact that it can be very, *very* uncomfortable was a realization for me. I didn't have it long—only half an hour. But it was enough. You begin to squeeze somebody's arm, like when they put the blood pressure cuff on, and it gets uncomfortable. But you don't realize that if you take it up a few more notches, it gets more and more uncomfortable. The overtone is: "Oh, my God, is this healthy? What's going on?"

The possible meanings of pain—uncertainties as to the problems it might indicate—thus add to its distress. Yet the discrepancy between his professional training and his disease experience shocked Albert; he had not recognized the depth of this chasm before.

He was surprised, too, that his providers did not ask or care about the details, the qualities of discomfort or pain.

> Nobody asked me what kind of pain I was having. They asked me if I felt better after the nitro. But not "Where is it, exactly?" Nobody cared. As soon as your t-waves on your EKG are abnormal, the doctors don't care very much about the clinical quality.

Albert was disturbed that, to his doctor, his test results became far more important than his feelings.

His experience was important to him, though only fellow sufferers could fully appreciate it. Hence, Albert became eager to share it, as a "war story." Others, who had not endured it, could not relate.

> If you've had it, you find someone else who has been through it: you know that blowtorch feeling going up and down your arm . . . having to walk around bent. . . .

As a result of their treatment, only now did some of these physicians question their definitions of "clinical significance." Suzanne, the psychiatrist who started lithium treatment for bipolar disorder, said, for example, that clinicians are not sensitive enough to the impact of weight gain as a side effect that can cause profound social and self-image problems.

> It really bothers me how definitive psychiatrists are: "Patients can handle the weight gain on a medication. Let's just throw them on that. It doesn't matter that she's twenty-three. For the weight gain, she can exercise." That's *bullshit*. Don't put her on it: she's not going to take it because she's going to gain fifty pounds. She'll never get a boyfriend, and in this society *that's* more important than anything.

Indeed, for Suzanne, weight gain was the hardest aspect of her treatment. She continued, "That's the main problem: I'm fifty pounds overweight. I'm a former athlete, a skier. I just can't go on the ski slope now: I'm exhausted."

Weight gain as a symptom can cause enormous psychological distress, in part because it is stigmatized in both medicine and broader society. For example, Ernie found his change in body shape more disturbing than either his Huntington's disease (HD) or depression. "There are no obese doctors," he observed. He felt that both colleagues and patients viewed overweight doctors with suspicion: Why had these physicians not taken better care of themselves, given the health risks involved?

Similarly, ill doctors realized more fully the extent of difficulties associated with nonspecific symptoms (e.g., of fatigue): the extent of the burden of decreased energy from disease. For Suzanne, on lithium, "everything is a hump to get over." She added, "My therapist said, 'The first thing you should do at home is put your gym stuff on. Don't even go home—go right to the gym.'" But she felt she simply couldn't.

For physicians, decreased energy can be particularly hard, given the profession's competitiveness and ethos. Suzanne continued:

> I run out of gas more quickly—not just energy-wise, but everything-wise. I tolerate life less—don't get as much done as everyone else. I'm just not as functional. *Everybody else's car has a larger gas tank.*

Many become more sensitive not only to patients' complaints of "minor" symptoms such as "tiredness," but also to how hard these feelings were even to *describe*. Paul, an internist who lost a job offer due to his HIV, said, "I now have a huge respect for people when they say they're *tired*. You have no way to *define* it, but getting to the end of the day is really a challenge."

Lack of mental and physical energy, and feelings of being overwhelmed can profoundly impede professional and personal lives in unexpected ways. Roxanne said, "I realized that nothing is simple when you are sick. *Any little thing isn't little.*"

Organization and planning take mental energy more than one imagines. Suzanne added:

> I require a lot of support to have a life. I don't go to the market because you have to pick everything out, pay, make sure you have the money, bring it home, put it away. That takes a lot of patience. Organizing meals is a lot—just too much.

Yet physicians may discount patients' reports of these frustrations. For example, Jeff could no longer jog because of illness. His physician, however, trivialized this problem.

Running meant everything to me. It was how I got out my frustration and anger. I got a runner's high. It was an escape. But my aerobic capacity went down. My internist didn't take that as seriously as I wanted. She'd say, "You're such a jock!" I often felt that if I couldn't run, I'd just as soon die. In childhood, I felt bad that I couldn't do anything athletic.

Such symptoms may thus be nonspecific and unimportant to *providers*, but carry highly significant meanings to *patients*.

As a symptom, *insomnia*, too, proved much more distressing than anticipated. For months, Pascal, the Lebanese internist with HIV, couldn't sleep, which disturbed him far more than he had envisioned.

Ever since I was diagnosed, I've had insomnia. It became a constant problem. I did all the stuff a physician would tell a patient with insomnia: not drinking caffeine, not doing anything else in bed but sleeping. I went to hypnosis, even took antidepressants—but nothing helped.

Consequently, Pascal learned not to dismiss this symptom as he and other physicians often had.

These ill doctors newly appreciated such symptoms as ongoing nausea, tingling, and itching. Paul now better understood, and could teach others about, these:

It's so much easier now to understand what a patient is saying. Instead of just discounting "My feet tingle," you truly understand that. I try to frame it to medical students so they can understand: "Remember your worst hangover. That's what you're doing to people with these medications—headaches, nausea, vomiting, diarrhea."

Questions emerged, too, of how to view and weigh the benefits of treatment versus the risks of rare but severe side effects. Physicians at times discounted or ignored these adverse events, even if permanent or fatal, given the rarity. Nonetheless, a potentially fatal side effect, even if a clinician thinks it is uncommon, may deter patients from treatment. Suzanne stated:

A colleague did a whole presentation about one drug, and not once mentioned Stevens-Johnson syndrome. I had decided that Stevens-Johnson was too much of a risk for *me*. I asked, "What about Stevens-Johnson syndrome?" He said, "It's so rare that they don't even think about it." I thought: "No, people really *do* think about it. Patients have almost died from it!"

Suzanne's sensitivity was heightened by having just seen such a patient in the ER with this syndrome. As a fellow patient, she took that patient's experiences to heart.

> Her doctor had never told her that it could happen, and given her the option of taking it or not. Her arm was ripped up. It was horrible. I told her to get a lawyer.

Yet when the treatment in question was for themselves, as opposed to a patient, these doctor-patients now often altered their views of the associated risks and benefits. They realized that they may not only have underestimated the relative importance of a side effect, but also, as a result, have calculated risk-benefit ratios differently.

Physicians overvalued disease symptoms compared to side effects, partly as a result of their training and socialization. For instance, many doctors considered bipolar disorder very severe, while as a patient, Suzanne felt otherwise.

> Every time a doctor says, "With the more severe patients, like the ones with bipolar and schizophrenia, ..." I roll my eyes. Doctors say with surprise: "I had a bipolar patient, and in fact she's doing really well!"

She felt that such comments reveal physicians' underlying attitudes and prejudices about these patients.

Physicians may focus to such an extent on the need for a cure that they feel it justifies almost any cost. In addition, physicians may feel guilt about inflicting adverse symptoms on patients, and hence may pay less attention to these side affects. As will be discussed later, some thought pharmaceutical companies contributed to physician minimization of side effects. Fine print can deemphasize side effects in physicians' minds. Paul commented:

> All the people making the decisions about clinical guidelines have attachments to drug companies—speakers' bureaus and research dollars. One big name was talking about Norvir, and didn't know if it was taken two or three times a day. Obviously, he doesn't see patients. So how can he be making these decisions?

Currently ill themselves, many physicians appreciated their patients' side effects more, factoring in not just the effects, but also the psychological and social suffering involved. These physicians now realized how colleagues often underestimated such costs. Sally, the internist with cancer, said:

> I knew that if I didn't get my anti-emetic before I got my IV antibiotic, I was going to throw up for hours. So I was very insistent on it. Now, I am a little more demanding that those things be done for *my* patients. I try to do more now: to stress to trainees that it's important to look at not only the effects of your medication, but the *side* effects, and how to reduce them. Also, make sure that things get done when you've asked them to be done.

Problems with Adherence

These physicians also became more aware of other obstacles in adhering to medication regimens, such as sticking to a schedule. Countless patients fail to adhere completely to treatment, perceiving the advantages as less than the disadvantages of providers' recommendations. Once they became patients themselves, however, physicians tended to view these options differently. Adherence is important, particularly with certain medications, since nonadherence can lead to viral or bacterial resistance. It took becoming patients themselves to realize the potential difficulties.

These doctors now often failed to adhere fully to prescribed treatments. Neil, the HIV-infected neurologist, said about the need for strict compliance with medications, "I'm so busy during the day, and my denial is so high, that I don't take medicine. I take it in the morning and at night when I'm not at work. Taking it breaks my ability to deny."

Though some physicians continued to insist that their patients fully comply, a few now shifted their expectations and became more empathetic, giving patients more slack. To be more sensitive to their patients' difficulties and failures, many tried to use their own experiences confronting these obstacles. Steven, the suburban endocrinologist with HIV, at one point went so far as to consider changing his diet, to learn firsthand what diabetic patients had to endure.

> I was going to put myself on a diabetic diet, just to know what my patients had to go through. Now, I'm forcing myself to go on a structured medication regimen. It's similar: you have to structure your day and mealtimes.

In the end, Steven did not actually try a diabetic diet; it appeared too onerous. Efforts at complete empathy can be hard, if not forced by disease.

These ill doctors observed, too, that patients who did not adhere sometimes got blamed. The physician was not blamed, even if he or she had failed to educate the patient about the potential side effects. Jeff, the adolescent specialist, said that Latino patients often didn't question authority figures. If a patient was not compliant, the doctor might simply fault the patient, whereas the patient might not have understood the regimen, and feared asking.

These ill physicians often became more aware as well of colleagues being overly "cavalier" about prescribing medications. In part, physicians may too readily follow clinical guidelines that incorporate researchers' recommendations more than patient experiences. Paul, the internist who lost a job offer due to HIV, thought doctors pushed HIV medications too aggressively.

> These physicians don't have any sense of what the medications really do to you. For many patients, starting medications means declaring your diagnosis to your insurance company, and as a result, losing jobs, developing new symptoms, being sick at work, and reminding yourself of the disease every day. Doctors just don't understand that. I would encourage patients to go see a doctor who's HIV-positive, who'll have a much better idea of what patients are getting into.

Though patients do not necessarily have to consult only physicians with their same illness, Paul's comments highlight deficiencies in medical education.

Psychiatric Symptoms

"I now know what it's like to be frightened," Charles, the internist with HIV who had become an "underground researcher," sighed. These physicians had frequently downplayed and overlooked psychiatric difficulties, and now became far more sensitive to symptoms of anxiety and depression that can accompany physical disease. They revealed biases concerning these symptoms that are important for both lay patients who experience the symptoms, and fellow doctors to bear in mind.

The prospect of future physical symptoms can itself generate anxiety— far more than expected. Charles now came to see these issues "in a way I never could empathize with before."

People fear the unknown: I now know what it's like to have a pounding heart and a dry mouth, waiting those three, four, or five days until I get a blood test back. As the day approached, I would get more and more frightened and apprehensive. And I'm a doctor, *a scientist!* But I'm also just a scared patient.

Here, Charles identified differences between his dual conflicting roles: scientists are not *supposed* to be afraid. Yet he simultaneously occupied roles as biomedically-trained provider and fearful sufferer.

The experience of psychiatric diagnoses differed dramatically from what these doctors had imagined. For the first time in his life, Bradley, the tennis player who had an MI, became depressed, which bewildered, confused, and altered him.

After the surgery, I had what I had to characterize as a depression. I recognized the symptoms. For five to six weeks, I felt like not doing much. But I was dumbfounded, *even having been prepared for* it.

Clearly, these experiences involved not just cognitive, but also deep, inner emotional and existential layers of the self.

The *disruptiveness* of psychiatric symptoms astonished these physicians. Ernie, who had Huntington's disease, was most surprised about his melancholia: how impairing it was, involving loss of memory and enjoyment of life.

I enjoy my clinical work, but was just not able to do it. I used to get 10,000 phone calls a day, and be able to copy the numbers down just by listening to them. But when depressed, I couldn't write down even one phone number. I just didn't remember it.

Luckily, antidepressant treatment improved Ernie's memory.

Physicians also underestimate the effects of certain conditions, such as premenstrual syndrome (PMS), that have been the subject of controversy and debate. Suzanne, with bipolar disorder, said:

A lot of psychiatrists pooh-pooh PMS. But being PMSed *really* makes your symptoms worse. I would just fall apart. None of my psychiatrists ever noticed that—that it really does happen. So when a female patient says to me, "I'm PMSing," I don't think, "Oh, she's hysterical."

Lack of training and experience may make physicians who are not psychiatrists particularly insensitive to mental disorders. Psychiatric disorders are inherently more subjective, and less quantifiable, than medical conditions diagnosed through laboratory findings. Suzanne, the psychiatrist on lithium, observed:

> Even psychiatric residents have problems when they talk to patients: "Why *don't* you take your medicine?" As if it's easy taking seventeen pills a day! A delusional and paranoid person living on his or her own, trying to make it, not working, is not going to take six of one pill in the morning, four of another in the afternoon, and five of another at night. They're not going to remember.

Sadly and revealingly, shame and fears of stigma and discrimination led many physicians to hide their own psychiatric symptoms. Frank, the surgeon who had an MI in the OR, for example, saw other ill physicians he had treated as terrified, and embarrassed by their fear. "They're just like *regular patients*—frightened to death and superafraid. But they put on a *show* of nonchalance."

Losses of Dignity and Identity

Ill physicians heightened their sensitivity, too, to the indignities and losses of sense of self that patients endure. Patienthood radically altered outward appearances and self-images.

As suggested earlier, sick doctors literally found themselves clothed differently—forced to undress and to wear only flimsy patient gowns or lie naked—in ways that carried both real and symbolic import, signifying dramatic loss of power. For Brian, who had hepatitis, having to disrobe for his doctor marked the defining moment of his change in institutional status.

> To get undressed for the biopsy, and put on this paper gown—I'm exposed, not in my regular clothes. Even though they give me a gown, I feel impersonal exposure. It was awkward, knowing that people walk in and out of the room.

As mentioned earlier, many physicians resisted wearing such patient robes.

Deeper senses of loss of individuality and self ensued. The disappearance of hair due to chemotherapy disturbed many profoundly. For Nancy, loss of her hair robbed her of a significant part of her self and her identity.

I had very unusual blond hair, great hair—my best feature, by far. It was how people remembered me. Ironically, I lost the one thing that always defined me: my looks. It's a pain being bald. I have to wrap fabrics on my head, take them off and put them on. When I lie down, they make a big bump.

For Deborah, the psychiatrist with breast cancer, losing her braid was "more devastating than anything else," because it was her "mark"—a defining feature of herself. She no longer even recognized herself, and dreamed of having her hair again.

All my life, I had a very long braid. The first time I lost my hair on chemo, I was losing hair everywhere, and didn't want to cut it. Half my pillow would be full of hair. A friend who shaves his head said, "We're going to shave your head. I'll do it for you. Just forget you had hair." But that was more devastating than anything else: to shed my hair in the shower. Because it's part of you—*you are shedding part of you.* You get chemo and feel pain, but still keep *you,* yourself. But when you lose your hair, suddenly you become a totally different person. You don't recognize yourself. My hair grew back, but curly. Everybody thought I had a permanent. Then when I had radiation to my head, I lost my hair completely. I didn't know that after radiation, you can't grow your hair back at all. I still dream that my hair is back—a real stupid dream, but I have it.

As a scientist, Deborah tried to dismiss her unconscious desire for her hair. She had to change her self-image to that of a cancer patient. But she found this transition hard, and felt she now looked "unhealthy":

When I look in the mirror, *it's not me.* It's not my hair. My eyebrows now are very light. They used to be thick. My face looks round, and used to be skinny. In the mirror, *I don't see myself. It's a different me: a cancer patient.* That's my image of myself now. I don't know if other people know my diagnosis. Sometimes I feel they do. At a café, a woman had a wig. I said to a friend, "She's a cancer patient. I'm sure!"

Deborah suggested how radical transformations in outward selves shaped senses of inner selves as well. Theories of social construction suggest that identities are socially built. Yet here, more complicated, dynamic processes emerge: biological processes can play roles as well. *Inner and outer selves shaped each other.*

Often, physicians-of-record did not comprehend the difficulties caused by scars remaining from procedures. Jessica, the pediatrician with Hodgkin's lymphoma, said that every doctor should have her procedure done to know the extent to which needles hurt and can cause permanent psychic wounds. The psychological impact may be subtle, and therefore ignored by doctors. But for the patient, these marks can evoke disturbing memories and lasting emotional pain. Jessica said:

> Every doctor should have a bone marrow biopsy done just to see how it feels! People say, "I know how you feel," or "I know you're worried about. . . ." But *I* can say, "It hurts a little when they put the needle in. You'll have the scar." Sometimes I add, "Because I've had one of these." With older patients or parents I've had trouble convincing, I've actually shown them the scar: "This is where it is. It's not bad"—not with a patient I was first seeing, but with a kid I've known for a while who has gotten sicker.

Jessica raised the question of whether it is appropriate for doctors to display their scars to patients. It seemed overly intimate, but could aid patients. She felt this trade-off made sense, though other ill physicians felt the need to balance it with greater professional distance.

Ill doctors became more sensitive, too, to the dependency, uncertainty, and humiliation patients faced. Being left on a stretcher in a hallway for hours felt disrespectful and humiliating. Yet to striking degrees, professional training inhibited earlier realization of the impact of these deprivations and indignities on patients.

The uncertainties of patienthood took their tolls as well. Harry said:

> The patient has no idea what anything is, what's about to happen, what to be scared of—infantilized in an environment that puts you in a johnny gown, and doesn't even let you wear your own slippers, or ones that stay on your feet!
>
> Physicians come at 6 A.M., when the patient is fast asleep, and say, "How are you doing?" And before the patient has time to collect him or herself, the doctor is off and running. Patients want someone who can sit, listen, and empathize a little, and say, "Mmmhmm. Mmmhmm." It doesn't have to be very long—five or

ten minutes—but some sign of awareness of the helplessness, dependency, and questions.

These multiple sources of indignities accumulated, further reminding
patients of their relative powerlessness, and psychologically eroding them.

As suggested earlier, a hospital communicates to patients their relatively low worth in various ways. Walter said, "When you're the patient,
you feel that your life, *your actual life*, is going to be frittered away
because it didn't matter enough to someone."

Doctors were surprised, too, at the extent to which seemingly small
positive alterations in the quality of their daily life now loomed large.
After procedures, even being able to eat a meal again can be a major ac-
complishment. Roxanne said, "The first time I was able to complete a
meal was big: a major step!"

Clearly, doctors can be better trained to comprehend these aspects of
patient experiences. Patients can benefit from anticipating these obstacles
and aids as much as possible.

Silence and Codes: Communication Problems

Ill physicians became more aware of the importance, and yet the rarity, of
good communication, and the complexities of doctor-patient interactions.
These ill doctors now saw more fully how subtle cues and clues can either
facilitate or impede discourse. Many of these health professionals reported
indirect communication or noncommunication with their own providers,
particularly about socially taboo topics. Problems such as depression and
side effects were not only of concern in and of themselves, but also posed
substantial communication difficulties. Challenges arose not only in being
depressed, for instance, but also in being able to speak about it with one's
physician.

A few ill doctors felt that medical information had been sensitively
presented to them. Nancy, the internist with breast cancer, said about her
physician, "She has a magical way of giving bad news. Nothing shocks or
alarms her. I can get the worst news ever, and am upset, but after talking to
her, I think 'Wow, it's not so bad. I can handle this.' She has a great *talent* for
that." Indeed, this ability constitutes a clear and important skill that some
possess more than others. Here, too, stylistic elements prove important.

Yet far more commonly, these physicians became aware of the ubiquity of poor interactions. Sadly, inadequate doctor-patient discourse appeared far more to be the norm. Tom, whose lover died of AIDS, said, "I hear it all the time from patients: 'I went to a doctor, and he didn't talk to me.' "

Challenges arose concerning both the *form* and the *content* of communication. Doctors were often rushed, lacking time to answer patients' questions and, through verbal and nonverbal gestures, stymied potential discourse. Albert, who had an MI on the highway, saw an impediment in that doctors didn't sit down, but stood up during interactions at patients' bedsides.

> As a physician, I always sit now if there is a chair in the room. Standing at the foot of the bed talking to a patient is an important nonverbal interaction. *The cardiologist I liked best came in and sat down on the bed!* But most doctors came in with the chart, and would stand there. If the guy's sitting down, I thought, "He's committing to lengthening the interaction." I'm sure he probably sat there for all of three minutes. Maybe he was just tired. But it was important.

Albert's observation of the importance of sitting can help physicians with their patients more broadly.

Pressed for time, physicians may also keep exchanges with patients superficial, and fail to inquire about aspects of patients' lives that may help with diagnosis and treatment. For example, doctors may not ask about patients' future plans. Albert added:

> I was disappointed in the depth of the doctor-patient relationship. He was on one side of the desk; I was on the other. Whatever I ask him, he will answer. But he wouldn't say, "What do you think about this?" No one ever asked me what my plans were, in general. Then, we'd have had a dialogue, a candid conversation.

Doctors were often brusque, speaking to patients insensitively about critical areas such as prognoses, and the meanings and interpretations of medical tests. Even the nuanced details of how, when, and where medical information, particularly "bad news," was transmitted, proved meaningful. For example, Jacob vividly recalled the specifics of hearing his diagnosis: where, when, and what. He underscored the importance of each of these features.

While I was on jury duty, the dermatologist paged me. I remember his words: "The biopsy results came back, and they're not good. It's a melanoma." I was standing up in the telephone booth in the courthouse. I almost collapsed.

In conveying bad prognoses, doctors' *tones* may be particularly insensitive. Medical information—even a mere three to five words (e.g., "you have cancer")—can have terrible and lifelong implications for the individual patient. Walter, the politically-active internist, was disturbed by his doctor's matter-of-factness in presenting the options and the decision-making process.

He looked at the CT scan and said, *"There's nothing we can do."* I was devastated. He said, "You'll never be able to eat. You have tumor everywhere. If we get into your abdomen and there's tumor everywhere, what do you want us to do? It will hurt, and won't change the outcome. You'll be dead." *He didn't mean it to be devastating, but it was.*

Again, physicians-of-record may be oblivious to the emotional impact of their words.

Ill doctors also became more aware of the potential insensitivity of even *offhand comments*. Jessica, the pediatrician, was upset by what she perceived to be her oncologist's sadistic side remarks.

I had two moles on my arms. He said, "You should have those taken off before you start radiation. Because a few years from now, *if you're still around*, it could be a problem." I used to cry on the way home. Because I was a doctor, he would talk to me about his other patients: "I have another patient just like you. She looks like you: same age, and has the same exact tumor. She's in the hospital." So, of course I say, "How's she doing?" He says, "She's dying."

A physician's quick remarks may literally be matters of life and death for a patient, who weighs these comments very differently than the doctor does. Jessica became more aware of casual "offhand" statements by colleagues in response to bad news.

I told a colleague, "I have cancer." She said: "You're kidding!" I found that very offensive. People say that kind of thing and don't mean anything—it's an immediate reaction. But I thought, "Why would I kid about that? I'm going to die!"

For patients, these comments remained palpable. Even innocent comments had profound effects because of their implications.

Doctors varied as well in how much information about side effects they provided to patients beforehand. Some failed to explain important treatment complications. For example, no one had told Deborah, the psychiatrist with metastatic breast cancer, that her hair would never grow back after radiation. "I think they all thought that I knew. But how would I know? It's not my field."

As suggested earlier, her doctors may also have felt uncomfortable discussing these side effects with Deborah because of their implicit guilt at harming patients.

Questions arose, too, of when patients were "informed enough." The answer varied, and was not always clear.

Several doctor-patients were surprised to glean important facts not from their physicians, but from others. Such lack of communication from providers occurred about taboo areas, including not only death, but also mental health and sex. Bradley learned of potential post-op depression not from his own cardiologists, but from his doctor-son. Similarly, Tim, a young, recently married dermatologist, was not told by his physician that he might become sterile after radiation therapy for his leukemia. Luckily, a friend informed him.

Physicians-of-record not only revealed ignorance about the experience of psychiatric symptoms, but communicated about these topics poorly. Jeff, the adolescent specialist, described how his mental health symptoms were inadequately assessed by his physician, who, as a result, missed a diagnosis.

> I told her, "I think I'm depressed." She asked about appetite and weight change. But all these were negative, so she said I wasn't depressed. But she superficially skipped over it. She needed to really delve into it, to say, "I want you to see a counselor." I think my unsafe sex was depression-related. She should have found out why I said I was depressed, especially since *I'm not just some layperson*! She should have put down her pencil and paper... and figured this out. I'd go to the gym with tears in my eyes. . . .

Eventually, Jeff found a therapist. He started Prozac, but it was his own idea.

Faulty discussion also occurred concerning *sexual* dysfunction. Embarrassed, Jeff couldn't mention his impotence to his doctor, and only dropped hints. But his physician failed to grasp these clues. Poor communication or noncommunication can thus be *mutual*.

> For a year, I tried to tell my internist that erections were a problem for me. Sometimes I wouldn't bring it up. I wanted *her* to. Other times, I would *indirectly kind of say it*. I only dropped hints, because it's embarrassing: "I'm doing fine, but wish my libido were better." Her next response wouldn't be centered around the libido, but "What's your last testosterone level?" It would be normal, and she would drop it. A year and a half into this, for some reason, she said, "I'll send you to a urologist." In a month, I was back having erections. It could have happened a year and a half earlier.

Clearly, as patients, these physicians had difficulty being explicit about these stigmatized issues. Explicit communication was difficult. Jeff learned he had to be straightforward, not oblique. "I have to be very direct. A lot of patients just don't have that ability."

As mentioned above, poor communication about side effects stemmed in part from physicians' guilt, and focus on the benefits of treatments, both of which can also produce and result from hubris (as described below).

"They Think They're God": Physician Arrogance

"All doctors think they're important," Dan said, "critical to the survival of themselves and everyone around them." Such arrogance often abetted poor communication. Frequently, physicians resisted challenges to their authority, feeling they were right and patients wrong.

Such pride can prompt doctors to conceptualize successes and failures of treatment in self-affirming ways. At times, doctors overreported successes and downplayed failures, defining the risks and benefits differently than did their patients. Anne, the Swiss internist who had picked up her pathology results herself and had seen that her doctor had not removed all of the cancer, disdained oncologists, disagreeing with their judgments and definitions of "good" versus "bad" outcomes. In particular, they ignored side effects:

> What they call a success often is not, and is very ridiculous—
> they're giving someone three months more of a miserable life. But

medications have a lot of side effects that oncologists never explain. It pisses me off when I see them talking themselves up for something that is ridiculously minuscule.

Admitting negative outcomes, despite the promise of modern scientific triumphs, is to confess and confront medicine's limitations. Hence, doctors may frame prognoses and treatments in unrealistic and self-serving ways. Anne continued:

Doctors lie to themselves and their patients, because of the limitations of what they're doing. Medicine has made immense progress, but there's a whole lot more to do, and a lot of doctors, especially oncologists, just *mislead* patients.

Anne's feelings grew from both her patients' and her own experiences, each set sharpening her critique.

At the extreme, especially early in their careers, doctors may insist on upholding their power, even if patients receive poorer care as a result. The fact that doctors think they are more important than their patients may be a necessary conceit: this bravura and sense of confidence can maintain a distance that bolsters objectivity and, as we will see later, generates a placebo effect. Dan, the oncologist with chest metastases, said, "Everyone wants to be important. But getting away from *your own God complex* is important, but difficult: you need to prove how important you are."

Arrogance can hamper the quality of care provided. Deborah described physicians "playing the game of the doctor. It's really arrogance: 'I am the doctor, three steps above you.'" Indeed, such hubris almost killed her. When she needed oxygen, a resident neither gave it to her nor called a superior.

I was suffocating, coughing and losing my breath, and needed oxygen. I wanted to die. The resident walked in, and didn't know what to do. I said, "Go call somebody!" She refused: "I am the doctor. I'm not going to call anybody." I happened to know nurses on the floor. One walked in just to say good morning, and said to the physician, "You're out of your mind! She needs oxygen!" The nurse grabbed the mask and gave me the oxygen, and told the resident to leave. That nurse saved my life.

Physicians get trained to interpret patients' complaints, seeking underlying, known medical problems; but in so doing, they may discount patients' words. Consequently, doctors can block their own receipt of potentially valuable data. Pascal, the Lebanese internist, said:

> Some physicians treat me like an idiot. They don't consider me a physician, and won't listen completely. They don't understand that I need support psychologically. They blow me off: "There are support groups you can go to...." I had stomach aches that I knew were gallstones, because I had studied it. My doctor said, "That's impossible. You're a young man." I said, "Just do me a favor: do an ultrasound." It was very difficult for her. But sure enough, I had gallstones.

Such hubris can exacerbate doctors' insensitivity to patient's physical pain. Deborah cried because of her surgeon's gruff manner and the discomfort he inflicted, of which he seemed unaware.

> He used a very large needle for a biopsy, and no anesthetic. I couldn't understand why. It was very painful. He got enough tissue, but wanted to go back again. I said, "You're not touching me! I can't let you do this." He said, "Ok, I think I have it now." He sent it to the lab, and called two hours later, and said, "I have bad news for you." His manner was very rough. He was very arrogant. I never went to him again.

Are women doctors less arrogant and more compassionate than men? Deborah and a few others thought so—"at least to their women patients." She said:

> I had a male surgeon do the surgery, and it was the same story. Another man removed part of my parathyroid and did a very good job, and was very nice. But the other procedures I had were done by women. They are just more compassionate. I don't let men touch me anymore.

Deborah suggested a continuum, from utter lack of compassion to gruffness. Yet when she needed oxygen, it was a female, not a male, physician who wouldn't provide it. Here, gender did not entirely correlate with heightened empathy. Still, most complaints of physician arrogance reported by these doctor-patients were of male, rather than female, providers. Deborah's studied conclusions were consistent with stereotypes, and work by Carol Gilligan (1) on gender differences in moral decision-making—that girls address moral problems in relationships by dealing with people's feelings rather than more abstract principles. But among physicians, men continue to outnumber women approximately three to one (2). Certainly, many men interviewed here appeared warm and caring; and not all women are equally compassionate, or necessarily more so, than men.

Cultural differences can also exacerbate distancing from patients. Hubris can separate doctors, especially from poor or foreign-born patients. On the other hand, Deborah, for example, had attended medical school in Latin America: "So I've learned a lot about communicating with people who are poor and have nothing."

As described earlier with regard to medical errors, doctors received little feedback to challenge or counter this insensitivity. Indeed, the system and practice of medical education may facilitate or even exacerbate callousness. Deborah observed that faculty did not teach compassion or critique physicians who lacked it. "If somebody has a bad bedside manner, very few people will say anything. In my training, nobody ever told me *anything* about it."

Trainees found it especially difficult to give such feedback to senior doctors. A rigid hierarchy separates senior and junior doctors, mirroring that between doctors and patients. Peter, an HIV-positive medical student, on hearing a surgeon deprecating a female patient, felt, "I can't say to him: 'Hey, you shouldn't do that!' "

Pleasing Doctors: Dynamic Barriers to Communication

"You want your doctors to like you," Nancy observed. Many of these ill physicians now became aware of the extent to which, as patients, they sought to "please" their physicians, and the ways this desire interfered with discussions of clinical problems. Nancy, who had brain metastases, described how her physician-father told her she should be more assertive with her caregivers. But she justified her reticence: it resulted from her own psyche and her desire to get along with her providers.

> You want to be *a good patient*, and sometimes are afraid to rock the boat. My parents are always bugging me to be pushier. Today, they wanted me to call to see if I could get radiation this week. Since they bugged me, I did it. But I knew I was inconveniencing a covering doctor who doesn't really know me.

In social interactions more broadly, each party generally wants the other to feel positively, and doctor-patient interactions are no exception. Jacob, the religious radiologist, described how he wanted to bolster his physician's feelings. However, as a result, he avoided asking many questions.

> I know that the doctor feels good if I trust him. The fewer questions I ask, and the more he knows that I feel I'm in his hands, the happier he is, and the more positively he'll relate to me. *I want him to know he's a good guy.*

Dependent, and eager for as much assistance from their doctors as possible, even these ill physicians felt they needed to engage, and at times flatter.

This process of approval-seeking may take hold after an initial period, during which time trust in the doctor is established. Jacob continued, "I'll look for dents in the armor of his abilities, in which case I might switch providers." But once Jacob decided to work with a particular doctor, he remained, and tried to establish as strong a relationship as possible.

In turn, doctors provided feedback that encouraged patients' efforts to please. Patients may then realize and get "conditioned" that their doctors *seek* positive feedback. Lou, the cancer patient who had a plaque on his wall, elaborated:

> Patients protect doctors. When the doctor stops on rounds, and says, "How are you doing?" and the patient answers, "Poorly," the doctor has a long-drawn face. When the patient says, "Fine," the doctor smiles and waves hello. *The patient gets conditioned.* The question is, Who's protecting whom? And how do we get around that?

Lou suggested that physicians protect themselves partly from difficult interpersonal or potential medical issues with patients. He felt that in these interchanges, he and many patients implicitly sought to deny their illness.

Patients sought opening cues from doctors that affirmed the possibility of raising certain topics; conversely, the absence of such cues can impair communication. Stuart, the internist with HIV who was now teaching at the university, described how even hugging patients could unintentionally silence them. "I tend to be a hugger. But I realized that sometimes when I'm hugging people, I'm really giving them physical cues to *shut up*! So I tend now just to hold their hand or touch them."

Even when not understanding important risks or benefits of a procedure, patients may refrain from challenging their doctors, but simply trust them to provide all relevant information. Simultaneously, physicians may underestimate patients' capacities to comprehend data. Herb, the neonatologist with an MI, reflected:

> My doctor said, "I'd like to blast open these two vessels...." I didn't say, "Let's think about this." He had an air of confidence, and I liked his demeanor.

Herb, who treated infants, trusted his physician's full logic, though not understanding it.

These barriers to communication may be mutual, too, since patients may hesitate to talk about certain medical problems—desiring to minimize them because of embarrassment or denial. For instance, patients may not want to give what they perceive as "bad news" to their physicians. Mathilde's husband, for instance, understated his medical problems to his doctors. She explained:

> They would say, "How are you?" He would answer, "Oh, fine. I exercised twenty minutes." That's pretty good when the doctors hardly have time to get on an exercise machine. But I knew what it took to get him out of bed, and that his will was such that he would try to overcome any limitations.

As mentioned earlier, this passivity toward doctors may arise in part from familial models. Yet physicians appeared not to be wholly aware of patients' desires to please in these ways, or of these mutually reinforcing dynamics. Neil, the neurologist with HIV, liked patients getting better, and was surprised when one of them sensed, and tried to fulfill, this desire.

> I had a very sick patient who was given up for dead. Not that I have a God complex, but three years later, he's still alive. It's been a lot of luck. He is bed-bound, and smokes, and last month when I was on vacation, he accidentally lit himself on fire. When I got back, he said, "It was an accident. I'm sorry if I've upset you by this." *I'm sorry if I've upset you!?*

This patient felt shame and guilt at disappointing his physician. Yet Neil was struck by the irony that he himself felt bad about having been away when this event occurred. Thus, both doctor and patient tried to placate one another, though neither acknowledged the other's attempts.

Thus, doctor-patient communication emerged not as static, with each party conveying statements to the other. Rather, decisions on what and how to communicate were very much affected by perceptions of how each party (a) thought the other party would respond, (b) wished the other party would respond, and (c) thought the other party in turn wanted to respond. Patients often responded to what they *thought* their doctors wanted to hear. However, these patient perceptions may not be accurate. Patients may react to *their own misperceptions or misunderstandings* of what they think their doctors wish. Patients may fear physician replies that do not in fact occur. Such assumptions can further hinder optimal communication and care.

Patients tried to affect their doctor's reactions toward them, yet faced conflicts. The establishment of trust is a mutual process. Yet a desire to establish trust may compete with a mandate to disclose the whole truth. At times, ill doctors faced tensions as to whether to: please versus disclose disappointing news (e.g., about nonadherence or symptoms).

These doctors were surprised to observe these processes in themselves; previously they had been unaware of seeking positive feedback from patients. These physicians encountered conflicts, too, over whether to express versus conceal their displeasure or disappointment with their own providers and patients.

Doctors' and patients' desires can clash. Patients may want to disclose information and prolong or extend interactions, while physicians do not. Patients' desires to please doctors, doctors' desires to be pleased, and physician arrogance also can combine, further impeding discourse.

Such dynamic processes have been explored in other contexts. The French postmodern theorist Jacques Lacan argued that in psychoanalysis, four entities are always involved: the patient, the doctor, the person the patient thinks he/she is talking to, and the person the doctor thinks he/she is speaking to (3). Who each party thinks he or she is talking to may differ from whom he or she is in fact talking to. These multiple distinctions complicate subsequent interactions. The narratives here suggest that models such as Lacan's, highlighting the complex dynamics of provider-patient communication, apply in medical encounters beyond psychoanalysis.

Patient Time versus Doctor Time

After becoming sick, these physicians became more aware of conflicts between doctors and patients regarding *time*. Specifically, they became more alert to differences in availability, experiences, preferences, and definitions of time. Many of these physicians became disappointed with how the "timetables" of physicians and patients collided. In particular, many expressed surprise at problems with waiting to receive care, and at how much distress these delays caused.

Views and experiences of time have been examined in many social domains, but less in medicine. Still, the amount of time physicians have with each patient may be decreasing (4), though the implications of this change on patients' experiences have been underexplored.

In general, time is measured not only in standardized and objective units, but in sociocultural terms as well (5, 6). Cultural factors can shape, for example, the lengths of future and past time periods that are measured (7). In the workplace, types of tasks and social structures affect how individuals experience dimensions of time, such as its "flexibility, linearity, pace, punctuality, delay...urgency, scarcity, and future and present... perspectives" (8). The duration of time is also experienced subjectively (9).

Within medicine, the little attention that has been given to time has focused on long-term hospitalizations for psychiatric disorders and TB, before the advent of more effective medications (10–13). Patients and doctors seek timetables to shape expectations (e.g., for discharge from the hospital), and negotiate and bargain about when events such as hospital discharges occur. Timetables structure psychiatric training (10, 14)— specifically, how professional development progresses over months and years. Recently, how physicians make decisions concerning prognoses has also been investigated (15). Though doctor's visits have been perceived as getting shorter due to managed care (16, 17), some data have suggested otherwise (18–20), and physician visits may in fact be lengthening slightly because of increases in the number of elderly patients, many of whom require dietary counseling for hypertension (20). Lengths of hospitalizations have been decreasing, often due to financial and administrative factors (21–23). Time delays have been documented in receiving treatment—such as analgesia for acute abdominal pain (24, 25) and treatment for acute MIs—that can reduce treatment effectiveness (26). Long wait times may be associated with decreased overall satisfaction with treatment (27, 28), though other research has found that patients often misperceive time, overestimating more than underestimating wait times (29). Indeed, perceptions rather than actual wait times may predict patient satisfaction (30).

Still, the day-to-day timetables of doctors and patients, and perceptions and conflicts that may result, have been underexamined. Given that encounters between doctors and patients involve hierarchies, how do these two kinds of individuals within the same dyadic social interaction experience and view these issues relative to each other? Though doctors face multiple competing demands and have limited periods with each patient, it is not clear how they integrate such time pressures into their work and handle this conflict each hour and day.

Availability of Less Time

In recent decades, the advents of managed care and of technological interventions have exacerbated each other in diminishing the amount of time doctors have with patients. Sally, the internist with cancer who brought her laptop to the ICU, said about the past:

> When we used to make rounds, there was time for discussion, because there were so few things we could do. Now, procedures and tests totally fill the time and minds of doctors, so they're a little lost.

The decreased availability of time both causes, and results from, the availability of quick quantitative tests. Physicians may become very "procedure-oriented," pushing to get tests done rather than examine patients. This orientation has several other causes as well, including belief in "the objectivity of *the numbers*." Sally said, "An intern is just too eager to say, "Let's get another chest X-ray, another this, another that." They don't listen to my chest; they get a chest X-ray." Doctors readily substitute high-tech procedures for low-tech ones. As we shall see, often this belief in "the numbers" as powerful and predictive may be illusory. Still, patients may have little choice but to lower their expectations accordingly.

Differences in Experiences of Time: Waiting as Suffering

"Most difficult for me has been the process of waiting," Steven, the suburban endocrinologist with HIV, said. Previously, many of these doctors had failed to realize the degree to which patients experienced time differently—as *longer*, since uncertainty and disease loom over patients' heads. Waiting lengthens the experience.

Importantly, these doctor-patients suggested the existence of "patient time," "doctor time," and "institution time" that moved differently and conflicted—both long-term (e.g., with regard to prognoses) and short-term (e.g., in a waiting room). As Jacob said, "*A person waiting is a person suffering.*" Even when they understood the reasons for delays in waiting rooms, these ill physicians grew angry. Jacob came to realize as never before the importance of minutes, hours, and days, and specifically the painful uncertainty of anticipating a lab result: "The difference between being a doctor and not being a doctor was *the timing.*"

Conflicting notions of time implicit in their physicians' delays in returning phone calls or answering questions shocked and annoyed these ill doctors. These delays reflected the privileged status of physicians' schedules over those of their patients. These tensions impelled doctor-patients to become even more aggressive in their own care. One ill physician said, "I get and interpret my own lab results—otherwise I'd have to wait three months until my next appointment." Ronald, the suburban Connecticut radiologist, reported:

> My doctors never called me back, so I started using the physician assistants, and only using the doctor once in a while. The week before my doctor's appointment, I have my blood drawn. So when I go to see him, the results are right there. Otherwise, I'd never get a call back.

Insurance coverage limited Ronald's ability to self-doctor. In contrast, lay patients could not self-doctor to compensate for doctors' shortages of time.

Surprisingly, even on a smaller scale, these physician-patients repeatedly expressed frustration at not receiving appointments and lab tests *immediately*. Several physicians reported being astonished at their distress caused by these delays. Harry, the internist who had an MI, described his annoyance at this situation:

> I discovered an intense irritation that I had to go and sit in my doctor's office. I had an appointment at 11:30 A.M. and wasn't seen until 12:50, and was driven up the wall! I'm not different from anybody else. But why should *anyone* have to wait around? It is SOP [standard operating procedure]. Some doctors are pretty good at figuring out how to have people *not* wait so long, or get treated better. Rationally, I understood: they want to stack the airplanes up, so that whenever there's an opening, one can land. But it's very irritating.

Though Harry had practiced medicine for over thirty years, he only now thought seriously about why *anyone* should have to wait.

As mentioned, waiting can be one of the most difficult parts of being a patient. As fellow physicians, these doctors received more "call backs" than lay patients. Still, this special treatment did not fully alleviate the problem. Steven, the suburban endocrinologist with HIV, recognized that he faced fewer delays because he was "halfway" between a patient and a doctor. But he remained perturbed.

> I hate waiting for things that I know don't take this long—calling doctors and not being put through immediately. I struggle with being a patient and being a doctor at the same time. If I called just as *another doctor to a doctor*, to discuss a case, he'd come right to the phone. If you're *just a patient*, he won't. Doctors will call you back at their leisure. You play phone tag.

As alluded to earlier, these frustrations stemmed partly from the symbolic meanings of these delays: the diminution of status.

A few doctors admitted, "I know I've kept patients waiting, too," but most had difficulty resolving this discrepancy between having kept patients waiting and now having to wait themselves. Medical socialization impedes awareness of these concerns, distancing and disconnecting doctors, who then see and construct patients as the "other." Grueling hours of premed courses, med school, internship, and residency instill separation that helps physicians maintain professional distance. This distance aids doctors in assisting many patients over time, minimizing burnout, yet can diminish patient satisfaction and care.

At the same time, many of these physicians simply accepted that delayed timetables are "just how things are done." Pascal, the Lebanese internist, now understood these issues more clearly, but had trouble acting more swiftly for patients.

> I now understand a lot more how long things take to happen when you call my office and ask for something. But *that's just the system*, and how people are used to doing things. It's unfortunate, but *there's only so much I can change what I do.*

Pascal saw even his own office as part of this intractable "system"— seemingly beyond remediation. Yet his feeling of being unable to alter his own practice—his sense of helplessness—highlighted barriers, both real and perceived, beyond these individual providers. Some of these tensions may be inevitable, since the experience of being a patient may invariably involve both waiting and suffering. Indeed, the words "patient" and "patience" derive from the same Latin root, *patientia*, "to suffer" (31). Often, illness and treatment take unpredictable amounts of time. Unforeseeable courses of illness make needs for follow-ups uncertain. Emergencies are unplanned. Many patients miss appointments or arrive late. Moreover, health care workers and institutions frequently structure medical events around their own ongoing needs, demands, and priorities, rather than those of patients. These data illustrate how physician-, rather than patient-oriented, medicine persists. Hierarchies in medicine and managed care's competition for physicians' time compound each other, aggravating these problems.

Preferences Concerning Time of the Day

Doctors and patients conflicted as well over what hours of the day were most ideal or convenient for medical treatments. Physicians often forgot patients' timetables and sense of time. For example, these physician-patients became aware of the disadvantages of doctors—especially surgeons—visiting hospitalized patients early on "morning rounds," waking patients up. Deborah observed how surgeons visited at dawn, disturbing patients. "They put the light on, and eight people scream, shout, and drop things. They don't give a damn that the patient in the next bed is half-dead."

Moreover, some physicians may prescribe medications for times of the day such that side effects harm patients more than otherwise. Sally, for example, was given medication at night that gave her explosive diarrhea. The drug could have been administered much earlier in the day. She complained to the hospital staff, but in vain. Eventually, only by going "on strike" could she change the hours of dosing.

> I felt like a test tube, not a patient. I was on kayexalate, which gives you massive diarrhea. They gave it to me in the morning, and I got "my business" finished before sleep. But then, only because they didn't think about writing the order until 9:00 P.M., they gave it to me at 10:00 P.M. It was the first day I was allowed out of bed to use the commode. I had all these IV lines, and an oxygen mask, and it was a big production to move six feet to the commode. I knew how explosive the diarrhea was. So I was up until 2 A.M. waiting for it to happen. I talked about it with the house

officer: "I'm going to wait till tomorrow to take it." But that caused a whole big fuss, so I just took it. The next time, I went on *strike*! Eventually my attending wrote a better order.

These ill physicians' providers frequently failed to grasp the importance of timing in patients' lives and quality of life. Sally continued:

> One doctor tapered me off steroids too quickly before Passover. I said, "Can't we wait a week? I have sixteen people coming over for Passover." He said, "No, I want you to do it now." He went into this whole thing about his own family's dynamics—he grew up in an Orthodox Jewish home, and it was awful. I said, "But that's not our house. I really treasure it!" I followed the taper, but it was too fast. I had to be readmitted. My kids came to the hospital and we had the seder there. They brought a few things I had made, and we set the table in the hospital. My doctor had no remorse. It wasn't a medical necessity to taper me then.

Thus, the medical profession does not follow *patient time*, but *physician time* and *hospital time*. Increased physician appreciation of these differences could help improve patients' quality of life and care.

Defining "the Future"

These competing timetables led to different, frequently contrasting definitions, and hence understandings, of prognoses. In discussing the future, doctors and patients regularly communicated about time, but disagreed about the precise meanings of descriptive terms. How long is "long"? How short is "short": hours, days, weeks, months, or years? Doctors and patients may define "fast" and "slow" very differently. A doctors can say, "We have plenty of time," but both objectively and subjectively, for a particular patient, the disease may progress much faster. Walter reported:

> My doctor said that Hodgkin's doesn't spread *that quickly*. . . . But once you're told that you have a serious illness, it's very hard to have that overall perspective.

Moreover, competing views of time can be hard to address or reconcile.

Physicians' arrogance may lead them to defend their predictions and interpretations of the durations of periods. Walter continued:

How does he know that it's not going to spread to this or that group of lymph nodes within six weeks? He says, "Oh, I've seen the course. You're just anxious!"

The average natural history of a disease does not apply to everyone. But it is simpler for physicians to believe in and follow these means, despite often wide individual variation, rather than try to determine the degree of uncertainty inherent in any particular patient's prognosis. Yet Walter found that his own view of his timetable was pathologized by his physician as due merely to anxiety.

In part, these incongruities arose because doctors are mandated with a threefold mission of providing diagnoses, treatments, and prognoses, yet the future cannot wholly be predicted. Hence, physicians may want to hedge their bets by speaking in ambiguities. But doctors' and patients' different experiences and approaches regarding time exacerbate distress. Why do doctors nevertheless prognosticate? Their clinical experience enables them to do so because they have observed numerous cases of a particular disease, and lengths of patients' survival. Yet, countless unpredictable factors can alter these periods.

Falling Between the Cracks

Physicians' lack of time had other effects as well, contributing to patients' tests and follow-ups "falling between the cracks." Due to managed care, primary care providers, though "gatekeepers," are swamped by deluges of data and detail, and have less freedom and flexibility in their schedules. Nancy, the endocrinologist with breast cancer, said:

> It's unusual to have a primary care physician who is going to take care of *all* the details. Mine gives me referrals, but it's too much work to keep him informed about what my oncologist is doing.

Nancy and others came to realize more than before how details got lost or forgotten.

> As a doctor, I often let the ball drop, and did not follow up on details. *Now, being a patient, I realize that's awful.* Doctors don't go out there and actually check if the secretary ordered the tests. You don't necessarily know when the patient gets a lab test done. The results don't necessarily come to your box in a timely fashion. The results could be available, and you don't know it.

Nancy had never before either looked at her own office procedures from this alternative perspective, or realized the extent and implications of the problem.

Overworked, many physicians were too overwhelmed to remember or follow key aspects of patients' treatments. Ill physicians now sympathized with their providers' plight. Ronald, the radiologist, said his doctor regularly forgot critical parts of the medical history. "He's a sweetheart, but burned out."

Still, physicians' lack of ongoing attention generated dismay. In particular, several complained of surgeons who did not even visit postoperatively. Nancy continued:

My neurosurgeon never came to see me. He obviously thought: "I am working for an academic salary. My fellows can see the patients. It's safe, they know what they're doing." But *that is so unprofessional: he's teaching his students and fellows to blow patients off!* I was angry. I'm sure he thought it was this little harmless procedure. And he thought I was pushy. I was probably being a little pushier than a normal patient, but they hadn't really taken a history, so they didn't know I had problems that could affect anesthesia. They were totally being surgeons, and putting things off.

After surgery, Nancy's covering doctor never even answered his page to see her, and the staff did not know what physician was responsible for her.

The surgeons didn't come by, and gave very confusing orders. It took the nurse six hours to figure out who was covering me. We paged him several times and he never answered.

Harry was told by his surgeon, half-jokingly, "I never need to see you again." As a result, Harry "sent him a postcard every year, on the anniversary of my operation!"

In fact, such decreased attention may be spreading. Faculty used to read through all the charts in the past, but may no longer do so. Nancy added:

The generation before us was stricter. The chief residents used to go through every patient's chart and leave little sticky notes. Now, I don't think the attendings even *look* at the charts of their patients. It's very lax.

Given competing time demands, doctors often had to triage, and give less time to some patients, commonly poorer ones seen in clinics. Roxanne, the gastroenterologist, reported, "Doctors say, 'This is just a clinic patient.' It's not right to have *two systems*." Within each of these two tiers, doctors routinely provide patients different amounts of time.

But lack of time with patients can jeopardize the quality of the care. Getting to know a patient well initially can mitigate later problems. Roxanne said:

> I had a depressed accountant as a patient. She had liver disease and
> wanted me to know that she had gone to a university, even though
> she had lost her job and had come to the clinic because things
> had gone badly for her. Then she went elsewhere, and they treated
> her for hepatitis C, and messed it up. She got depressed from
> the interferon, became suicidal, and came back to see me. Had I
> not taken out time, and had a sense of her, I might have missed
> the causal connection—that her depression was due to her
> medication.

What Are Reasonable Expectations?

In voicing these disappointments and dissatisfactions, were ill physicians expecting too much, raising the bar unrealistically high? A critic might argue that the shortcomings they perceived did not necessarily constitute "bad medicine." After all, these physicians possessed increased knowledge and ability to criticize their own doctors' behavior. What *is* the appropriate amount of time that patients should wait at a doctor's office? These complaints often reflected larger frustrations and rage at the onslaught of disease. But are these physician-patients justified, or simply acting entitled?

Certainly, an ill doctor may tolerate and accept his or her physician's alibis less. Dan, with chest metastases, said:

> I wouldn't buy the excuses: the surgical intern said that she was
> in the OR and couldn't get away. I said: "I know what surgical
> interns do, and I am sure that in reality you were not essential in
> July for a thoracic surgical procedure."

Many ill physicians anticipated obstacles, and knew full well the competing demands that their doctors experienced. Deborah said, "You can't expect to feel well taken care of all the time. They have other patients.... It's a very busy breast cancer floor, always full."

However, the goal here is not to criticize health care providers, but to pinpoint areas that can be improved. Indeed, these doctors often understood and acknowledged colleagues' imperfections. Providers may fail to "make the right decision" as a result not of "medical error," but of the inherent uncertainties of clinical care. The "right thing to do" may be clear only in retrospect. Consequently, certain problems may be inevitable.

Still, some of these doctors felt that often patients simply wanted too much. Jeff, the adolescent specialist with HIV, commented, "We just don't know everything, and can't be expected to."

But even as fellow practitioners, these doctors felt that their expectations were reasonable, and their disappointments valid. Even if a critic might argue that these doctors were asking for too much, *they* did not think they were doing so. These physicians also generally took as a standard of comparison their own behavior—not abstract or platonic "ideal" care. Sally, the internist with cancer who brought her laptop to the ICU, recognized that "we all make mistakes," but that doctors have bases for assessing the care they receive. "Doctors are more aware of errors because they have a database from which to judge. But I've learned to be forgiving. I know I've made mistakes... we all do."

In sum, in entering the role of patient, these physicians faced a wide series of internal and external problems. Professional socialization fueled a sense that they wore "magic white coats" and could not get sick. In part as a result, they displayed symptoms of "post-residency disease," marked by various types of denial—from delaying initial diagnoses to ignoring progressive markers of illness, verging at times on magical thinking. Some felt they exercised "good denial," but the definitions and boundaries of "good" versus "bad" denial can be hard to see and assess in oneself.

They frequently relied on "insider" status, yet nonetheless confronted obstacles due to insurance and bureaucracies, which surprised them. Though a few received VIP treatment, many more experienced screw-ups in care. They recognized their own past mistakes, but were still astonished at others' errors—even those of colleagues whom they respected.

Through their odysseys, these ill physicians became more sensitive to patient perspectives, concerning the difficulties of side effects, treatment adherence, and inexpressibility of even "minor" symptoms such as pain, fatigue, nausea, anxiety, and depression. Losses of dignity, selfhood, individuality, and identity devastated them, and illness taught many the costs of dependency, uncertainty, and humiliation. They learned how patient time, doctor time, and hospital time conflicted; how "a person waiting is a person suffering"; and how poor access to a doctor can reinforce disturbing feelings of dependency and loss. They complained, too, of indirect or nonexistent communication, particularly about taboo topics such as mental health and sexual problems or side effects, as well as of verbal or nonverbal insensitivity and trivialization of problems. Physician hubris facilitated poor communication, and precluded self-awareness.

Yet these doctors had trouble reconciling their new experiences as patients with the fact that in the past they, too, had sometimes kept patients waiting and had not promptly phoned patients back. The profession hampered awareness of many of these concerns, further highlighting the degree to which it viewed and constructed patients as unequal, distant "others."

These doctors became more aware, too, of how *definitions concerning time varied* widely (e.g., what it meant for disease to progress "slowly" or "rapidly"). Moreover, as a result of competing time demands, test results and treatments fell "between the cracks."

Doctors structured time in ways that patients had to follow (e.g., in the waiting room), reflecting and reinforcing authority relationships within these settings. What happens when disagreements resulted? Sally felt compelled to go "on strike," exercising what she felt was her only option. As a doctor, she felt empowered to refuse her doctor's orders. Presumably, lay patients would not feel as empowered to do so.

Within a culture, time is socially constructed, but clearly may be experienced differently by various groups (i.e., doctors and patients). Surprisingly, heretofore these doctors were not aware of how much their patients' experiences clashed with their own. One's experience of time helps shape, but can also limit, one's point of view.

Though questions emerged of whether these ill physicians' complaints and expectations were reasonable, these doctors felt their standards were fair. Still, it remains unclear how to reconcile their expectations with the "reality" that the profession has difficulty meeting these standards. Professional and public education needs to find more effective solutions to address these discrepancies, obstacles, and dilemmas. As we shall see, increased awareness of these barriers can help.

5

"They Treated Me as if I Were Dead"

Peripheralization and Discrimination

"When I came back to work, some colleagues wouldn't even look at me," Deborah, the psychiatrist with breast cancer, said, shaking her head in dismay. "People passed me in the corridor as if I wasn't there—as if I hadn't come back." Ill physicians faced obstacles due not only to internal psychological states, and interactions with providers, but also to relationships with bosses and other staff at work. Colleagues had to decide how to act toward sick doctors, and did so in a range of manners, approaching them as either doctors or patients. Fellow physicians had to decide whether to reduce the status and standing of these ill colleagues, and could support or avoid them. In turn, these ill physicians' senses of self were profoundly shaped by perceptions of how others viewed them.

From Subtle to Overt: Types of Discrimination

Frequently, physician-patients faced and felt stigma and discrimination. A few with treatable, nonstigmatized conditions faced little, if any, bias against them, though at times even they encountered resentment from colleagues. Harry, the war refugee with heart disease, did not think he had confronted any stigma per se, but faced annoyance from colleagues who had to cover his practice. He raised a question of what, exactly, constituted stigma.

> Doctors who covered for me resented that they had to put in extra time. Was that stigma? No. It was part of their job, but still

annoyed them. Did I have fewer referrals afterward because people said, "He has heart disease, we shouldn't stress him so much," or "Is it safe to send him a patient when he might get sick next week?" I wasn't aware of that, but it might have entered someone's thinking.

In fluid, complex work settings, Harry illustrated the difficulties of pinpointing discrimination per se, separating it from colleagues' other potential motivations. Yet these ill doctors reported and feared very real loss of employment and job offers, failures of empathy, and subtler peripheralization or marginalization. Trainees and those with new jobs or particular stigmatized diseases—psychiatric diagnoses, cancer, or HIV—confronted particularly negative reactions.

At times, outright discrimination, such as retraction of job offers, occurred. HIV-infected physicians encountered these concerns starkly, in bold relief. As a result of his HIV infection, Paul lost a job offer—it "disappeared."

I worked for an HMO, and chose to have health care outside of the system, through Blue Cross. When I called the HMO to find out if there was a preexisting waiting period, they said no. But it turns out that they meant no for *their* insurance, not for Blue Cross. So I was out of insurance for a year! When I talked to the person that told me there was no preexisting waiting period, he kind of understood that I was HIV-positive. They hired me, but then I got an offer to work for the Public Health Service. The HMO continued to recruit me to come back. So I reapplied. I didn't get reimbursed for my travel, so I had to turn in the documentation again. The person I was supposed to give it to was on vacation, so I had to turn it in to the same person with whom I had talked about the preexisting illness. Then, a week later, mysteriously, there was no position for me. The head doctor said, "I think you should get a lawyer." I assumed he thought it was because I was gay. A memo stated their policy: HIV-positive health care workers were not limited in any way. But then *this* happened. I didn't have the strength to fight it. I didn't want to be in the press as an HIV-positive physician suing this HMO.

Battling such discrimination is hard—public and potentially humiliating.

Doctors with HIV may face particular stigma. Early in the HIV epidemic, health care workers' concerns of becoming infected with HIV from patients received media attention, and many health care workers opted not to practice in high incidence HIV areas. But the well-publicized case of Kimberly Bergalis, allegedly infected by her family dentist, refocused public attention on the risk infected health care workers could potentially pose to their patients. The U.S. Senate voted 99 to 0 to require testing of health professionals engaged in invasive procedures, and mandated ten-year prison terms and fines for health care workers who knew they were HIV-positive but failed to inform patients on whom they had performed such procedures (1). This bill did not become enacted, and the CDC subsequently advocated that individual states and health care institutions make their own decisions as to what procedures were "exposure prone" ones from which HIV-positive health care workers should be barred on a case-by-case basis. Yet HIV-infected health care workers may continue to face the possible loss of their jobs, and discrimination (2, 3, 4). Still, it is important to note that only twice have health care workers ever been documented to have infected patients—once in the U.S., and once in France (1). Nonetheless, some courts have argued that patients have the right to know a physician's HIV status or alcohol history (5) because it is "material" to a patient's informed consent decision (i.e., posing possible risk, no matter how small). Most patients have said they would change physicians if their physician had AIDS (5). Some county medical associations have arranged to have all patients of an HIV-infected physician HIV-tested after learning of the physician's positive status. Patients have sued infected doctors, claiming "emotional distress" from learning that the physician was positive—even when the patient remained uninfected.

Physicians with other diseases routinely encountered, or feared, discrimination as well. Such bias varied in directness and intensity. For instance, at times, doctors with other disorders experienced not clear, overt discrimination, but "inflexibility" from colleagues who failed to show empathy, or to acknowledge their colleague's disease and decreased function (even if only temporary). As a resident, Deborah experienced a lack of accommodation, if not discrimination per se, when her schedule changed.

> I was starting radiation therapy every day for six weeks, and had to juggle time. So I went to the head of my new unit and said, "I'm having radiation. I may be late in the mornings." He got very angry: "I don't care what you do, or how you do it. But you have to

be here at 9 A.M. rounds." I said, "I may not be able to do that.
I may be half an hour late." He said, "I'm really not interested." So
I talked to the head of the radiation department, and asked to
have radiation at 6 A.M. For my whole four months on that unit, I
was never late. That was not discrimination, but *very harsh*. I
wasn't sure if I should confront him. I decided it wasn't worth it.
But I used to get up at 5 A.M.!

As Deborah indicated, addressing this bias can be formidable, and thus is
avoided.

Colleagues expected each other to perform their *full* duties. No room
was allowed for filling only part of the role. *The doctor role was all or
nothing*. Thus, at times, colleagues treated an ill physician still as a physician, and refused to make any allowances for sickness. These colleagues
might have been expected to show compassion, and treat an ill physician
as they would any other patient—with empathy and concern. Instead, due
to work demands, colleagues could expect ill doctors to maintain complete or almost complete responsibilities.

Many of these ill doctors experienced subtle and not so subtle forms
of *peripheralization*: being passed over for promotions, or no longer either
being asked to be on committees, or getting fellows to assist with research or clinical duties. Brian, who had hepatitis, said, "My illness im-
pacted my competition to become director of the clinic. Someone else
was chosen." Once they were perceived as sick, these doctors lost status
and power. Illness might not impair a physician's ability to function, but
was nevertheless *seen* as doing so. Ill doctors were perceived as somehow
not being full or whole physicians.

The implications of these altered views can hurt. In the competitive
world of medicine, where trainees must be driven to succeed, ill physicians commonly envied colleagues receiving promotions or extra resources. Scott, who had an infected foot, saw newer colleagues receive
more patients.

I'm jealous: the department got some new hotshot genetics fellow.
She's good, but doesn't know more than me. But they're giving
her all these cases. Whenever they want to ask a genetics question,
they turn to her. I've been there for five years!

Peripheralization can manifest itself in small, but still disturbing,
ways. Bradley, who became depressed after his MI, found that colleagues

did not consult with him as much on their research. He noted, "People don't give me their papers to review, or talk to me about protocols. I get left out.... I need to accept the fact that at this point they don't need me."

Bradley wavered between sadness and acceptance concerning his plight. He attributed the problem to "getting old," not to the threat from his illness per se. Yet these changes occurred following his heart attack, after which others perceived him differently.

Discrimination could also be subtle or nonverbal, and hence difficult to prove or redress. Neil, the neurologist, described how attendings did not reject him, but nonetheless treated him as "different."

> Nothing was said, but through their *tone of voice,* they treated me as if I were sick: "Poor child." They didn't reject me per se. The director of the program became inappropriately very motherly. On rounds she would touch me, just grab me—she'd be talking about patients. It was not sexual, but "Dear, dear...." They were giving me too much sympathy. *I didn't want it—to feel anything had changed.*

Alternatively, staff may fail to take into account or may misinterpret a physician's symptoms. In many ways, doctors were not allowed to enter the sick role. Colleagues may misunderstand the effects of mild, non-specific symptoms, such as low energy and pain, seeing these as voluntary rather than unwilled. Dan, the oncologist with chest metastases, described such misapprehensions.

> From time to time, I would need to go into my office and sit down for fifteen minutes because of significant pain. The nurses viewed this as inattentiveness. From time to time, I also told them, "Just leave me alone, I'll take care of this problem with the chart," or "This patient needs prescriptions? Leave it, I'll take care of it." As a result of that, and of two not unexpected complications of procedures, I had my privileges suspended.

Dan's account may have been one-sided or incomplete, but nonetheless underlined a clear problem.

The institution's need for manpower may block compassion for ill employees. Ill physicians were all the more surprised by such failure of empathy, because they expected fellow health care professionals to be caring, and to "know better" than to reject sick colleagues.

Occasionally, individual colleagues could personally be consoling while institutions as a whole were not. Dan continued:

> The administration is not very supportive—not interested in anyone with a problem. They want all their docs not only to *think* they're God, but to *be* like God—physically perfect, able to work 28 hours a day, 380 days a year. Anything less than that makes administrators' lives very complicated. They want simple, not complicated, lives. Most colleagues have tended to be sympathetic, even protective—even more than I'd like: "Take it easy. Are you taking your medication? You look tired; did you get a good night's sleep?" But the hospital as a structure is very uninterested in anything but its self-preservation. It is a mammoth administrative entity with thousands of employees. It looks at what it considers to be a global picture, and wants no problems out of the norm. "If you're not feeling well, don't bother us." I'm not sure hospitals are different from other big institutions, like General Motors.

Dan and others noted the implicit irony: "You expect the medical field, committed to caring for the sick, to be better." Yet hospitals clearly have conflicting missions of healing the sick and operating efficiently as organizations. Organizational needs can override those of individual patients, though such priorities are never explicitly stated. Staff members can thus separate their human compassion from their professional demands and expectations of each other.

Peripheralization may be more implicit and indirect, and thus harder to prove than many forms of discrimination. Often it was unacknowledged, even by "enlightened" colleagues who saw themselves as merely trying to "help" the ill physician. Sally, the internist with cancer who brought her laptop to the ICU, said:

> People aren't necessarily aware that they're doing *peripheralization*. They are aware of discrimination in general—they have categories that one might talk or file a complaint about. But peripheralization is a lot more subtle in terms of getting people to acknowledge that it's really happening, because it's really an accumulative experience, not one item. Colleagues put me in a different category. Partly, they think, "I don't want to overburden her." But part of *my* "therapy" is working.

Quandaries arose about how much leeway to give sick doctors. As we shall see, these conflicts were negotiated and resolved in complex manner.

While observers might hope that laws protect against such discrimination, these ill physicians remained wary. Discrimination can occur in subtle and intricate ways. Moreover, those who are ill, but still functional, are not covered by the Americans with Disabilities Act (ADA). One HIV-infected radiologist said of current legislation, "I wouldn't be protected by the law because I'm not disabled at this point. My doctor advised me not to tell anyone at work because I'm not covered by the ADA."

Additional laws, even if existent, may not be well-enforced. Tom, the internist whose lover died of AIDS, felt that added legislation simply could not effectively shield one against discrimination.

> Laws protect me from discrimination, but that doesn't make me feel any better. I know how discrimination works: *it doesn't work by the law.* You can sue people, and maybe get what you want. The law can't guarantee they won't discriminate. If they're not employing me anymore, how do I prove it's because of HIV? Enough laws are in place.

Public policy may simply be unable to stop certain *subtle* forms of discrimination, such as losing patient referrals.

Indeed, some well-meaning physician-patients themselves reported having referred less to doctors whom they perceived as impaired. Harry, the war refugee with heart disease, said, "It depends on the illness, of course. I discovered some of my colleagues were alcoholics, and I sent them fewer patients. Anything that impaired reliability—being forced to take time off—could be a mark against you."

Specific types of diseases, symptoms, and jobs increased this bias. Infectious diseases can elicit especially negative responses. For example, Peter, the medical student, felt he could not be as open concerning his HIV infection as he could be with his other diagnoses.

> My diabetes is not life threatening. HIV is. Both are chronic. But with HIV, you're living in a bowl. With diabetes, you're out in the world—you don't have to worry about who you tell or sleep with. You're not going to transmit diabetes!

Psychiatric symptoms were particularly taboo, since colleagues frequently saw these as volitional. Jessica, the pediatrician, felt that mental illness could generate more discrimination against her than carcinoma, because she could be blamed for the symptoms.

> Cancer's not your fault. You can't help it. But doctors view mental illness as my own fault. I felt it in conversations about other people: a lessening of respect for the person who had it.

In many ways, being held responsible for one's diagnosis heightened stress. Hence Ernie, for example, felt discrimination more due to his depression than his HD, since the latter can produce psychiatric symptoms, but is clearly genetic.

> I have not faced any discrimination from HD. But the hospital was not nice about the depression: they actually were going to fire me! They sent me a letter saying they were not going to hire me for the next year.

Coworkers differentiated psychiatric symptoms somewhat on the basis of perceived voluntariness, yet these underlying assumptions were not always accurate. Physicians, though empirically trained, did not always think scientifically about this issue of causality—particularly when they had other, invested reasons for not doing so.

Conversely, just as certain diagnoses elicited bias because patients were blamed for them, physicians with other disorders sensed that they encountered *less* stigma because they were clearly "not at fault" for their illness. The drug company researcher, Jim, thought that his lymphoma was seen as less blameworthy than certain diseases such as lung cancer.

> If you have lung cancer, people say, "You used to smoke." Lymphoma is from blood cells dividing billions of times, and one mistake getting made. You happen to be unlucky. Colleagues have appreciated that I've done whatever I can: going back into the office as quickly as I could, starting to work hard, picking up where I was before.

Jim and others eschewed the sick role, and sought to prove to colleagues that they were not "at fault." When hospitalized, Jim even bought a cell phone, in order to stay in contact with his office. Indeed, ill physicians can overcompensate, working harder than necessary to return to full work capacity, but potentially inducing added noxious stress.

Psychiatric illness could further fuel discrimination due to fears that it would prevent the patient from fulfilling work responsibilities. As a result of her depression, Jessica feared that others would view her as unable to be a "good doctor," which in turn could jeopardize her job. "People might see me as *defective* in some way. I don't admit my depression to my colleagues—they would have a strong prejudice against me."

Colleagues' miscomprehensions about mental illness reflect long-standing historical and social prejudices, arising from fear and discomfort from perceived loss of control of the mind. Yet these misunderstandings among doctors have disturbing implications: these providers might inadequately treat psychiatric symptoms in their patients.

As suggested earlier, physicians can become very *judgmental* toward psychiatric illnesses, particularly drug or alcohol abuse, reflecting wider societal prejudices. Suzanne, the psychiatric trainee with bipolar disorder, said:

> A lot of times when a doctor is getting a history about drugs and alcohol, you hear a little bit of judgment—subtle, like "When did you start doing *that?*" or "In addition to snorting *all* that cocaine, do you drink alcohol?" Whereas *I'll* say to a patient, "So, when you get really tweaked out from the coke, would you use heroin or alcohol to come down?" I'm very nonjudgmental. An ER resident says to patients, "You're still living with your mother?!" Many mental patients live with their mothers. He used to say, "How long has it been since you haven't been *normal?*" He'd shout at them. With a bipolar patient, I'll say, "So after you're really, really manic, and you crash, do you ever feel like you want to kill yourself?" It's like I'm just chitchatting with somebody about the flu.

Suzanne's approaches, based on her own experiences and revealing empathy and intimate knowledge, can aid other physicians, too.

HIV-infected physicians encountered particular problems, given fears of potential provider-to-patient transmission. Due to such fears, some institutions scaled back activities more than required by universal precautions. For example, an HMO told Jeff not to perform pelvic exams. When he protested that these procedures were not invasive, he was told he "could do pelvic exams, but only if using double gloves"—which are not part of universal precautions, and would decrease the sensitivity, and hence the efficacy, of the exam.

Though at first glance, HIV may appear to be a "special case"—given fears of provider-to-patient transmission—other diseases, such as hepatitis, can also be spread from physicians to patients. Moreover, HIV transmission from physicians to patients has occurred only twice in the world.

Colleagues' perceptions that a physician is not merely sick, but *dying,* prompted added obstacles. Some doctor-patients were implicitly written off entirely—as "dead"—and had their patients reassigned. *Thus, the state of dying itself can be a stigmatized condition,* causing awkwardness and discomfort among colleagues, and in turn abetting stigma. When Deborah had metastases, everybody gave her the "signature of death. . . . Colleagues didn't think I was going to make it. They treated me as if I were *dead."* When she later returned to work, coworkers ignored her, unsure how to approach her.

> It took me a while to put together my patients' charts. People
> put them in a box, and didn't tell me where it was. We
> keep dummy charts—the real charts go to the chart room. Some-
> body had taken all my dummy charts, after they distributed
> all my patients, and put the box somewhere and never told me.
> I found out just two months ago. Somebody said, "This box
> belongs to you." I said, "What are you talking about?" So here
> came this box.

Physicians felt stigmatized by institutions in symbolic but painful ways. For example, Deborah's voice mail was taken away.

> When I came back, I had no voice mail. There is a list of every-
> body's phone number, and my name doesn't appear on it—things
> that may seem unimportant. It took me three months to get my
> voice mail back. I had to fight, so people thought I was very rude. I
> applied for it, and nothing happened for three months. I went
> back, and said, "It's not fair. I'm seeing patients. I need voice mail."
> They still haven't come up with a new list, even though I'm seeing
> patients again in the clinic. I don't understand.

Indeed, a "death role" or "dying role" appeared as a specific subtype of the "sick role." At a certain point, ill physicians realized that they were treated not merely as "patients," but as "dying patients." Colleagues may simply not know what to say. Medicine, the profession most affiliated with death, in certain regards maintains an aversion against it. As Jessica Mitford wrote in *The American Way of Death* in 1963, the U.S. health care system, too, attempts to avoid, rather than confront, death (6). As a result, Americans tend to view death as a taboo subject. Only when these physicians were threatened with being forced out of their professional role did they see how much their field failed to address fully the issue of death. Deborah herself did not understand the problem—she didn't view herself as dying, even though colleagues did. As we shall see, her denial may have in part been healthy.

In addition to the kind of diagnosis, the type of job can also shape discrimination. In medicine, job security can be precarious *a priori*, often based on verbal, rather than written, contracts. One radiologist's position depended on "a gentlemen's agreement: that once you make it to 'member,' you're a member until you decide to leave."

Trainees were particularly vulnerable to discrimination. Suzanne had disclosed her bipolar disorder to her medical school dean, which helped reduce overnight call. But the information threatened to impair her future career when it almost appeared on her school's letter to residency programs.

> I told one of the deans. So they all knew. I never could have gotten through medical school unless they *did* know, because we had to do a lot of call, and I had a lot of episodes. In one, I was out of school for six days. I got *a lot* of support from them. All the overnight call I was doing in surgery, ob-gyn, and pediatrics was precipitating symptoms. They knew I wasn't going into any of those fields, so they said I didn't have to do overnight call anymore. But when I applied for residency, they were going to put that in my dean's letter. I argued that they never told me that it would show up down the line: "I'm going into psychiatry. I've chosen this career specifically because it doesn't require much overnight call— I have enough sense to know that. So please do me the respect of not putting that in my dean's letter and sabotaging my career. If I had known that you were going to put this fact in there, I probably would have just forced my way through, and gotten sick a lot." They decided not to put it in.

The dean appeared unsure of how to handle this situation, feeling awkward accommodating a disability and maintaining confidentiality versus following the school's usual requirements and standard operating procedures.

For a trainee, even partial disclosure (e.g., of the existence, if not the name or nature, of a diagnosis) can engender reproach. Earlier, Suzanne had faced unpleasant reactions, if not outright discrimination, from her pediatrics supervisor, whose comments might even be actionable.

He said, "This one here has some *mysterious* illness where she can't take overnight call." He was very mean to me throughout the rotation. "It's obvious that you're running at a slower pace than everybody else. I hope you're not considering pediatrics." His section of my dean's letter stands out from all the rest: "Her performance is: good. Interacting with her was: fine." No actual words.

Suzanne indicates the potential subtleness of discrimination—that it can even result from silence, from what is not said (e.g., in letters of recommendation). As a result of these experiences, she decided not to disclose her illness at the hospital where she was now a resident.

Trainees faced particular problems because they were beholden to supervisors and evaluators, and hence had less power or autonomy to defend themselves. Peter, the HIV-positive medical student, said:

I had to tell my dean why I was leaving. But I was a guinea pig in policy-making. A cloud always hung over me. What restrictions would be put on me?...Supervisors weren't told that I was positive, but that I had "a blood-borne, communicable disease," which is one of very few things. If they pushed, they could figure it out. My classmates didn't know. So when I had to refuse to do a procedure, my classmates didn't know why. It looked like I didn't *want* to learn. Residents would say, "Why doesn't *he* go do this?" The attendings would say, "He can't." My resident would say, "*Why* can't he?" I was constantly walking on eggshells. Sometimes I did things I probably shouldn't have, according to their rules. *I wanted to show them that I wanted to learn!* My intern used to say our medical school was very lax. The attacks were indirect. If it weren't for my status, I wouldn't have had to deal with this. It always made me look like the bad guy.

The secrecy made it hard for Peter to counteract this antagonism. Even in the absence of disclosure of a specific diagnosis, partial information or silence could provoke discrimination. In the competitive world of medicine, colleagues reacted to illness-based work excuses with hostility, not sensitivity. Yet to abandon the field entirely as a result was hard, in part because medicine bolstered self-esteem.

These forms of discrimination occurred, too, because of blurrings of boundaries and conflicts of interest. Supervisors and coworkers who knew about a colleague's illness could hold it against him or her professionally. Deborah, the psychiatrist with breast cancer, said:

I was going to do a one-month cancer ward rotation. But after he had accepted me, the head of the ward said I could not do the rotation. I was very angry. He was very nasty, cruel, and inhumane. He said, "I don't think you're capable." He thought my judgment was poor if I wanted to come and work there: I couldn't work with cancer patients because I myself had cancer. I really felt discriminated against, and pleaded with him: "I don't think my judgment is poor. I think I could manage it. I'm stable." He said, "No way. You're not a survivor. You're still being treated."

Though she might lack objectivity on the ward, Deborah felt that he did not handle this situation well.

Moreover, when she was a patient and this ward chief attempted to consult with Deborah in the hospital, she declined. She felt he had a conflict of interest:

He tried to see me in the hospital, because he sees many of the patients on the breast cancer floor. I refused. I didn't want to see anybody. Three times, he sent his fellows to see me. But I didn't request to be seen by a psychiatrist. I didn't want one.

Still, he perused her medical record, raising profound questions of invasion of privacy. "I know that he read my chart, because I saw him on the floor a couple of times, and avoided him." She tried to fight, but in the end, felt she couldn't "be a martyr."

Types and settings of medical practice could affect vulnerability as well. For example, with regard to HIV, some practices and practice settings were felt to be more HIV-friendly than others. Specifically, physicians in academic and administrative jobs felt more comfortable disclosing at work, and feared repercussions less than physicians in private practice who saw predominantly heterosexual patients. Certain geographic areas appeared more HIV-friendly than others—in particular, urban more than rural environments, and certain cities (those with large, visible gay communities). A few doctors felt confident that disclosure would not precipitate discrimination; some selected specialties and posts where that was the case. Pascal said, "I chose this job because if I work with HIV-positive patients, there would be no question of who got what from whom."

Views of Self as Contributing to Fears of Discrimination

Deeply-seated feelings about oneself can enlarge the wound that others'
perceptions cause. These self-views can exacerbate fears of discrimination. At times, sick doctors may feel shame, and their concerns about
possible discrimination can reflect their own worries and psychological
projections—their own views of themselves as flawed.

For example, fears of subtle cognitive deficits can warp self-
perceptions. Belief that one's mental functioning is declining could result
from actual processes (i.e., caused by side effects of medications or symptoms of disease) and/or mirror long-term anxieties about the future.
Wilma, in her eighties, still worked in her lab, and was horrified at the
prospect of colleagues viewing her as physically disabled. However, her
fear partly suggested her own projection, her terror of possible cognitive
slippage.

> I hate being seen in a state of cognitive disability—having to use
> two canes or a walker, more for safety, so that I don't fall. I have
> to admit: there must be a certain element of depression. I am
> tired. It's hard to go to work, and I really am not getting things
> done as I should. I don't like to be seen using a cane and a walker.
> They might think the brain might not be working, an uncon-
> scious association in their minds.

Wilma intimated, too, an element of distancing—referring to "the brain"
rather than "my brain." Still, the fact that sick doctors' fears of discrimination may reflect projected feelings about themselves does not lessen the
very real instances of discrimination that can surface.

Physicians' beliefs in their own invulnerability can increase the shame
they feel if they do in fact become sick. Especially with diseases to which
their own behavior may have contributed, physicians often thought they
"should have known better" than to become ill at all. Stuart, the internist with HIV now teaching at the university, criticized himself:

> Being a doc, *you're not supposed to get sick. You're supposed to know
> better.* It would be like coming down with lung cancer from
> smoking: "I should have stopped." I think back to the two episodes
> when I could have been infected. I should not have taken those
> chances.

These doctors reveal the degree to which they, too, are aware of, and might be influenced by, blaming patients for disease. As suggested earlier, Stuart and others also felt doctors should somehow be held to a higher standard—to have used their medical knowledge to alter their own behavior. Here again, physicians may differ from lay patients, and have more difficulty.

Magical thinking can exacerbate difficulty accepting one's illness. Despite scientific training, one doctor wondered at first if HIV was in fact a punishment. "I can remember thinking: 'Why me? Am I a bad person, am I evil?'... I prayed the test would be negative."

All-too-human rationalizations can hamper optimal use of one's own medical knowledge. Kurt, who had used crack, felt he "deserved" HIV. These doctors employed rationalizations based, too, on other aspects of their lives. Kurt continued:

> Because I'm a doctor, there is more shame. Not only should I have known better, because I was a doctor, but I grew up in L.A. My best friend died of AIDS at twenty-five. I'd buried many people. But my partners were generally young. I could feel lymph nodes. I knew what high-risk people looked like. I could see whether these guys were in the high-risk group. It was a fucking game: Russian roulette.

Kurt made numerous assumptions (e.g., that he could visually diagnose HIV in his partners) over many years.

Some of these physicians feared that their sense that "they should have known better" would be shared by their colleagues. As will be discussed later with regard to mechanisms of coping, such apprehensions may impede obtaining care and beneficial services.

Entering and Exiting the Sick Role

These concerns about colleagues' responses in turn molded decisions about whether, when, how, and to what degree to enter and exit the sick role. Ill physicians faced dilemmas not only about adopting this role, but also about relinquishing it. The sociologist Talcott Parsons and others have written extensively about entrance into this position, but much less about decisions on when, how, and to what degree to *leave* it—who does or does not do so.

Often, these doctor-patients disagreed with coworkers as to whether to work or not, and if so, to what degree—from part-time to full-time—and who should decide. Overall, four scenarios arose (conceptualizable as a 2 × 2 table), based on whether the ill physician did or did not want to work, and whether colleagues felt he or she was or was not ready. Occasionally, an ill physician and his or her colleagues concurred as to when and to what degree to reduce (and later increase) his or her workload. Other times, conflict ensued.

For both work and personal reasons, many tried to exit the sick role as quickly as possible, and return to healthy or "normal" functioning. Yet some did so too hastily. Innocently, peripheralization may start with the doctor-patient willingly entering the illness role. Later, problems can arise of *how quickly* to leave it.

Conversely, other ill physicians may feel physically unable to work at full capacity, even though institutions may be unable to function optimally without personnel (especially leaders) working full-time. Initially, colleagues may want to "spare" a sick doctor the burden of work. Yet the sick role could be a double-edged sword, relieving some duties but taking away others that one may in fact want. Frank, the surgeon, had an MI in the OR after he rushed a patient down on a stretcher when he felt hospital transport personnel were taking too long to arrive. Once in the OR, he experienced chest pain, and within an hour or two received an emergency coronary artery bypass graft. He reported:

> Afterward, I started delegating more, because I found it convenient. But in the first year or two, I lost some of my influence. I was treated as very fragile, which had both advantages and disadvantages. They wanted to see whether I was going to stay alive. When I was out of commission, they started a new program that was my idea, but it didn't work. So I was left cleaning it up. They wanted to spare me a lot of work. They were afraid I would overwork.

Colleagues—as friends and as health care providers—may be concerned about and monitor an ill physician, whether or not he or she wants this extra attention. Being closely observed can feel overbearing. The nurses now watched Frank carefully, concerned about the possibility of another heart attack. "When I get really temperamental in the OR, the older nurses say, 'You'd better take it easy. *You don't want to have another one!*' "

Over time, problems arose over exactly *how much* leeway to provide physicians who are or have been seriously ill. Many doctors at first wanted some allowances made, but then desired to resume their former duties. Some wished to proceed too swiftly. Others wanted to reenter at what they considered an appropriate pace, while staff and colleagues were wary or not considerate enough. Questions arose of how these decisions should be made, who should make such determinations, and when such allowances should end. Tensions emerged between being placed in the sick role and wanting to see oneself as healthy.

In sum, ill doctors faced a range of forms of discrimination and subtler peripheralization: losses of job offers, referrals, fellows, and requests to consult on papers and grants. Discrimination can be verbal or nonverbal. When they were becoming ill, doctors often wanted colleagues to give them some slack, but conflicts then surfaced over how much, and for how long. Over time, some doctors wanted less, and others, more. Certain diagnoses—psychiatric ones and those perceived to be the doctor's own fault—attracted particular discrimination. Types of settings influenced degrees of discrimination, too, and trainees were particularly vulnerable. Some sought jobs in which they might face less bias. These physicians' own shame could also aggravate perceptions of such negative reactions from others.

The narratives here move beyond much of the current literature on stigma, to issues of how it is *mutually* negotiated in dual directions over time. Sadly, many doctors felt laws would at best only partially alleviate these problems.

As we shall see, against this vivid backdrop of forms of discrimination, these doctors had to make critical decisions about disclosing their illness and treating their own patients.

6

"Coming Out" as Patients

Disclosures of Illness

"I felt we were living *double lives*," Mathilde said, "as if we were prisoners twice"—because of both illness and secrecy. Through decisions on whether, what, when, and to whom to divulge their diagnosis, sick doctors could alter or maintain others' views of them. Some ill physicians chose to lead double lives and live with secrets. Others went public. They illustrated the degree to which *information about one shapes how one is viewed*.

Clearly, doctors have a right to privacy concerning their personal health information. Yet patients, and potentially certain colleagues, may have a right to some of this information *if* it pertains to risks and benefits of treatments that patients undergo. Thus, if a physician's illness can potentially harm a patient significantly, physician privacy can conflict with patients' rights. For example, for HIV, some have argued that a physician's disclosure of his or her illness may be relevant in exposure-prone procedures (1). But what about in other situations? Do continuity of care and trust ever warrant disclosure of a doctor's illness? Do these decisions affect doctor-patient relationships, and if so, how? These doctors viewed and approached these issues in varying ways. They spent most of their waking lives with colleagues from whom they at times hid secrets. Importantly, *information bestowed power—either for or against the individual*. Given threats to medical privacy more broadly, due to the burgeoning electronic storage and transfer of information, many aspects of these issues are taking on increasing urgency, but have been underexamined. Doctors' disclosures of personal, nonmedical information have been probed, focusing on casual remarks regarding their own attitudes and feelings toward treatment (e.g., "I wish I could sleep standing up") (2). Physician divulgences of health behaviors (e.g., diet and exercise) can also motivate patients concerning these behaviors (3). Psychotherapists' disclosures to patients of personal characteristics (e.g., religion and marital status) have been probed as well, and remain controversial. A psychotherapist's pregnancy, for instance, can evoke a wide range of psychological responses (4). In psychotherapy, doctor-patient relationships, transference and countertransference, can be critical. Impaired physicians (e.g., due to substance abuse) have received attention, as such impairments may potentially interfere with patients' receiving optimal quality of care (5). *But physicians' disclosures of their own serious or potentially fatal illnesses or explicit medical problems*—more sensitive areas that may threaten the stability of the doctor-patient relationships—*remain relatively unexplored.* How does medical information about an individual affect how he or she and others view that individual? As Erving Goffman described in *The Presentations of Self in Everyday Life*, each day, we all shape how others see us, as if we were actors performing on a stage (6).

Disclosures at Work: Weighing Pros and Cons

Ill physicians and their colleagues disagreed not only over whether the physician-patient should still work, but also over whether and to what degree he or she should even *discuss* the illness. Four scenarios emerged that can be conceptualized as a 2 × 2 grid, in which the sick doctor did or did not want to talk about the disease, and colleagues did or did not wish to do so. These four situations were those in which (1) both parties wanted to discuss the disease; (2) the ill physician did not want to talk about it, but colleagues or staff did; (3) the ill physician wanted to discuss it, but colleagues did not; and (4) neither party sought to discuss it. These four basic patterns were further shaped by whether the sick doctor *knew* that colleagues knew of the diagnosis (i.e., that it was a rumor); and whether colleagues knew whether the sick physician knew that they knew (i.e., whether the sick physician was aware he or she was being talked about). At times, colleagues knew, but were unsure whether and how to discuss it.

Several doctors were surprised that "others don't know you're sick unless you tell them"—that their own private trauma, so disruptive to themselves, could be utterly invisible to others.

As we shall see, each of these roles—doctor, colleague, friend, and patient—involved varying norms, desires, and expectations of truth-telling that could clash.

Tell Why?

Despite the potential dangers, for several reasons these doctors decided to disclose their illness to colleagues. Some of these ill physicians simply could not hide their disease; the severity and symptoms were too obvious. Jim, the drug company researcher, disclosed his lymphoma to everyone because he felt he had no alternative. "I was so sick, and knew I was going to be dealing with this for a long time, and be out of work. To try to conceal this just never would have worked."

Long-standing relationships with colleagues could instill *expectations* of disclosure, particularly about less stigmatized disorders. Bradley disclosed his MI to his boss, since they had known each other for over four decades. "I'd been in the same place for forty-five years. The flow back and forth is pretty high about personal as well as professional things." Hence, over time, professional and personal boundaries can blur.

Others chose to sacrifice some privacy in return for certain benefits, making risk/benefit calculations about disclosure. David, the psychiatrist with HIV, worked for a government clinic, and knew he could not be fired because of his illness. Initially, he disclosed to avoid being on call. ("My boss said, "If there's anything that we can do...." I said: "Yeah, get me off call!"")

But those who disclosed had to decide, too, *how much and what information to provide* concerning prognoses over time, and when and whether to reveal test results that marked worsening disease. A physician may divulge the "basic problem," but not later test findings that show a worsening prognosis. Between the two extremes, gradations of information existed. For example, Lou, who had an award on his wall, didn't tell coworkers when he had follow-up studies. "I had CTs every six months. They were negative. But I didn't say anything because people might say, 'Well, they *could* be positive!'" He feared that colleagues would see even his need for follow-up as evidence of his continued high risk for disease.

Illness might be discussed *only indirectly, in code* or euphemistically. These ciphers might or might not be correctly interpreted. Albert, who had an MI on the highway, reported that he disclosed information only allusively. "I don't say, 'I have health problems'—that's not the way I like to think of it—but 'I've had *events.*'" To acknowledge health problems to both himself and others remained hard, ever since he first experienced and ignored symptoms on the highway and continued driving. Yet he felt uncomfortable remaining *wholly* secretive or silent with others.

Colleagues may know certain features, but not others, about a doctor's disease. Deborah felt "The less I say, the better." She did not mention the results of tests to colleagues, and even lied about them, vigorously trying to separate her professional and personal lives.

> I'm usually very talkative. But my illness can really jeopardize me. I try not to say anything. People ask me how I'm doing. People know I go for tests, but I don't tell them what my tests show— good or bad. When people ask, *even if I am doing bad, I say "good."*

Deborah thus dissembled, but felt she had to. She told people only what she felt they needed to know—not more—because of fears of gossip. "I keep a façade. People talk a lot. If they ask me questions, I just say it's not important. I'm not going to get support from here."

Deborah and others assessed carefully where it was safest or best to seek support. However, colleagues may be genuinely concerned, and resent these barriers.

Those who considered telling colleagues struggled, too, with *when* to disclose. Most difficult was whether and when to tell when applying for a job. Like many others, Roxanne, the gastroenterologist with cancer, wrestled with the pros and cons of when to inform her boss. She finally did so only after she had been definitively hired.

> After I arranged to have this position here, I came to give a talk. That's when I told my new boss. I did not want to hide it. He's a good guy. If something did go wrong, I wanted him to know. I didn't mention it during the negotiation, though. I had thought of it, and now regret that I didn't. I didn't want to be deceiving. I'm an open person. But it might be a problem in terms of confidentiality and security. I haven't told anyone else here.

Such professional secrecy can rub against one's general openness as a person, a trait that many value in themselves. Hence, silence now can cause added conflict.

Choosing Silence: Not Tell Why?

"For a long time, I remained closeted in my professional career," Alex, the HIV-infected gay dentist, said. Terrified by the potential repercussions, many of the practitioners here chose *total concealment*. These providers often denied experience of any stigma or discrimination, because they purposely hadn't told anyone. The potential loss of future job opportunities or insurance made privacy valuable in and of itself.

In general, norms mitigate against the disclosure of personal information in the workplace. Indeed, many of these providers remained "closeted" about other facts about their personal lives. Secrets are, after all, an integral part of life (7). Many concealed not only their health, but also other aspects of their personal or professional lives (e.g., that they were looking for another job). Sexual behavior, in particular, was kept concealed. For some, disclosure would have to be *dual* (i.e., of homosexuality, drug use, or sexual activity, as well as of illness).

Colleagues might want to know about a physician's illness, then hold it against him or her. *Loss of information through leaks could diminish and weaken one's institutional power.* Hence, many chose not to disclose diagnoses at work because of fears of such leaks and their negative repercussions. These doctors worried, too, about the growing lack of privacy overall in society. This wider phenomenon disturbed Roxanne:

> There's nothing you can keep your own. Medical records get subpoenaed. It's out of control. It's like being a priest or a rabbi. The information they hear can be violated. No one deserves this information about me.

Roxanne drew parallels with the confessional seal, intimating the *sacredness* of personal information. She wondered whether people "deserved" such information—and if so, to what they owed such privilege. For her, personal data had a special status as an integral part of the individual.

Yet inevitably, leaks occurred. Jennifer said:

> When I became infected, I only told a couple of coworkers and my husband, an ER physician at the hospital.... But within a month, it became pretty obvious that quite a few people knew. Nurses came up to my husband and offered condolences.

Her experience reveals much about lack of institutional confidentiality.

Gossip can spread—even if it is inaccurate. Brian, who had hepatitis, said, "There were rumors about me. I lost weight, looked exhausted, and wasn't as sharp. A nurse asked one of the other physicians if I should be tested for HIV."

Some understood that an individual they informed might feel upset and then tell others. To avoid this possibility of wider diffusion, some chose utter silence. Peter, the medical student with HIV, felt his career depended on strict confidentiality, but he faced conflicts as a result:

> It puts the question of confidentiality on anyone I tell, because once they know, they're going to need support. I can't let them *not* do that. But if they tell someone, that person tells someone else....

Peter felt caught in these binds, recognizing the degree to which *information*—specifically medical information—*is by its nature social.* Others wanted, sought, and spread it to lessen their own distress about it.

At times, a complicated choreography resulted, as a doctor-patient learned through indirect comments or innuendos that others knew that he or she was ill. Paul needed to tell someone in his residency program, and did so. He then sensed, based on subtle cues—how they would ask questions—that others had learned of his infection. These others knew, but didn't say anything *explicitly* to him about it.

> I really needed to confide in somebody in my residency, and talked with the behavioral science director—a very loving and kissy-touchy-feely person. But afterward, it became apparent that people knew. *It was never discussed. It just was understood by the questions they would ask:* "Are you feeling ok?"

Here again, awareness of the lack of rights to this information can prompt others to reveal their knowledge only indirectly.

In the era of HMOs, computer files, and the Internet, many simply resigned themselves to the loss of medical confidentiality. Yet the implications of such lack of privacy were not always known, even if nonetheless feared. Paul, whose job disappeared, said that in his office, confidentiality simply required too much effort.

> Ten people work in this office, and have husbands and children. In most cases, I don't think it's intentional. I watched another doctor try to prevent her infection from going public—it just wasn't

realistic. It takes too much energy. It just happened so fast: rumors were building.

These doctors also observed hospital coworkers overtly violate each other's confidentiality. Brian, who had hepatitis C, saw colleagues searching for each other's medical information for gossip. As a result, he and others sought treatment at other institutions.

> I see doctors and nurses go into the charts and electronic system and look up other employees. They'll say, "I heard so-and-so was sick. They've been admitted to the hospital." They're looking to see what's wrong—because they don't know—and so they can gossip. I'll say, "You shouldn't be doing that." They'll look at me and say, "Oh, it's nothing. I was just checking up on them, making sure they're ok."

These employees rationalized these violations of privacy as altruistic—out of concern for the patient on whose privacy they were infringing.

Conflicts surfaced because, within the culture of a medical institution, staff may commonly discuss milder medical problems among themselves. These social bonds among coworkers can clash with the need for privacy. Whether to see ill coworkers as colleagues or as patients can then compete. Harry, the refugee, said:

> For better or worse, physicians talk about their colleagues in the lunchroom—not maliciously, but because everybody's interested. You want to know who's in the hospital, and go visit them.

Such curiosity may be an instinctual human trait. Some scholars have argued that gossip confers evolutionary adaptive advantages, teaching one about dangers already experienced by others (8). But in civil democratic society, privacy remains an important right.

Often, these doctors' friends were fellow health care professionals, a situation prompting particular difficulties, and disclosures to very few, if any, friends. Tina, an HIV-positive pulmonologist, for example, informed *none* of her friends, as most were other physicians, and she feared that word about her infection would leak back to the hospital where she worked, and that she could lose her job. She contracted HIV after sleeping with a gambler who often went to Atlantic City. She feared that disclosure would increase her shame at having been sexually involved with "someone like that."

Even in research that necessitates signed informed consent, privacy is never fully guaranteed. Harry stated bluntly, "Confidentiality doesn't exist anymore. The government can look at the chart, as can the drug company, the investigators, and the Institutional Review Board."

Potential limits to confidentiality could result, too, because of medical transcribers, who type medical chart notes and information that physicians dictate onto tape recorders. Surprisingly, several ill physicians volunteered this concern. Transcriptionists were invisible, but nevertheless firmly present in the minds of those at risk for discrimination. Mathilde said:

> I had a patient whose wife was a transcriptionist here. One transcriptionist transcribed my doctor's dictation, and I panicked. So I went to tell my doctor. Then, he specifically requested that his dictations only be done by certain people. But more people out there may know!

She still wondered how many others knew her husband's diagnosis.

Especially in a small community, social and professional networks may mingle, thus *facilitating leaks*. Employees in a doctor's office may know patients socially. Pascal's confidentiality was breached when his dentist hired a patient's girlfriend.

> She got a job in my dentist's office, and found out about me. This patient was losing his mind, and started seeing me in the hospital, saying in the hall, "My girlfriend talked to the dentist you go to. *So you have it, too?*"

Moreover, growing numbers of organizations ask about medical disorders. Managed care companies, state licensing boards, hospital administrations, malpractice companies, dentists' offices, and even scuba shops now inquire. Ronald, the HIV-infected Connecticut radiologist, said:

> The state licensing board used to ask about your incapacities. Then, the malpractice company asked. Then, every managed care company asked. They never asked if you were HIV-positive, per se. But it would be on a list, and it was pretty clear what they were asking about.

Consequently, physicians had to weigh whether to tell the truth or not, at times concealing if they felt the information was not truly pertinent.

Tom said: "Do you lie, and say to the dentist, 'No, I'm not positive,' because you figure it's ridiculous, and you're not putting anyone at risk"? These dilemmas proved difficult.

Pharmacies can also infringe on privacy. Tom, whose lover died of AIDS, felt pharmacies provided *no* confidentiality. "They shout out, 'Zoberex for Jones!' Everybody around, including my patients, then knows." Though the 1996 Health Insurance Portability and Accountability Act (HIPAA) has increased awareness of the need for privacy, significant concerns remain.

Another risk of disclosure is that one can never "untell." Once it is out, information can never be reconcealed; rather, it takes on a life of its own. *Information soon becomes an independent entity, separate from the initial owner and intended recipient.* Once divulged, the information can no longer be truly owned, controlled, or contained. Steven, the suburban endocrinologist, needed to tell someone, but now regretted having done so. He informed two coworkers from whom he was now estranged. He had considered sharing it with others, but was glad he had not.

> My natural inclination was to share it with somebody. I needed to do that. In retrospect, I wish I hadn't. It hasn't resulted in any bad consequences *yet*, but that's always lurking in the back of my mind— that people I told ten years ago will not use that information in my best interests. I told two friends. We've since parted ways.

Interpersonal relationships can wax or wane unpredictably with time, complicating these disclosure decisions. Yet most of these doctors hadn't considered possible changes in relationships over time as potentially threatening privacy.

In addition to discrimination concerns, ill physicians decided not to disclose diagnoses because of fear that others would see them as "patients" and "ill," rather than as "doctors," or "whole". Lay patients, too, often feel that their physicians treat them merely as "diseases." Yet an ill lawyer or accountant may still be seen as a lawyer or accountant, while these ill physicians feared no longer being seen as doctors.

Physicians also may hide symptoms because of embarrassment at incapacity, loss of control over their body. Eleanor reported about her ill husband:

> People called me: "I stopped by, and he refused to see me." He'd say, "I was too tired; I wasn't feeling well." But his debility

embarrassed him. He was weak, had urinary incontinence, lost a tremendous amount of weight, and had that typical cancer complexion.

Individuals may also refrain from disclosing their illness because they have trouble accepting it themselves, minimizing or denying it. Denial is difficult to define. Used by Freud to denote a psychoanalytic defense mechanism, it has since been widely and more loosely adopted and employed in society at large. Many of these ill physicians used the term in describing their own behaviors and reactions.

Being "Outed"

Though a doctor may seek secrecy, nonverbal communication or visible symptoms can occur. Those who display apparent, "public" symptoms may be particularly vulnerable to discrimination.

Codes and gestures can indirectly disclose diagnoses. Deborah did not tell anyone until her symptoms became evident: when her hair fell out. She then wore scarves, only to have people ask her about them. "I didn't want to wear a wig. Everybody said, 'Is this a new style?' People knew, but didn't say much." People may "know" but feel awkward talking about it, either because it makes them uncomfortable or because they are not "supposed" to know.

Medication can also expose. Consequently, some felt compelled to divulge their illness only at the point at which they started treatment. Jerry, the surgeon-lawyer, feared that filling prescriptions in the pharmacy would unveil his diagnosis, so he "came out" and retired at the point he needed drugs.

> I was getting my T-cells done anonymously. But once I needed to start getting prescriptions filled, the only way to do that and still work would be by disclosing, because people in the pharmacy would see. Someone would find out.

Medications that involve complicated regimens (i.e., dosing during the day, ingestion with or without food, or refrigeration) forcefully challenged the maintenance of privacy. Fears of these logistics can delay treatment initially. Steven, the suburban endocrinologist with HIV, started meds, but in his office he had to hide them. Unfortunately, *secrets assume power in one's life.*

It's a dirty little secret. This is the first week I've been in my office, having to take pills. I do it secretly, and those secrets hold power. When you have a secret, it means something: there's unpleasantness to it. I had a little pillbox with me this morning, and as I went down the hall, my pills rattled. I wondered if anybody else heard. At 4 P.M., I'm ready for my second dose, and go back to my office. I don't shut the door because that will raise even *more* problems. I turn my back. Yet the staff is notorious for creeping up on me. So that's stressful: wondering if I turn around, are they going to see me pop these pills, and want to know why. I almost never shut the door because I haven't really had any secrets—even if I get a personal phone call. If I shut the door every day at 4, they're going to wonder. So I just look around, make sure nobody's coming down the hall, open the box, and pop in the pills.

Steven illustrated here how much difficulty and psychic energy clandestinity involves. Such furtiveness burdened him far more than he anticipated. He added:

I didn't think it'd be this hard, interviewing patients, thinking, "When's my next dose? What do folks in the office think about this?" Constantly worrying someone's going to find out.

At night, these fears awakened Steven.

Use of insurance or lab tests could also permanently expose. The need for insurance potentially sacrificed privacy—most painfully with stigmatized conditions, including mental illness. Still, many felt they had no other options. Suzanne and others used labs outside, rather than inside their medical centers. Here, as elsewhere, in the complexities of medical institutions, violations of privacy and confidentiality occurred due to blurring of roles—as employee, patient, and even at times family member.

Lying About One's Illness

Other ill physicians felt unable to disclose their illness, and rather than remain silent, felt compelled to lie. They dissembled in particular settings when the risks of divulgence appeared to outweigh the benefits of disclosure. Though society views lies as morally reprehensible, studies have shown that college students in fact admit to lying, on average, twice a day (9). Some ethicists condone falsehoods that protect another individual.

But when, if ever, is it permissible for physicians, sworn to uphold the Hippocratic Oath, to fib? Pascal, the internist, decided to lie about his HIV diagnosis during a physical exam for residency. "I had to say 'No,' or 'I don't know,' when I was asked during my physical for my residency. I lied about it." He felt that in this particular setting, the truth was neither necessary nor relevant, and that the risks of truth-telling outweighed the benefits.

Particular revealing events, such as hospitalizations, may prompt deceit. Some anticipated that they would have to dissemble about their diagnosis in the future (e.g., if ever needing to be an in-patient).

Many felt that malpractice and health insurance companies compelled them to be dishonest. Consequently, they didn't answer truthfully on applications for staff membership or privileges or malpractice questionnaires. Steven, the suburban endocrinologist, confessed:

> It comes up on applications: "Do you have any problems? Anything that could interfere with you practicing medicine?" If you really wanted to be very truthful, you might answer: yes. But who's going to?

Yet those who deceived then feared that *such lies might later be unearthed*. Dishonesty and attempts to protect confidentiality can backfire. Mathilde feared her office staff would learn of her husband's illness *because of* efforts at concealment.

> My office manager saw the test. I had put on it the name of a patient, Larry. But Larry didn't pay the bill. So my manager called Larry, who in the meantime had died, and said to the wife, "Why haven't you paid the bill?" She said, "We never had the test." I thought my manager might figure something out. She might even have known.

The office manager never spoke to Mathilde further about it, either knowing and respecting Mathilde's confidentiality, or remaining unaware.

Not surprisingly, such falsehoods caused enormous psychic burdens. Friends and colleagues may sense they are not being told a full or accurate story, but refrain from questioning apparent half-truths. As Mathilde continued, her friends implicitly agreed to let her falsity remain undisturbed.

My friends might guess. They look at my eyes, and there is a common understanding that I might not be telling the truth. I might describe my husband's neuropathy as a complication of the chemotherapy, not HIV. But I think there was a sign of agreement between us: that I would say what I wanted, and they would not ask.

In essence, Mathilde communicates: I know that you know that I am not divulging the whole truth.

In various social contexts, norms prevail against prying. Boundaries and mild violations are recognized; and a certain level of trust remains. Still, prevarication required constant vigilance, and even performance. Mathilde continued,

We were great actors. I could put on such a face! My dearest friend would sit next to me, and I found myself saying things that might raise a suspicion, and immediately had to put the defense up. I gave the most incredible explanations about what was going on. I needed to tell people that this was happening to me, but I had to *hide*.

These doctor-patients thus revealed a wide spectrum of approaches to disclosure, shaped by a range of factors. In general, those who disclosed diagnoses fully had fewer fears of discrimination, because of the severity or type of the diagnosis, the type of workplace, or the sense that they had less to lose. Other doctors faced troubling moral choices, and often opted for closetedness—though at a cost.

The Costs of Silence

Silence could serve as an alternative to disclosure, but carried a high price. As suggested, concealment of an illness could hamper seeking care. HIV raised these concerns dramatically, but was hardly unique. Those "in the closet" about a diagnosis encountered difficulties going to medical appointments during the day. Psychosocial stresses could increase. For example, as a surgeon with HIV, Jerry could not ask for time off when his partner was sick. Jerry worried he would lose his job, and didn't even call in sick during a crisis—when his lover became acutely ill on an out-of-state vacation.

On the plane, he was very sick. He went to the hospital. I came in
to work at 9:00 A.M. At 9:30 A.M. he died. I couldn't take the
day off, and worked that whole day. I couldn't say, "Can I have
another week off?" I was angry: if I had a wife with breast cancer,
I wouldn't have had to go back.

Both gay and HIV-infected, Jerry faced double stigma.

Secrecy may impede the start or maintenance of needed treatment.
Since Larry, who had HIV, was starting a fellowship, he feared that ini-
tiating treatment through his insurance would "out" him, so he did not
take meds. In the OR, he feared he would be unable to hide side effects.
"Things are stressful enough without having to deal with diarrhea...."

Yet, in the case of disorders or treatments that cause immuno-
suppression, nondisclosure can prompt situations in which one is ex-
posed to potentially lethal infections. Such exposure led Roxanne to disclose her cancer, but left Larry working in constant fear. He felt helpless,
scared of discrimination and added disease. He highlighted tensions between professional responsibilities and personal needs that extended
well beyond HIV alone.

Hepatitis C and TB are my two main concerns. One patient needed
to be intubated because of multidrug-resistant TB. I just put my
mask and gloves on. What am I supposed to do? I can't sit there
and say, "We have to call someone else because I'm HIV-positive,
and am putting myself at risk." I showed up. This person was dying
of TB, looked terrible. Under my breath, I said, "fuck!" Patients
who need a lot of transfusions or have hepatitis B are my other
concern. I try to keep my gloves on at all times. But powder from
inside the gloves gets everywhere. It sounds silly: hepatitis B or
dry skin? But after I've been in the OR for twelve hours, powder
covers my hands. That can drive you crazy.

Fears of being outed led some ill physicians to hide their diagnosis even
from the doctors who treated them. Larry was hospitalized at his institution when he developed a blood clot, but he felt he couldn't tell the
physicians there that he was HIV-infected, so he didn't. A colleague recommended such silence. Before Larry was admitted, this friend and coworker paged him to warn him:

He said, "Unless you're convinced that the HIV has something to
do with this, don't say anything." He knows this department better

than I do. It would take only one senior professor to say, "I'm not going to work with him in my OR." That would be the same as getting fired.

Larry felt that he had little choice but to conceal, and that, in retrospect, his decision was right. A senior professor later read Larry's chart.

One of my professors came to visit me and said, "Oh, I went through your chart and everything looks ok." I still haven't told the clinical director that someone went through it.

Larry felt *he had to remain silent even about this violation of privacy*, illustrating again colleagues' insensitivity to the lack or distortion of boundaries.

Still, as a result of his reticence, Larry underwent a "fancy," costly diagnostic workup that yielded nothing, even though he knew that HIV caused his problem.

Fears of the consequences of disclosure led some to forgo all insurance coverage, despite the potential jeopardy to one's health. For a year, Paul had no insurance. At a previous job, he had had to divulge his HIV infection on an insurance form.

There was documentation of me being positive through my previous insurance, so I couldn't lie. There was a preexisting waiting period, so I had no health insurance for a year with T-cells of 200!

Regardless of their diagnosis, these doctors feared the increasing loss of privacy in society generally. Erosion of job stability in medicine exacerbated apprehensions of future denial of insurance. Jessica, the pediatrician with Hodgkin's, said:

There were subsequent jobs where I couldn't get insurance because of a waiting period, or having a "preexisting condition." I'm paranoid that some day if I change jobs I will be denied insurance. I just have a general angst—from the media and Big Brother. The less that people know about me, the better.

A nationalized health insurance system could potentially ameliorate these problems, though ill physicians remained skeptical about the likelihood of such a policy being adopted in the United States.

Silence also precluded support or help from colleagues. Several physicians arranged for colleagues to monitor them for subtle symptoms that could influence work performance. But due to closetedness, not all sick doctors could have themselves watched in this way. Suzanne, with bipolar disorder, said sadly, "It would be nice if somebody knew, because it could really take a load off me: What if I decompensate" (that is, become significantly less able to function)? "It'd be so much easier if someone knew."

Colleagues ignorant of a physician's diagnosis could unknowingly be insensitive. For example, colleagues commented harshly to Suzanne about her weight gain. "One resident is a real pain in my ass. Every day: 'Did you go to the gym?'" Another supervisor thought Suzanne was just slothful. Again, she felt powerless to unveil the truth. "I was sleeping fourteen hours a day, and was hypothyroid from the lithium. He just thought I was lazy, and treated me poorly."

Silence about one's diagnosis can be used against one. Suzanne wanted to tell her supervisor that she was dealing with other stresses besides those of residency. But she felt she could not let him know.

> Sometimes it's right on the tip of my tongue. The program director says, "You've been a little impulsive." I want to tell him that my level of functioning is actually pretty miraculous.

Reticence can also foster isolation. By not disclosing to his coworkers, Ronald, the suburban Connecticut radiologist with HIV, felt "separated" from them. Ironically, this distance became reinforced—partly self-imposed: "they don't really know who I am."

Maintenance of secrecy consumed enormous energy. Mathilde described the devastating fallout:

> It *erodes* you: You have to hide it, as if you had committed a sin.... There was a *curse* upon us: we couldn't tell our friends. Keeping it hidden stressed our kids, too.

Again, the information, as a secret, assumed a force and life of its own.

"*Secondary secrecy*" can result, keeping others' awareness of the concealment itself hidden. At his hospital, Larry now had to make sure that people were not cognizant that a coworker knew.

> Just one person in my department knows. I go out of my way to protect him, because if people find out, they could go after him: "How could you encourage him to join our department, knowing his diagnosis?"

Fears of disclosure led some to stay in jobs they would otherwise leave—"stuck," wary of job or insurance discrimination if they moved. Others avoided particular jobs because disclosure would be necessary. Thus, the need for secrecy can limit one's type of practice. Pascal, the internist with HIV, felt trapped because if he were in private practice, he would have to try to purchase his own insurance. If not for his illness, he would have been "more aggressive" in his career.

> I might consider doing private practice. I want to be my own boss. But I'd have to buy insurance. . . . That's why I work for an institution. I don't like it, but can't move.

Blurring Boundaries: Colleagues' Reactions to Disclosure Decisions

"Don't tell me too much," Anne's boss told her. Within the tight subculture of the workplace, colleagues may not want to know about or discuss a coworker's illness. Colleagues may be aware of, but not speak of, a colleague's disorder in order to preserve and respect privacy and "professional" norms. About his colleagues, Peter said, "They want their privacy. We've never even sat down and had a meal together!"

Yet an ill doctor's right to privacy could potentially conflict with his or her patients' rights to learn the physician's diagnosis. Coworkers—particularly superiors—may "not want to know," since disclosure at work can raise liability concerns. Divulgence to a boss can complicate subsequent interactions. Roxanne, the gastroenterologist with cancer, said, "I told my boss. It adds an extra level of complication to the relationship. He doesn't want to think, 'Here is a liability. She could die.'"

Professional aspects of a relationship can hamper not only disclosure to colleague-friends, but also the ability of these individuals to offer support, especially if they occupy different levels in the medical hierarchy. Colleagues who have specific political influence over one's career may not want to know much about an illness, since it can precipitate a conflict of interest. Anne, the Swiss internist, was explicitly told by her boss: " 'It's not good to say too much.' That was painful for me. I don't think I was asking for more than support.' " Clearly, definitions vary of what is "too much." Evidently, Anne's boss felt he had to separate his personal and professional roles as much as possible in order to avoid a conflict of interest. He had to ensure first the best interests of the clinic, not of individual employees within it. Hence, he tried to separate his knowledge of Anne personally from his professional decisions.

Awkward situations emerged, too, if colleagues asked each other about their health status "just as friends," since over years at a workplace, personal and professional boundaries soften. Steven, the suburban endocrinologist with HIV, worried about colleagues inquiring if he'd ever been HIV tested. He decided he would answer, " 'Everything is going ok'— which is not a lie." Here, he distinguished between full and partial truths and lies. Steven felt he would be comfortable giving *truthful, but only partial and incomplete, information.*

Yet failure to disclose can cause tensions, as some colleagues may know, and *disapprove* of the dissembling. Given the consequences, Tom did not list alcoholism on a form, but was confronted about this prevarication by a fellow Alcoholics Anonymous member and colleague.

> A hospital application asked about substance abuse. I knew one of the guys on the credentials committee from AA. He's an asshole, and had his secretary call and say, "Are you sure you don't want to answer 'Yes'?" I said, "I'm quite sure. Have him call me if there's a question." He called: "I'm confused." I said, "It's none of their business. I've never been in treatment, and frankly, you're violating my confidentiality by bringing it up! He was overstepping his bounds. I would prefer to be 100 percent truthful. I like it when they ask, "Do you *currently* have a problem with substance abuse?" That's easy: No.

Tom illustrated the intricacies of different moral and psychological calculations.

Perceived intentions underlying others' questions about one's health shaped perceived responsibilities to tell the truth. Some of these ill doctors felt lying was permissible, depending on who was asking, and why, and whether the questioner really needed to know. They felt that the potential harm from truth-telling could outweigh the benefits and possible moral censure incurred through lying.

Colleagues may suspect, even if they do not definitively know, a physician's diagnosis, but be unsure *how* to discuss it or offer support. Nancy, the endocrinologist with metastatic breast cancer, reported:

Colleagues said, "I don't feel I know you well enough to say anything." I remember feeling that way, too. People just don't know how to bring it up. Another colleague, when I confronted her, said, "Well, I didn't want to *remind* you." *As if I forgot?*

Here again, unstated workplace norms of privacy outweighed those of camaraderie, closeness, and support. Colleagues may have information, but not the *right* either to have that knowledge or to share it with others. Implicitly, the consent of the person who is the subject of information may be critical in determining who has the right to the knowledge. Perceived rights of ownership of information thus vary, based in part on how one came to possess the knowledge.

Colleagues may be aware, but not feel comfortable discussing the topic because to do so is socially too awkward or painful. Ernie, with HD, felt that none of his superiors at work—only friends—said anything to him about his lethal HD diagnosis.

To ask a colleague about his or her illness, and risk being upset or re-buffed, can take courage, too. Deborah, the psychiatrist with breast can-cer, described a conversation with a colleague about this very topic.

She said, "All along I wanted to ask you, and just didn't have the guts. I don't know how to approach you." They're not sure if the ill person is going to reject them.

Deborah's clear reserve no doubt contributed to her colleagues' uncer-tainty about how to raise the topic with her. She cautiously weighed in-quirers' interest against her desire for privacy.

As suggested, colleagues may question the exact boundaries of when professional relationships should or do evolve and become personal as well. Does a professional relationship have enough intimate, and few enough political elements, to make illness discussable? Colleagues may broach the subject and test the waters. Or awkwardness can make personal issues utterly off-limits. Colleagues did not ask Deborah much about her illness until she returned to work—resulting from, and causing, tensions.

One of the attendings never called me at the hospital, or sent concern via other people. When I got back, she said, "I want to talk to you. Come to my office." I did. She said: "What's wrong? Can you tell me what happened?" I said, "I appreciate your concern, but am really not interested in talking." I had never really had anything to do with her, so I didn't feel I could confide in her. She was insulted. To this day, I haven't had a good relationship with her. I felt that she was doing it more to feel good about the fact that she is concerned about the residents. But I didn't appreciate the way it was done—that it was really *true*. Maybe I'm wrong. I felt I was very brusque. I wrote her a note: "I really appreciate that you called, but I really don't feel I'd like to speak to you about my personal problem. I have a support system already." If she had called me in the hospital and just said, "How are you?" that would have bridged the distance. She just ignored the note.

Prior closeness can facilitate disclosure, and disclosure can promulgate further closeness. Previous literature has mentioned professional silence, but it emerges here in part as a *dynamic* process. At times, these individuals pushed and pulled against explicit and implicit workplace boundaries and norms.

Physician-patients may want colleagues to know, but to respond to the news only in particular ways. Nancy wanted people to ask, but she desired that they see the information she gave only as positive. She also hesitated bringing her illness up, "afraid I might upset them." She wanted people to ask how she was doing, but only "in the right way," further underscoring the dynamic nature of such interactions—*responding to others' responses to oneself*. Lou thought that colleagues "should say, 'I heard you were sick, how are you feeling?' When people do that, I usually say, 'Thank you for asking. I'm not doing that well, but I'm sort of hanging in there.'" He did not answer their question directly, yet stymied further discussion, closing off openings for additional queries.

Efforts by ill physicians to be upbeat about their illness could encounter resistance from colleagues. Lou felt colleagues responded to illness in a professional rather than a personal way.

Colleagues put an arm around me and said, "Isn't that terrible? I feel so sorry for you." They have a funereal affect, which is not helpful. Better are those who react more naturally: "How are you doing?" *We don't teach doctors really how to respond to sick people on a personal level!*

Doctors learned how to respond to illness as professionals (based on medical science), but not as human beings (based on genuine empathy). The two approaches differed in whether and what emotion was expressed, and how information was framed. Only since being a patient himself did Lou realize the need to be positive with sick coworkers.

> With other colleagues who are patients, I try to be upbeat, and more cheerful. "What are you doing for fun?" I ask, "How are you doing?" *if* they want to talk about the illness.

Lou's comments raised dilemmas as to whether and when such attempts at positive framing may verge on denial.

Either conflicts or mutual enforcement concerning disclosure may ensue. At one extreme, both parties may be ambivalent about discussing a coworker's illness, leading to mutual silence. Deborah said colleagues avoided her, and she then eschewed them as well.

> They often ignore me, and I kind of ignore them, too, because I don't want to get into it. Or they just don't know what to say. I don't ever call them on it—go up and say, "Hi."

Preferences for or against disclosure can thus collide. Doctors, colleagues, and patients may benefit from being more aware of the implications of these contrasting preferences and needs. No doubt, patients who work in nonmedical fields encounter similar complex interactions and potential tensions. Yet the experiences here reveal critical attitudes and insensitivities of doctors that can shape their views of patients more broadly.

Telling Patients

Ill physicians struggled as well with dilemmas of whether and what to disclose concerning their health and personal life to their *patients*. Should patients ever know about a providers' illness, and if so, when? Do patients have a right to such information? Who should decide? Divulged information can shape a professional relationship. At core, these physicians faced difficult quandaries of what is professional in these matters.

These issues arose prominently among doctors with HIV, but also appeared among doctors with other disorders. HIV is infectious, carries particular stigma, and constitutes an epidemic, affecting many others. Though the infection could potentially harm a patient's safety if an HIV-infected surgeon worked in a closed, not visible, body cavity, the HIV-positive doctors here all rigorously avoided such a possibility. Yet ill doctors, particularly those with potentially life-threatening disorders (e.g., cancer), confronted similar and related questions, even if at times to lesser degrees. Bill, the Southern radiologist with HIV, said he'd prefer to know if his surgeon was intoxicated more than if he had HIV. "I'd much rather know if my doctor's had three drinks that morning before he takes me to the OR, than if he's got HIV. And surgeons who drink: *that* happens all the time."

Yet in day-to-day interactions, principles can conflict with practice. Often, the social contexts of relationships with patients created expectations and pressures for candor. At times, patients observed outright evidence of disease in physicians, and then had to decide whether to inquire. When Lou, the internist with cancer who had an award on his wall, became bald, patients asked about his health, which led to more of a human-to-human, as opposed to doctor-to-patient, relationship:

> Since my hair was gone, patients were aware of it. I couldn't hide
> it. They'd ask how I was, and it deepened the relationship. I
> didn't tell everyone. I didn't want them to worry. But if they
> seemed to notice, I would tell them: "I'm on chemo."

Given the complex interpersonal dynamics of these relationships, though ethically not obligated to disclose, Lou did so, responding to patients' queries.

To help patients put their own symptoms into perspective, other doctors divulged, if asked. Brian, who had hepatitis, sometimes felt sicker than his patients, and said so to them.

> At times, I've felt sick, and said very jokingly, "Now don't think *you*
> have an overwhelming illness. In fact, right now, I've got fever
> and am probably sicker than you." A few weeks ago, I had a really
> bad cold and headache, and had to work a night shift. A patient
> actually said, "You look like you don't feel well." I said, "You're
> right. I don't," and in a joking sense: *"You're better than I am right*
> *now."*

For others, questions lingered of what to tell patients who probed. Deborah, the psychiatrist with breast cancer, said, "Patients were asking, 'What happened? Where is she?' Nobody would say anything. That was a dilemma: what to tell patients."

The complexities of the pros and cons involved left some doctors utterly unsure and confused about what to say. Simon, a radiologist with HIV who refused audiotaping, terrified that others might somehow learn of his infection, did not want to disclose to patients, and was taken aback, unprepared, when they inquired. "A patient asked me if I'd been tested, and *I went blank*. I don't remember what I said. A technician was there. I suppose I said something that was inappropriate."

The profession itself may impede disclosure, as colleagues may not want a physician's patients to know. For example, after returning from her hospitalization, Deborah wanted to see her first long-term patient, who "was taken away from me. I really wanted to tell her what happened—I never had the chance." Institutions can erect structural barriers to decrease physicians' revealing their disease.

Patients might be told *only* if they asked. Pascal, the Lebanese internist, informed patients only if they inquired.

Yet patients may also ask inappropriately. For example, a patient once rudely interrogated Mark, the internist with HIV whom I interviewed in a diner over lunch.

A straight woman in her late thirties with the flu walked in off the street with her boyfriend—white-trash type. But regardless, I wasn't just going to give her antibiotics and send her out; that's not the way I practice medicine. She was having some difficulty breathing, and I was thinking about the possibility of pneumocystis. So I asked her if she had ever been tested for HIV. She got indignant, and said, "Yeah, about three years ago." Her boyfriend was there, and maybe she was bothered about discussing it. I said, "And it was negative?" She said, "Yeah," and... she turned around to me and said, "And you?"... I said, "Yeah."... "And?" I said, "...I'm positive." Her mouth dropped....I thought: this could come back to haunt me.... But I'd already decided I'm not going to live like that....I'm sure she'll never come back, but that's fine.

Patients may wonder about a physician's health, but be afraid to inquire or feel that to do so would be inappropriate. They may feel awkward and uncomfortable asking, and hence wait to be informed. Stuart, the internist with HIV now teaching at the university, said another physician's patients would not inquire, but hoped to be told. They refrained from asking due to both their sense that such personal inquiry was "taboo," and their own fear and denial of their physician being ill or dying. About one colleague, Stuart said:

This doctor had K.S. [Kaposi's sarcoma, an AIDS-defining diagnosis, consisting of large purple splotches] on his face, and patients

wouldn't ask. They were just waiting for him to tell them. After
he was hospitalized, people started to come forward and ask.
But the staff wouldn't answer. It might have been their denial, too,
even though the guy had lost thirty pounds and looked like hell.

In fact, Stuart continued, this hospitalized doctor went so far as to lie
to everyone about being sick. "He denied all this: 'Why do people keep
thinking I have AIDS?' He had been hospitalized for CMV, a fairly AIDS-
specific opportunistic infection."

Patients, sensing implicit norms and taboos, may reveal their concerns
only indirectly. Ronald, the suburban radiologist with HIV, reported,
"People have said things without asking. One woman said, 'Doctor, I'm
so glad: you look so much better. We were really worried that something
really bad was going on!' " Here again, this case elucidates broader issues:
that patients may know or suspect a physician's illness, but feel that
unstated professional-client rules deny them the right to possess that information, or even to broach the topic. Patients acquire their own sense
of professional norms, even if physicians do not explicitly communicate
or instill these.

Patients want to feel they can depend on their doctors, and generally
desire to establish long-term relationships with providers. They wish to
assume their physician is healthy, and can't quite imagine he or she is not.
Indeed, when Stuart retired to teach, he sent a letter to patients to inform
them of his HIV. Many utterly misconstrued the message.

I wrote a letter to introduce the subject that three months later, I'd
be leaving, and that my associate was going to take over. . . . I
thought: the next question they're all going to ask is "What are you
going to do next?" So I just wrote that I'm going to retire, spend
more time relaxing and traveling, and . . . spending some time
teaching at the university. In my mind, that meant that I was going
to be volunteering . . . to teach. Almost universally, that phrase got
interpreted as "He is a professor at the university now. He doesn't
have weekend call." They did not scratch their heads over this
forty-five-year-old guy going from working ten to twelve hours a
day to sitting in a cabana with a lemonade. They answered the
question themselves by filling in the teaching at the university as a
full-time job, with some free time to travel. . . . They'd ask, "Can we
still come and see you there?" I'd say, "Well, I won't be seeing
patients." I found it easier *not* to challenge their concept of what

was going on. Suddenly, it solved my problem. I dreaded the next three months, of people saying: "What are you going to do?" Instead, everyone understood.

Occasionally, doctors disclosed to patients in order to motivate the latter to improve the therapeutic alliance, and start or adhere to treatments. Physicians then had to gauge when the information would be useful (e.g., "if it seems to serve a purpose").

Others told when they became frustrated at patients' complaints about relatively minor matters. To a patient who complained all the time, Nancy, with metastatic breast cancer, disclosed in utter frustration. Again, quandaries arose as to the appropriate boundaries between doctor and patient—specifically, when, if ever, the doctor may be shifting these too far by divulging too much. Nancy explained:

> I became exasperated with this man, because all he did was complain: He had a horrible wife, was overweight, had diabetes, was depressed, his wife was having more children, and he was $300,000 in debt. He felt that everything we suggested was not going to work....I lost my patience and said, "Look, you want to know a *real* problem? *I* have a real problem." He was shaken, and I admit it was not very *professional* for me to do. But it did take him aback a little. I said, "*You have the ability to make yourself better, and I don't! You should do that. I wish I could.*"

Nancy saw her display of emotion as unprofessional, but felt that in the end, it benefited her patient. Physician anger and frustration may not be appropriate to express, but are *all* such displays of emotion or personal issues taboo? Should physicians *always* remain cool and detached? Doctors may in fact hide behind façades. Questions arose as to the degrees to which physicians did hide, and the costs involved. Perhaps a physician's display of emotion can at times motivate or otherwise benefit a patient, though when and why need further clarification. As the field becomes technologically more effective in treating disease, perhaps the norms of professional demeanor among physicians should change to permit more human interactions and emotion than some doctors now allow.

Some physicians disclosed their illness to impel patients to continue to work and not retire on disability. Mark, the internist with HIV interviewed in the diner, disclosed to discourage a patient who desired to leave work prematurely.

With 450 T-cells, he was totally well, but wanted disability. I
said, "You've got more T-cells than I do! There's no reason
you can't work." He said, "You don't have HIV." I said, "Yes,
I do."

In addition, as Nancy and Mark both indicate here, and as will be discussed later, physicians with serious illness can feel frustrated, angry, and
even envious when treating relatively healthy patients who nonetheless
complain and don't comply with proven treatments.

Physicians who *did* disclose to patients encountered a variety of reactions. On the one hand, the revelation could foster trust and closeness. For
example, Walter, the activist, divulged his Hodgkin's lymphoma to help a
patient make a treatment decision.

His life came out better. I was a human being with him. He feels
privileged to be privy to my secret, which says something about
his value: that I trusted him to know.

Physicians and patients can reinforce their trust of each other (e.g.,
through a positive feedback loop). A sense of camaraderie can develop.
Jacob, the radiologist, added, "I deal with cancer patients a lot, so it's been
a big plus rather than a negative to have cancer. I show them my big scar."
Illness itself can increase intimacy.

Yet such closeness has potential problems. Patients' knowledge of a
physician's illness can skew the relationship. With patients, Paul thought
it was best not to have his own health be a major topic in interactions.
"The patients that do know. . . are very concerned. It's good, but seems to
take the focus away from why *they're* here."

Half-truths, half-lies, and misrepresentations can occur. Alex, the dentist with HIV, worked in a small town, and many of his patients attended
the same fundamentalist church as he and his family. When queried, he
responded that he stopped work because of an auto accident—a misrepresentation.

When they're talking around the issue, and you're talking around
the issue, and obviously by their questions, they know: Well,
just be honest and tell them. I've only done the dance a couple of
times and I realized how stupid it was. "You haven't been looking
very healthy lately. How come you really did quit practice?" I said,
"Well, I had an automobile accident. . . ." I do have back problems
and allergy problems, and would use both those excuses. All of

those are somewhat true. The car accident was minor. But misrepresentation like that is akin to lying....

Hence, these physicians raised questions of definitions of sins of omission
versus sins of commission, and of "partial" truths. Some have decided to
fib to their patients. When asked, Stuart dissembled to a patient: "...he
said, 'I just want to know: You're going to be around, right? You're not
sick or anything?' I tacitly lied: I'm not sick.'"

In part, Alex feared that patients might sue; and disclosure could hurt
his field as a whole. "I would cause sensationalism in the papers. It would
not be good for my profession."

Still, generally, many patients found out last, often "only after the
doctor dropped dead."

In all, these doctors shed light on the intricacies involved in balancing
ethics against interpersonal aspects of doctor-patient relationships and
communication. Patients faced dilemmas of whether to comment on a
doctor's condition either implicitly or explicitly. Doctors had to decide
whether, and what, to disclose.

Across diseases, similar quandaries arose of whether, what, when, and
whom to tell. Yet with HIV, given its infectivity, patients wondered if
they had a *right* to know. Still, they sensed that to ask directly might be
taboo.

These narratives raise larger important questions (e.g., how ethical
issues are approached and handled within the social and psychological
nuances and complexities of the doctor-patient relationships that are often built on fragile trust). Doctors felt that a patient did *not* have a right to
know the doctor's health status generally, unless it in some way threatened the patient's health. But what felt psychologically appropriate could
conflict with what was considered ethical. Even if disclosure were ethically unnecessary, trust and closeness could make nondisclosure awkward.
Silence can foster distance and tension. Hence, doctors may disclose, even
though they are not ethically required to. At times, physicians disclosed to
help patients cope. Divulgence may be more beneficial for certain diagnoses or types of disorders than for others. For example, former substance
abusers often treated substance-abusing patients, and drew on personal
experiences to be more effective (5). Physician disclosure can potentially
strengthen patient-provider bonds, and thus treatment alliances. Yet even
here, clinicians faced dilemmas of *how much* and *what information* to

reveal. If a doctor divulged a positive HIV status, should he or she reveal the mode of viral exposure (e.g., sexual activity)? Physician nondisclosure or misrepresentation may also skew and dampen the doctor-patient relationship.

Currently, physicians make these decisions by themselves, since at least initially, they alone possess this information, while their patients do not.

Patients may want, or feel they have a right to, this knowledge, and may indeed have such a right, if it is pertinent to their health (10). But these determinations can pose complications (e.g., whether such patient concern should ever trump the physician's right to privacy). Patients' claims involve their physical or psychological health, while physicians' rights may involve protection against potential stigma and discrimination. Here, the *degree* of threat to a patient's health may be key. Patient death or serious physical harm clearly could trump a physician's right to privacy, yet patients may claim, without merit, that they suffer psychological distress from knowing that their physician is ill. Even if they remain uninfected, patients have attempted to sue—though unsuccessfully, given the low degree of actual harm—HIV-infected physicians who had not disclosed that information (11). Moreover, discrimination and stigma of physicians could impair *their* psychological well-being.

Questions also arise of whether and when a doctor should tell patients that he or she knows that he or she may not or will not be able to provide long-term care to patients (due to retirement or change of job). Especially in psychiatry, the loss of a physician can distress fragile or vulnerable patients, exacerbating symptoms, and possibly decreasing patient adherence, and hence health outcomes. Patients who feel abandoned or betrayed may then decide to access future health care less. Hence, patients may argue that they have the right to this knowledge as well. But do they? How long before leaving their job should physicians disclose such information? These types of knowledge about a physician vary from job change to serious illness and short life expectancy. Arguably, physicians' symptoms of fatigue or decreased concentration could affect quality of care, too, necessitating disclosure, though the effects on care may be small. Nonetheless, dilemmas remain of who should make these determinations, and how these decisions should be made. Physicians and patients may hold conflicting implicit definitions of "appropriate" communication.

Physicians should not divulge all ailments to all patients, but should realize that patients may be anxious about these issues, and view pros and cons of physicians' decisions differently than do these doctors themselves.

Providers may decide not to disclose, but should then be aware of how these decisions may impact patients. Alternatively, despite ethical justifications of reticence, doctors may volunteer information. But they may not be as aware as they should of the potential risks and benefits involved. These discussions need to take fully into account the nuanced and intricate social contexts of suffering and emotional difficulties faced by doctors (e.g., when patients ask) and by patients (e.g., whether to ask). As suggested here, a physician who decides that disclosure is not appropriate could respond to a patient's query not by ignoring or evading it, but by acknowledging it and alluding to the dilemma involved—for example, "We could discuss my health, but I think it makes more sense to focus on *your* health here today." In any case, these concerns illustrate the delicate tensions involved in doctor-patient relationships.

Going Public

These doctors wondered, too, about disclosing even more broadly beyond the confines of the doctor-patient relationship—to the public-at-large. At times, larger groups, including the media, were interested in a physician's illness. To varying degrees, a few doctors opted to go public. Several announced their status widely for a range of reasons: because it might help others, or because the pressures of secrecy became too much. Yet, in retrospect, many who did so regretted it. In the fiercely competitive field of medicine, some wanted or planned to go public, but decided to wait, at least for the moment.

A few wanted to write about their illness. Deborah, the psychiatrist with breast cancer, considered doing so, but chose not to, because it could jeopardize her future.

> I decided to write about all these things. But at the last moment, I decided not to, because of discrimination: I was going for job interviews. I couldn't be exposing myself early in my career. Once I got established, it would be different.

Sadly, nine months later, Deborah died, never having penned her experience.

These issues of public announcement arose prominently, though clearly not exclusively, with HIV. A few with HIV dared to go public officially, involving the media, in order to make a broad political statement.

Varying degrees of going public existed. For example, John, a public health official, disclosed widely, though not fully and publicly, in a letter. "I sent a Christmas letter out to 100 friends, and told them I had HIV, and was taking a job with the health department." His disclosure was dual—of both diagnosis and job change—each legitimating the mailing.

Some told select circles of colleagues or coworkers that grew over time. These decisions may have been influenced by past experiences. For example, Pascal told the staff at his clinic, since a previous physician there had died of AIDS from a needle stick, but had delayed divulgence.

A few literally went national with news of their diagnosis, whether willingly or not. Infected with HIV by a needle stick, Jennifer "came out" widely because rumors about her had begun to spread. She then chose to go even more public because of her sense of broader professional and social obligations.

> Something struck me about my own responsibility to myself and others to hold my head up high and say, "Look, this is a disease we all have to deal with. *If we as physicians don't deal with it, how do we expect anybody else to do so?*"

In short, Jennifer saw physicians as providing role models to others in following health-promoting behaviors, a view that not all her colleagues shared. For her to do otherwise, she felt, smacked of hypocrisy.

> I worked with HIV patients because I had hoped that society would become more accepting. If I pretended my infection was a secret, I was a hypocrite. How could I encourage my patients to share their status, and then be living with this secret myself?

Jennifer thus went public *because* she was a physician.

Once doctors decided in principle to go public, they had to confront myriad choices of *how* exactly to do so—difficulties for which they were generally unprepared. Unlike other infected individuals who were neither celebrities nor physicians, to Jennifer's surprise, her announcement generated media attention, and panic.

> The decision part was not that difficult, but I was naïve about the telling part. I never really thought about how people were going to take this.
>
> I told a colleague who was a good friend that I wanted to tell our weekly hospital conference. She arranged the speakers. For some

reason, I told the hospital chief of staff. He told me I was crazy. I
said, "I don't care, I'm going to do it anyway." He said, "We can
keep this hush-hush." I said, "I'm going to do this, and would
like your support." He said, "We will support you. We're just re-
commending you not do it." Then he said, "You need to tell the
public relations people." I said, "Oh, please!" But as I was leaving
the hospital, I walked by the PR department, and went in and
told this woman. She was horrified: "You can't do that!" I said,
"It's what I'm going to do." So she panicked and sent out a press
release, and said, "You don't know what this is going to do to the
community." I thought she was nuts. I just couldn't see how
anybody was going to care. Lots of people are very public with this.
But I wasn't thinking that not a lot of *doctors* are public about it.

To Jennifer's surprise, her announcement generated national news
and a furor. Many physicians in her community, particularly those who
didn't know her well, shunned her. At the local medical society, a rumor
spread that she had been infected not through a needle stick, but through
sex.

There was this huge element of denial: this couldn't possibly
happen. There were a lot of rumors about how I *really* got
infected—that I actually had an affair with a patients' lover. A lot
of physicians just didn't want to be around me. They thought there
must be something crazy about me to want to work with HIV
anyway. In the grocery store, I'd say hello, and they'd literally turn
around and walk away.

In the end, Jennifer did receive a degree of affirmation. "Some of the
people who thought I was crazy before the fact, later came up and said
they thought it was right to do." In fact, she actually gained advantages
from going public, but only after switching jobs. "I then worked for a
company full-time, lecturing on women and HIV. It was great."

Still, on balance, Jennifer felt she would not recommend that physicians go public, as she had done. "They've really got to think long and
hard about it, and decide what kind of career they want." Altruistic
motives of promoting openness could benefit patients and other health
care workers, but had to be weighed against self-preservation.

In response to the reactions she encountered, Jennifer advised patients
to be more circumspect in disclosing to others. "Before, I pushed patients

to disclose more than I do now. I thought disclosure was great: Get this off your chest. But it's not always that way."

Nevertheless, coming out can serve political, institutional or social functions. John, the public health official, announced his infection for political reasons. He was more readily able to do so than Jennifer because he did not treat patients. During a controversy:

> Activists decried named-HIV reporting. They were not HIV-infected, but purporting to speak for the HIV-infected community. I said, "I *am* HIV-infected, and am offended by this." I decided to call a spade a spade. But the media decided that the story was not whether AIDS should be reported or not, but that *I* had HIV. That became the main news. Most people said: "I'm glad you came out about this issue." But going public made me more of a jeopardy to the political leadership.

Not surprisingly, many ill physicians immediately knew that they would never go public; they were too "private." Still others ranged between these two extremes, and drew lines as to *how "out"* they felt comfortable being. Pascal, for example, had been able to tell staff, but not the media. "I'm shy," he said, "not a public person."

Others wished to go public, but felt that for political or economic reasons, they simply could not. Tom disclosed that he was gay. He wanted to be public about his illness, but wasn't, because of the potential effects on his clinical practice. ("That would be a service to colleagues. But I feared my practice would dissipate.") He concluded that the risk was not worth it.

Telling Family Members

These ill physicians, particularly those with HIV, also had to decide whether, when, and what to tell their families of origin. They feared their identity would change, even in their family, from doctor to patient, and they often sought to avoid this alteration. These familial dilemmas both resembled, and at times differed from, those in other social contexts.

Often, physicians delayed disclosing their illness to their parents. Though they were successful professionals, many doctors now lived in large cities, far from their families of origin. At times, even these physicians felt shame about their disease. They wanted to maintain the image of the successful, healthy doctor, a source of parental pride.

The consequences of secrecy with families can be very costly. When his family visited, Charles, the underground researcher, had to "de-AIDS" his home and "hide my medicine." If they knew, he feared they would devalue him: "I have to imply to them that I am gainfully employed. To tell them would worry them. And I'd lose stature in their eyes."

In short, these doctors faced questions of whether, what, when, and to whom to disclose their illness, as they sought to shape how others saw them. Some readily disclosed, but others did so only indirectly, in code or nonverbally. Workplace norms mitigated against personal revelations, and many opted for silence. Broader loss of privacy in contemporary society, and especially in hospitals, compounded these concerns. Yet noncommunication also carried costs: reduction in potential support, increase in isolation, and impediments to care. Secrecy could require mendacity and psychic energy; prevent these physician-patients from entering the sick role with its attendant advantages; and lead to social awkwardness and feelings of being "stuck" in jobs. Disclosures could be difficult, too, as colleagues were fellow physicians, and could be friends—occupying *three roles* that at times conflicted. Supervisor-friends may "just want to know" a diagnosis—as friends. Coworkers may know a diagnosis, but not whether or how to talk about it.

These physicians struggled not only with whether to tell colleagues, but whether and what to tell patients—some of whom noted evidence of their physicians' disease, and asked directly or indirectly in ways that these physicians felt were appropriate (or not). These decisions—whether to prevaricate or not—could shift doctor-patient relationships.

A few of these physicians went public, though in so doing, taboo diagnoses such as mental illness and HIV posed particular hurdles. Going public required a high degree of acceptance of one's illness and an ability to tolerate the potential career costs. Many longed to go public, but felt they could not.

Disclosure often emerged here as a process less of strictly individual decisions, and more of dynamic, two-way interactions. Yet past literature on illness disclosure has generally not examined expectations of those who are disclosed *to*, and their reactions (12).

Expectations and pressures from others concerning divulgence were often powerful and unanticipated. These internal and external pressures intensified stresses with which, as we shall see, physicians then struggled to cope.

Part II

BEING A DOCTOR AFTER BEING A PATIENT

7
Double Lens

Contrasting Views and Uses of Medical Knowledge

"I'm not a 'pill wimp' like some of my patients," one physician said. "I'm more rational, because I know more." Illness affected how these doctors not only acted, but also perceived the profession, patients, and risks and benefits of treatments. After acknowledging their initial diagnosis to the degree that they did, these physician had to weigh and assess different kinds of medical knowledge, approaching it in varying ways. *In general, they assessed risks and benefits differently than did other patients*, drawing on professional experiences and abilities in evaluating research findings. Overall, they found that medical knowledge helped immensely in many ways, but posed potential problems, proving to be a double-edged sword. Their views and communication of such risks and benefits are important since medicine increasingly involves complex sets of often conflicting data. Doctors regularly present this information to patients who grapple to understand, but may not interpret it correctly. These physicians revealed how medical knowledge can take on magical properties, but be limited, too.

Varieties of Medical Uncertainty

Previously, these physicians had to confront these challenges of medical ambiguity only with regard to those for whom they cared. Now, countless uncertainties hovered over these physicians' own lives. Though they had handled medical uncertainty for others, facing it themselves was very different. They approached these vagaries in a range of ways—from treating themselves aggressively, as described earlier, to inflating or deflating risk, trying to view dangers in black-and-white terms.

In the positivistic biomedical model of medicine, uncertainty poses fundamental problems. The sociologist Renée Fox and others have described how medical students learn to handle the uncertainty inherent in much of medicine (1), but little if any attention has been paid to how physicians deal with these ambiguities later in their careers. The ways physicians cope with lack of predictability in their own lives as patients have not been examined.

Among these doctor-patients, three kinds of uncertainty arose: concerning medical *prognoses, personal lives,* and *professional lives.* Coping with these three kinds of unpredictability often constituted the most difficult part of being ill.

Uncertainties in prognoses and treatment responses threatened one's career and personal life. For example, John, the public health official, described this ambiguity about the future as the hardest aspect of his illness, due to his inability to plan appropriately.

> The most difficult thing has been the uncertainty: this total unpredictability. *What's going to happen?* Three years ago, I stopped my practice because my count had gotten low. Now, I'm thinking about going back to practicing full-time. That would never have crossed my mind.

Doubts about one's professional future—the inability to anticipate or imagine having a future at all—proved extraordinarily unsettling. Jerry, the surgeon-lawyer, felt that after his partner's death, this murkiness troubled him most.

> The most stressful thing, after getting over the initial shock, was the uncertainty of the future—the doubt. I look more toward the future than I used to. I just joined a national committee, a three-year commitment. Three years ago, I didn't have the optimism that I'd be able to do that.

These professional quandaries illustrated how important stable professional and personal expectations were to daily life. These doctors had to differentiate between short- and long-term plans, and decide on the exact length of appropriate time frames: just *how* long or short a period to anticipate.

Many physicians on disability due to HIV fantasized about retraining in another subspecialty or field, such as law. But such switches required high investments of time and energy, without clear returns. Jerry, the surgeon, became a lawyer, but wondered if all the effort was worth it. Now, he concentrated on shorter-term endeavors—immediate tasks and gratification on a day-to-day basis, tangible results—rather than any long-term projects.

The fact that medicine preselects for individuals who desire and seek certainty over unpredictable processes can compound these difficulties.

Dilemmas emerged, too, of how to alter one's time frame and expectations—not only at initial diagnosis but also later, as an illness became more chronic. With improved HIV treatment, for example, many physician-patients who faced changing prognoses were not sure whether to readjust the ultimate time frame for their lives—whether to plan to live or die. Jeff, the adolescent specialist, said, "The biggest issue is: Am I living like I'm going to be living, or like I'm dying soon? I've never been able to figure it out."

Grappling with uncertainty was hard because ill doctors and others often had trouble handling it, and readily dismissed it. Deborah, the psychiatrist with breast cancer, said that one of the hardest aspects of her illness was that *others* saw uncertainty as shadowing her life. "My program director keeps saying, '*If* you finish your residency, I'll be very happy. . . . *If* you survive the rest of it . . . . *If* you're alive . . . .' " His pessimism may have proved justified—she died 9 months after this interview—but she perceived insensitivity that deeply disturbed her.

For years, these doctors had vigorously followed a rigorous career path, and now, with the possible end of their life in sight, they had to decide whether to detour or deviate, and if so, how. Physicians who had gained personal rewards from their professional work now struggled with whether and how much to surrender these ambitions, and focus more on their personal lives. Many now placed personal goals over professional ones far more than before.

Though many strove to focus on simply living day-to-day, others went even further, and tried to "seize the day" to the maximum. Yet such "accelerated living"—traveling, and living as fully in the moment as one could—incurred many costs. Jeff, the adolescent specialist, said:

Accelerated living is very expensive. If you try to see all your friends around the world, and new countries, you go into debt. Debt is ok if you're going to die in six months. But if you're not, you have these credit card bills!

To live purely in the moment, as if each day may be one's last, may also be infeasible for extended periods. "Living in the moment" all the time may not be practical if one lives for many years. Planning for the future confers benefits, especially financially. As Paul said, "What may be good for a twenty-year plan might not be best for five years. It causes incredible tension."

A few attempted to live with this unpredictability by incorporating it as part of their lives (i.e., by having the uncertainty itself become the given, the norm). Jerry, for example, said he eventually became comfortable with his hazy horizon—to the degree that, after getting ill, he completed law school. Yet at the same time, he described the attendant mental costs.

> The uncertainty just becomes a part of your life. But it *is* tiring. I've thought, "I wish I could just get sick." I just didn't have the energy to keep living, waiting to get sick. It takes energy to be optimistic: I run out of steam.

Stoically, others attempted not to think about the future at all. Due to the unforeseeable, Nancy, the endocrinologist with metastatic breast cancer, stopped pondering the future, though even *that* decision pained her. She maintained a striking acceptance and calm, born of courage. Her response evoked the writings of Seneca, the Roman philosopher, who argued that humans should live each day as if it were their last—because it might be (2).

> I try to stop thinking about the future. Because just when you think you see how it's going to go, something changes. That's traumatic. I have some trips scheduled til June, but not beyond. When things happen, they will be dealt with. We'll be on top of it—do as much as we can. Hopefully, I won't suffer very much.

In the face of such ambiguity, others bargained for particular ends. Larry, the anesthesiology trainee, hoped, given his unclear prognosis, to be well enough to finish residency—seeking some certitude, justice, and order.

Assessing Risks and Benefits

Ill physicians changed how they viewed and approached statistics concerning the risks and benefits they faced. Increasingly, subjective factors affecting perceptions of statistics have been explored in economics and other fields, but have been less examined in medicine. The psychologist Daniel Kahneman received the 2002 Nobel Prize in economics for describing how individuals commonly use "biases and heuristics"—for example, overvaluing the odds of bad events and undervaluing the probabilities of good outcomes (3). Several psychological studies have probed such misperceptions of statistics, generally among college students and in regard to hypothetical situations. Interpretations of statistical information are affected by how it is framed, either positively or negatively (4). Among medical students, numerical estimates have been found to be more effective than verbal ones. Rather than being wholly disadvantageous, these seemingly illogical heuristics and biases may offer certain advantages. Gerd Gigerenzer's book *Simple Heuristics That Make Us Smart* argues how evolutionarily, unconscious cognitive strategies allow humans to very rapidly draw intuitive conclusions about complex situations (e.g., the likelihood of escaping predators in one direction or the other, given the distance to forest, etc.) (5).

Yet how these intuitive, but subjective and "illogical," factors affect physicians and patients in their assessments of risks and benefits remains much less clear. Donald Redelmeier, an internist, outlined categories of biases and heuristics that distort patients' perceptions of risks in medicine (6). Health care professionals present risks in varying ways, for example, using a wide range of verbal descriptions (7). Though different groups of medical personnel assign similar quantitative probabilities to qualitative descriptions of odds, providers may differ from patients in interpreting the words used (e.g., " 'likely' " versus " 'unlikely' ") (8). Even when numbers rather than verbal descriptions are used, patients may assess risks differently if presented with rates rather than proportions (9). The sequential order in which risks and benefits are presented can also influence responses (10). Many questions persist as to the implications of these issues among patients and doctors. Though aspects of these issues have been explored, particularly in genetics, these issues of interpretation of statistics have been probed less in other areas of doctor-patient communication. Psychological experiments have been conducted using hypothetical scenarios with students. But it is not clear how these results apply in the real world. Hence, understanding how doctors who have become patients view these issues and change their perceptions can be helpful.

The Advantages of Medical Knowledge: Knowing What
the Statistics Mean

Routinely, in confronting their own disease, these doctors drew on their
medical training and found that possession of medical knowledge provided distinct benefits. Many cited how they had "learned from clinical
experience," and used this background in evaluating research and interpreting statistics concerning prognoses and side effects. Generally, they
thought they "knew what the statistics meant" (how to interpret them).
Compared with many other patients, they felt they understood relative
risks.

Many believed they were less wary than their patients of medications
and statistically improbable side effects. These doctors saw lay patients as
frequently getting hung up on risks of complications, fearing that unlikely
complications might nonetheless occur. Such patients may be overly re-
sponsive to negative possible outcomes, even if these are improbable.

In processing information, many of these doctors thought that patients
often felt that a percentage likelihood of a complication happening meant
that it would occur—that patients did not understand how to interpret
and weigh the relative risks of disease progression. Walter, with lymphoma, said:

> Patients don't understand statistics—if you get a complication, you
> get it 100 percent; if you don't get it, you don't get it at all. When
> we start patients on a new medication, we give them lists of all
> the complications. It's very important to explain that it doesn't
> mean that they *will* get it, but that there is a *chance*. It's amazing
> how many times I have to go over it—which means that most
> doctors don't discuss it. Patients are much more aware of side
> effects than of the fact that they have a fatal disease that, untreated,
> will be fatal.

In patients' minds, detailed and explicitly presented side effects loom
large.

As a result of their clinical training and experience, these doctors have
experience in calculating and weighing relative risks against relative benefits, developing "gut feelings" and intuitions. In comparison, they thought
that media attention and hype about findings of particular studies influenced lay patients' risk perceptions more heavily. Harry, the internist and
war refugee, added:

Patients read the PDR, and if they find "thrombocytopenia" and look it up, it doesn't convey anything to them. They know it means low platelets. But what that *implies*, what the risks are, don't mean anything. They don't have any *gut feeling* about it. A doctor *knows* what thrombocytopenia is and can do. He has much more knowledge, and leaves aside his emotions. *He can be much more rational in appraising risks.* Patients are concerned over what their best friend *thought* she heard.

These physicians are more critical of purported treatment benefits that may in fact prove elusive. They felt they were more wary than nonphysician patients of "hype" about medications. These doctor-patients were able to critique reports of medical findings in several ways: for example, how much the data actually supported the conclusions. Peter, the medical student, said:

When they put something out in the media, I don't take it at face value. A lot of people do, but I have more knowledge. I investigate things. I look at it from more of a medical viewpoint than just an Average Joe.

Still a trainee, he was proud to possess these skills.

Relative to doctors, lay patients have difficulty, in part because of the mass of information available on the Internet and elsewhere. This morass of details may make it hard even to know where to start or what questions to pose. Rochelle, a surgeon with breast cancer, said:

A friend had just been diagnosed with cancer, and clearly had no idea what the big picture was. He was bright, but going to Internet sites. It was too much information. He was talking about levels of chemo protocols, which was just not on track. Some pieces were missing. I was explaining what kind of cancer this was. He was asking, "What does '-oma' mean?"

Contexts are needed for optimal comprehension of information, but may not be provided by Internet searches, or even journal articles. In contrast, medical trainees learned not only from books, but also from clinical experiences, providing structures and ways to make sense of isolated facts. Lay patients lacked this education, scaffolding, and context, built over years of experience, that allowed these facts to be optimally weighed and applied.

Dangerous Knowledge: The Disadvantages and Limitations
of Medical Information

As patients, these physicians came to realize not only the advantages, but
also the potential limitations, of medical knowledge. Frequently, they
came to see medical information as overrated, open to wide and varying
interpretation. Many had previously seen medical science as straightforward, and now perceived ways it fell short—often painfully so. They realized how doctors and patients differ in tolerance of, and needs for, data.
At times, even for these doctors, information now became "too much."
Possession of medical knowledge had downsides, as it included information about poor prognoses, possible complications, and errors. One aspect
of illness that may be more difficult for a physician is knowledge of the
eventual severity of a diagnosis—knowledge that providers ordinarily
might minimize or not communicate to a patient, "the things the doctor
doesn't say." Physicians knew the complications and problems of their
own diseases. "I knew what it was like to watch a lot of people die,"
Jennifer remarked. "I couldn't pretend I didn't know."

Doctors had witnessed the horrors of possible differential diagnoses,
the worst possible symptoms and complications. These experiences
shaped fears and observations in ways that did not extend to the same
degree when these doctors treated other patients. *With regard to themselves, they were far more subjective.* Many feared negative outcomes more
for themselves than for their patients. John, the public health official
with HIV, pointed out:

> I know all these horrors that can happen, and it's very easy for
> those to prey on my mind. Whole differential diagnoses go through
> my head. When I had knee surgery and a fever, I had been doing
> a lot of autopsies, and was worried about the worst complica-
> tions. After I had HIV, I got a rash, and was convinced it was thrush
> or yeast. Then I had herpes, and was convinced the HIV made it
> worse. But it could have just been the stress of *worrying* about
> whether it *was* HIV. People who aren't physicians experience that,
> too, but I think it's harder as a physician.

Still, as John intimated, such comparisons with lay patients are difficult
to make.

Doctors are aware of not only bad prognoses, but also possible medical errors. Nancy said, "I know more about the bad mistakes that can happen. That's scary."

Some of these physicians "worry about every little thing," tending toward "medical student's disease," in which no "real" medical condition exists (11). Pascal, the internist, found it more difficult being a doctor, knowing the possible meanings and interpretations of minor symptoms. ("The littlest things set off alarms: 'Maybe *this* is going on.'")

Though they commonly also "fear the worst," lay patients have fewer established categories for handling medical information. Doctors have *themselves witnessed* "the worst" cases.

As suggested earlier, spectrums emerged of how much information individuals wanted. As patients, most physicians desired more information, and some ordered a surfeit of tests for themselves, thereby complicating treatment decisions. Tom, whose lover died of AIDS, felt that being an MD made it both more and less difficult to be a patient, because of the amount of medical knowledge.

> The more information, the more confusing it is. The more data I
> read, the more conflicted I am. It would be easier to be a non-
> physician, go to a doctor, and have them make the decision for me.

Yet what, exactly, constitutes "too much" information? At what point does "enough" become "too much"? Why, exactly, is some information too much or too confusing? How can these points best be ascertained for each individual? Clearly, in the real world, one weighs not a single set of probabilities, but complex sets of multiple statistics—the effects of drug A versus drug B versus drug C versus drugs A *and* B versus A, B, and C versus no drugs, and so on, with side effects and benefits of each. At a certain point, such determinations become too complex to make for oneself, because they involve too many competing variables and factors. Yet the points at which different individuals become "overwhelmed" vary.

At times, physicians used their "understanding of what the statistics mean" to deny the likelihood of rare, dangerous events occurring, and to counter their own best interests. Their training could facilitate their minimization of the severity of certain risks. When they did not want or like the possibility of an outcome, they could negate risks that may in fact transpire, using their professional training to support their psychological desires. For example, Jeff, the adolescent specialist with HIV, "got comfortable with risk," feeling that the existence of dangers did not necessarily mean that the untoward event in question would occur. He played a mind game with himself that in the end proved detrimental.

> Being a physician *screwed* me. I play the scientific mind game. I know that each act of sex is not going to transmit HIV.... It takes maybe eighty episodes of sex to get pregnant once. I played the numbers game with myself. After an unsafe episode, I could always say to myself that the risk of getting HIV isn't 100 percent. I've heard it's as low as 1 in 300 episodes of unsafe sex. I didn't think it was going to happen. It had *no chance* of happening. I didn't see the risk as being as high as lay people do.

Hence, Jeff used his medical knowledge *against* his own efforts to maintain his health. Medical knowledge not only can be ignored, but also employed in the service of maladaptive denial.

Jeff went on to cite a common adage of medical training used to temper subjective biases that overvalue the possibility of negative outcomes: "Common things happen commonly. Uncommon things happen uncommonly. You see zebra diagnoses"—medical conditions that are rare, but nonetheless described in detail in medical textbooks—"only once in a blue moon."

As a result of their professional training, many also distinguished, and felt comfortable dismissing, small or negligible risks as "theoretical," ignorable in day-to-day practice.

Thus, ill doctors, in facing knowledge of their disease, may either over- or under-diagnose themselves, worrying too much or too little in evaluating the risks they face. As described earlier with regard to self-diagnosis, the difficulty of maintaining objectivity can lead to either of two extremes: "medical student disease" or "post-residency disease."

Yet even these doctors reported that despite their training, they were not always clear what "the numbers" on diagnostic tests meant in terms of clinical implications or prognoses. How much should one worry about a 40 percent risk of an event? These doctors, too, sought subjective interpretations of quantitative data (e.g., conclusions that a particular percentage of risk was "good," "bad," or "great," or that tissue was "dead" or "injured," a more definitive status). Albert, who had an MI on the highway, wondered how to interpret percentages, and was surprised that doctors didn't anticipate his routine inquiries about such interpretations. For example, did a 10 percent occlusion mean a high or low risk of arrhythmia? "I tend to show images to patients," Albert said, referring to radiographic photos. He explained:

It creates an image of candor, which is good. But as a patient, I didn't say, "Show me exactly where the lesions are." If I went through it again, I would tell my doctor: "I don't know anything about coronary circulation. My big concern is: How bad is my heart disease?...I know certain segments are not at all good, but what's the more general impression?" Radiologists should say, "The left anterior descending is clear, it's great. Unfortunately, on the periphery there are a couple of lesions." But instead, radiologists say, "sixty percent occlusion of your left marginal." I have to ask specifically, "How likely is a sudden arrhythmia? Is this an area of the heart where lethal arrhythmias are likely to occur? What about sudden death on the treadmill? Is everything downstream from these lesions nonviable?" They should have anticipated questions of that nature. You expect them to say, "Most of your circulation is good." They could have told me, "An area about the size of a half dollar doesn't contract the rest of the heart. We assume it's dead or injured...." But instead, they just said, "You've got these two lesions we're going to treat medically, and follow in six months."

Albert's doctors sought to avoid committing themselves to *specific meanings* of statistics.

Hence, physicians use an argot, a coded form of language with which they feel comfortable and that serves several functions, giving them senses of certitude, of providing an answer, and of "covering themselves" against error due to misinterpretation. At times, doctors "hid behind" the numbers, in part reflecting the reality that unknown factors may play key roles in treatment. Ultimately, ambiguity still haunted these statistical pronouncements.

Researching One's Own Disease

"We know very little," Roxanne, the gastroenterologist, said, referring to the medical literature on the causes of cancer. As suggested above, once ill, many of these physicians came to reassess the role of research in individual medical decisions, and became more critical in their evaluations of research as a whole. Roxanne, for example, became more sensitive to the elusiveness of "the truth," no longer thinking there was just one answer. "People base things on the literature and on one paper that's not been duplicated. I'm skeptical. There's a lot of literature, but also *fashions*—things used in the past. Now we're into other treatment approaches. We can't cure anything." Indeed, these ill physicians appeared previously to have paid little heed to the implications of this pattern.

In general, over the course of their careers, doctors—even if healthy—may increasingly come to be wary of scientific data, and to rely more on their own ever-growing clinical experience. With passing years, a few of the physicians here had become more cautious or even nihilistic about medical knowledge. John, the public health official, became more skeptical about much of what the profession had to offer, appreciating the limitations.

> As doctors get older, they recognize the shortcomings of their profession more. I don't have rosy glasses on anymore. Medicine gives you a lot of power, for good *or* bad.

Yet diagnosis with a serious illness deepened and accelerated this process of reassessment, compelling these doctors to challenge their assumptions even more.

Given this wariness, doctors then had to decide how much to seek research and statistics related to their disease. One approach for handling the intense anxiety of having a serious disease was "trying not to think about it." However, most sought rather to gather as much scientific data as possible about their diagnoses. Only a few did not look up articles on their disorder. Jacob reported, "I don't avoid it, but I don't *get into it*. I'm at a very good psychological state, so why mess it up?" He exercised conscious avoidance. His wife also actively pursued information for him.

But most physicians eagerly pursued additional statistics and information. Many immediately checked the literature and researched their illness extensively through Medline searches. Jim, the drug company researcher, for example, had regularly investigated other medical topics as part of his job. He currently did the same for his own disease.

> I've got files of articles on leukemia and bone marrow transplants now, the way I do about clinical trial designs. I search and keep on top of things. You can't avoid that.

The physicians drew on their research skills, critically reading and noting limitations of any one study, the complex variables involved. Jim continued:

> Being a *researcher* helped me as a patient—knowing that treatments and experiments don't always work. A simple thing—a tiny hidden variable—can confound a very complex molecular biology experiment.

Particular skills and experiences as a physician could prove especially valuable.

At the extreme, some felt that, in fact, "the literature lies." Jacob thought so, since, he felt, only confirmatory findings got published. Consequently, he challenged the reliability of the literature as a basis for making decisions. Yet his attitude may also reflect rationalization—part of his decision to avoid reading the literature concerning his diagnosis. Many felt disappointed by the limited generalizability of much of medical research. For example, in estimating prognoses, medical literature spoke of group means, but not individual patients. Juan, a clinician, felt frustrated that prognoses were based on medians not specific to him.

> They've got all these statistical estimates of survival, but they're just estimates. I've said to patients, "I can tell you what percent of people are alive so many months or years after their first pneumonia. But I cannot give you the information for *you*."

He saw researchers as "they"—separate and distant.

Criticism arose, too, of how, increasingly with the growth of medical research, trainees learned from computerized literature searches rather than from patients. Physicians also often consulted medical literature only *superficially*, performing literature searches, but reading merely the abstracts, not the articles themselves. Sally, the internist with cancer who brought her laptop to the ICU, said about her own traditional medical training several decades earlier:

> The patient became your thesis, one a week. You learned an awful lot.... It was patient-based. Now, a patient comes in and the first thing young docs do is a Medline search, and spit out abstracts, and don't read the articles themselves. The docs don't even *get* the article—they just look at the abstract!

Cold Hard Facts: The Roles of Cognitive and Emotional
Expectations in the Receipt of Information

"The night before my surgery, I was told I had a 5 percent chance of
dying," Herb said. "That night I couldn't sleep. If I had been told instead
that I had a 95 percent chance of surviving, I would have slept better."

Many of these doctors became more aware of, and sensitive to, how
statistics were *framed*. Repeatedly, issues arose not only of what the
statistics were, but also of how they were *presented*. In particular, their
physicians provided medical knowledge in ways that often failed to acknowledge or address patients' emotional needs. These ill doctors now
realized both the degree to which providers did not present information
with a full sense of the patient as a person, and the elusiveness of receiving information "objectively." Rather, they became more cognizant
of how inevitability data are subjectively framed.

These doctors saw colleagues as thinking that provision of medical
information in fact obviated the need to support patients emotionally.

Not uncommonly, practitioners conveyed diagnoses and other medical information with little sense of the patient's consequent emotional
state. In fact, they sometimes provided medical information in ways that
not only lacked empathy, but were brutal and harsh. Herb was told he
had an MI without any sense of how he might respond emotionally to
the news.

> A resident said, "I'm really sorry to say that you infarcted." I didn't
> hear that from the cardiologist. Nobody said, "That's a bum
> break," or "That's a surprise—I wouldn't have thought...." No-
> body sat down and said what the implications would be. The
> cardiologist only said, "On the basis of this, we're moving on to this
> next procedure."

Against the emotional distress caused by disease, medical information
often did not shield as much as doctors had assumed. As Mark said, "I
was surprised that I was as shocked and numb as I was when I found out I
was HIV-positive." Routinely, he had told patients who tested positive,
"We don't know what the test means, exactly, and many patients do well
for many years." But now, having been diagnosed with HIV himself,
none of these approaches helped him. Previously, he had seen these
prognostic statements as beneficial in themselves. Now, he felt that many

physicians overvalued medical knowledge as almost "magically" therapeutic in and of itself.

Once ill, these doctors often made decisions about their medical care,
not as doctors, but as emotional human beings—based not on "science,"
but on subjectivity. From different experts, Walter received conflicting
recommendations about treatment. In the end, he based his final decision
on his own sense that he just was *not emotionally prepared* to undergo a
bone marrow transplant.

> From three very bright doctors, I had three different opinions
> about what to do. One said his instinct would be to monitor care-
> fully, and not do a bone marrow transplant. I was going to be
> scientific, think it through. Then, I realized *I just wasn't emotion-
> ally ready* to do the bone marrow transplant: I was convinced I
> would die, because I had been so sick. It may not have been very
> rational, but *it wasn't science for me.* All that science later, I realized
> I was scared to do the transplant.

Walter was surprised that he adopted a nonscientific approach and that
his doctors, too, made recommendations based in part on their "instinct"
(i.e., not wholly rational logic). Medical training had schooled him that
doctors proceeded otherwise.

Recommendations based on quantitative medical tests might in fact
conflict with patients' physical and emotional states. Despite his work as a
drug company researcher, Jim came to recognize the importance of
weighing not only "the numbers," but patients' affective states. "If I was
feeling really tired and knocked out, a lot of times the doctors would have
transfused me. But I said, 'I don't want to be bothered with it now. I'm ok.'
Sometimes I don't know *how* I felt those things. I just did." Jim implicitly
weighed the risks and benefits, including the affective costs that he valued
more than his doctors did. As a patient, he acted much less like a scientist
than he thought he would. He now experienced these decisions far differently than heretofore.

Many of these doctors became more aware not only of the critical role
of psychological factors in the desire for and receipt of information, but
also of the *disparity* and dissonance between information and needs for
support and reassurance. These physicians now perceived, as they had not
before, how emotional needs overlapped with, but were distinct from,
"technical" information. Jeff, the adolescent medicine specialist, added:

I think about a friend who's a pediatrician and a single mom and had a baby, and her perception of what it's like to be a mom with the baby crying at 2 A.M., calling her physician with basically what she, as a physician, would think is a stupid call, but she's living it. Being a patient, you're able to relate so much better to what people go through.

At the same time, despite increased awareness of the degree to which fears shaped patients, these physicians described the competing pressures they nonetheless faced to provide their own patients with quantitative data rather than emotional reassurance. As mentioned earlier, doctors may be becoming more procedure-oriented partly because of decreasing amounts of time they have with patients, and higher rates of reimbursement for high-tech procedures than for low-tech physical exams. In many situations, tests provide ready answers. Harry, the internist and war refugee, said, "Nowadays, when you have ten minutes per patient, you send patients for complicated technical tests that tend to solve your problem much more rapidly." Dan, the oncologist with chest mets, described interns as very "procedure-oriented," because they had less clinical experience, and hence less confidence in their clinical observations and interpretations. Yet these hi-tech tests were inherently limited, too.

Ill physicians also received "cold" presentations of data as a result of dynamic interactions and collusion with their treating physicians. Specifically, their own doctors often did not frame prognoses as optimistically as possible because of assumptions that these physicians-patients wanted only "the cold, hard facts." These ill doctors were commonly presumed to know more than they did about their own disease by their physicians-of-record.

Yet at times, *ill physicians themselves actively contributed to such assumptions* by wanting to be perceived as fellow physicians rather than as patients. For example, as a patient, Jennifer found that her physicians treated her as a colleague, not as a patient, and presented "the facts" to her unadorned, rather than with emotional sensitivity. Yet she recognized that she fueled their impressions.

I wanted somebody to be warm and fuzzy with me. But I wasn't saying, "Hi, be warm and fuzzy with me." I just assumed they would know that's what I wanted—somebody to hold my hand, and say it was really going to be ok. But nobody was doing that. In fact, my doctors had a very pessimistic outlook for me. They said,

"Oh, just read this article," and assumed that I just wanted very objective information. But I didn't. I just wanted to be taken care of like everybody else. They thought I could sift through all the data and make my decisions. Maybe I presented that image, but *I was just as scared as anybody else would be.*

These sick doctors had trouble reconciling these two responses (scientific and simply scared), suggesting the degree to which two different parts of the brain appeared to be involved: one part believed "the numbers" can comfort patients, and the other part sought, as a patient, emotional support—not numbers alone. Indeed, functional MRI research has illustrated how different neurological areas are engaged in varying cognitive and emotional processes (12). At times, wide gaps separated these conflicting approaches.

When seeing their own physicians, other psychological defenses and social interactions prompted ill doctors to cling to the role of physician rather than yield to occupy the position of a "weak" and vulnerable patient. Jennifer continued:

I make it sound like it's all these doctors' faults who didn't treat me like a patient. But I probably participated in that, too: I may have gone in there like "I know everything." *I was in my own denial.*

Moreover, a number of ill doctors at first wanted "hard facts," but then found these difficult to accept. Walter wished to see his X-rays, yet found himself then resisting their interpretation and the diagnosis. It was one thing to want to be told "the truth" matter-of-factly, but another to acknowledge it. He said:

Because I was a doctor, the technician showed me my X-rays. I actually carried them to the radiologist. It was stupid: I didn't think it was tumor. My denial was such that even though this was my fourth go-around, I thought it was an obstruction from adhesion. I was totally aghast when the radiologist showed me the scan and tumor was everywhere.

Walter's hope overcame his intellectual appraisal of his own medical history.

The approach of some treating physicians—to provide only the "brute facts"—suggested, too, both their discomfort with having colleagues become ill, and their misunderstanding of patients' needs.

Accepting Versus "Defying" the Odds: Optimism Versus
Pessimism in Framing and Interpreting Statistics

Ill doctors varied widely in defining, specifically, "good odds." How
should one interpret risks, especially those that are less than 50 percent
(e.g., a 40 percent chance of death)—present, but not probable? Uncertainty affected these doctors differently. Overall, psychological tendencies toward "optimism" or "pessimism," and over- or underestimation
of odds shaped risk assessments. Often, *tripartite views*—as emotional
human beings, as doctors, and as patients—interacted, combining or
clashing. Again, these views underlined the inherently *subjective* nature
of much of medical discourse and information.

A few tried calmly to "accept" the possibility of bad outcomes, seeking a variety of reasons to support their views. Brian, who had hepatitis,
said, "I had a one-in-three chance of the medication clearing up my
infection. It was a long shot. But those were the odds." He felt he should
not fret, since he had limited power to alter this fate. He thought he did
what he could to shape the outcome.

> I didn't think about it much. My biopsy showed I have mild dis-
> ease. Presumably, it's been there twenty years. So I am good to live a
> whole bunch more. It could change, but why worry about some-
> thing you have no control over? I have *some* control. I take care of
> myself, eat well, and don't drink much alcohol. But I don't fret.

In supporting this attitude, Brian thus cited five factors that he took into
account (e.g., his disease was mild, and his prognosis was not bleak).

Others struggled to be optimistic. Jim, the drug company researcher
with leukemia, wrestled with how to view the fact that his chance of a
good prognosis was significantly less than 100 percent. He routinely assessed the odds of treatment effectiveness for other patients, but was unsure how to evaluate these for himself.

> Even with a "favorable" prognosis, my chance of being alive five
> years later is between one third and one half. Maybe treatments and
> supportive care are a lot better than they were, but the odds of
> them being successful depend on a lot of factors, and are good, but
> not 100 percent. When you get a cold, you get better 100 per-
> cent of the time. *There's no guide to thinking about how "good" odds
> are not always good.*

The definition and criteria of "good" can be unclear, and ultimately illusory.

Despite efforts to remain "objective," emotional biases in interpretations of data and pessimistic beliefs—at times irrational—crept in. Common cultural beliefs about luck and fate conflicted with scientific perspectives on the occurrence of random events. Scott, the physician with the infected foot, for example, felt he had "bad luck," and had to remind himself that chance events occurred independently. Even doctors could at times believe they were somehow "cursed."

> I'm not a religious person, but how could all these things happen? *Why me?* Bad luck. I don't know if that's true. Maybe it's one of those old wives' tales: if you have a negative perspective, small events can become bigger. If you start flipping a coin, you can get 100 heads in a row. But the odds of the next one being heads or tails will still be 50–50. So there's an aggregate of events, but that doesn't change the odds of what the next event is going to be: they *are* random.

Still, Scott had trouble believing that he had not somehow been fated to get sick. He grappled with his fears, though they conflicted with his rationality.

With patients, clinicians may contribute to optimism or pessimism. Doctors may underestimate and under-explain risks to patients—especially iatrogenic risks, about which providers may feel guilty or awkward. As one surgeon said, "Medicine systematically underestimates the complications we cause in messing with people's bodies." Such minimization of risks may reflect physicians' discomfort regarding the possibility of iatrogenic side effects. Anne suggested, too, that physicians' hubris biases them in defining their "success." This optimistic bias may reflect magical thinking, too. As we will see, doctors themselves may exercise an important magically-imbued *placebo effect*.

Questions emerged as to what constitutes an "appropriate" amount of fear, and how to make that determination. Certain physicians appeared pessimistic, overly afraid of bad but rare events in ways that appeared out of proportion to the likelihood of such events actually occurring. Perception of risks to oneself may be shaped by a variety of factors, from personal to professional. Walter said, "Doctors don't often understand statistics or bell curves. You may emotionally feel very compelled to treat. The people who most often opt for surgery say, 'Get this out of me.' " This tendency may contribute to these physician-patients seeking more ag-gressive treatment.

Trainees in particular seemed overly influenced by observations of rare but severe complications of treatments or disease in patients, though the odds of such events remained small. For example, Suzanne, who had bipolar disorder, refused to take a drug because of its risk of causing Stevens-Johnson syndrome, which she had witnessed in a patient.

> My psychiatrist suggested Lamictal, but my answer was 'no,' be-cause of Stevens-Johnson syndrome: I met one patient who can't move her arm now. That's enough for me!

Because she had less clinical experience, such an event may have influenced Suzanne more than it would older physicians. In fact, the statistical likelihood of Lamictal causing Stevens-Johnson is very low. However, as Tversky and Kahnemann (2) have described, individuals are biased in assessing risks, using, for example, an "availability heuristic" through which they disproportionately weigh vivid *personal experiences* of bad outcomes more than the actual probability of such outcomes occurring.

Trainees appeared to have particular difficulty integrating observations of rare but serious complications with epidemiological data that such extreme complications may in fact be highly unusual. It is not surprising that "medical student disease" results among trainees, who ignore base-line rates of conditions in assessing minor symptoms. The degree to which such misassessments hamper subsequent treatment decisions is not clear, and needs to be probed by researchers. But the fact that a rare but trau-matic event occurred can shape views among physicians (particularly if young) of the odds of its recurring. Indeed, extended, cumulative clin-ical experiences can counter tendencies to overweigh uncommon but traumatic events.

Some doctors felt fatalistic about their own condition, seeing their disease kill their patients. Stuart, the internist with HIV who was now teaching at the university, felt less sanguine about his own prognosis than he would have otherwise. "It was a problem seeing a lot of sickness with patients. So I was pretty pessimistic about my own outcome. I assumed that in five years, I'd be facing severe disease and death."

These doctors had strong views as to whether they would "overcome the odds" or fall victim to "fate." Some felt that despite high probability of a bad event, they would nonetheless *defy* the statistics. In contrast, others accepted the "numbers" as inevitable. Roxanne felt she knew how to evaluate research realistically, by which she meant not assuming that she would magically overcome the odds. "I look at the literature, whereas other people may think they will be the exception." She felt she knew better how to interpret risk. Indeed, she was brutally matter-of-fact about her prognosis.

Still, pessimism may confer psychological advantages. Bill, the Southern radiologist with HIV, said that since he was always expecting the worst, he never felt let down. "A pessimist is never disappointed, an optimist always is. So prepare for the worst and you're pleasantly surprised when it doesn't happen." He felt fortunate ("pretty lucky"), as he had outlived many friends and patients with his diagnosis.

Nonetheless, these predilections could change, due to subsequent research studies and one's own medical course. In viewing and interpreting statistics, Steven, the suburban endocrinologist with HIV, eventually switched from optimism to pessimism:

> I used to be very optimistic, but am becoming pretty pessimistic. I thought I wouldn't progress, but live in a symbiotic relationship with this virus the rest of my life, and it wouldn't destroy my immune system. That didn't happen. It was a real shock. So, as much as I try, I'm just not as optimistic as I was. My counts have fallen very quickly, and just keep going down.

Conversely, improved therapies can reduce pessimism. Jerry, the surgeon-lawyer, said that the first time he allowed himself to be optimistic was when new treatments for HIV were announced. Optimism cannot be wholly self-willed. Objective facts can also shape it.

Among these ill physicians, family histories of disease, too, influenced perceptions of risk. To live with even "low risk" (as opposed to "no risk") can be hard. In part, tendencies toward optimism and pessimism may be constitutional—ingrained components of personality. Nancy, the endocrinologist with breast metastases, had always been "fatalistic," expecting something bad to happen—even though she had had a "happy" life.

> I had this weird feeling that something bad is going to happen to me. I've been too lucky. I really felt like the other shoe was about to fall, because of how we lived. My father was a doctor; we had plenty of money. I had a very happy family life. . . .

She felt she got this predilection for fatalism from her father.

> I inherited his trait. He is the world's worst pessimist: everything is
> going to be terrible. Life is always bad. Yet nothing bad has ever
> happened to him either.

Yet, Nancy slipped slightly here, saying, "nothing bad has ever happened," when in fact, she had been battling cancer, now metastatic, for
two years.

At other times, Nancy had felt she might be "lucky," and an "exception" to the odds. Despite the statistics suggesting a bad prognosis,
she suspected she might have "slipped by." For her, "luck" meant defying the odds.

> In the beginning, I thought I had a bad prognosis, but maybe
> skimmed by—maybe I'll be lucky and it won't come back. I
> thought that until it came back.

Nancy tried to maintain a certain daily optimism, though having underlying fatalistic beliefs. On these matters, individuals can thus maintain
seemingly contradictory feelings, attitudes, and behaviors. Sadly, two
months after this interview, she died.

Others, too, verged on denial in automatically "assuming" they would
do well. Jessica, the pediatrician, felt that initially, she never "acknowledged" her disease. "I never really thought I was going to die. The books
said 65 percent of people have at least five years. I always immediately
assumed I was in that 65 percent. It never entered my mind that I wasn't."

Desires to minimize potential risks or believe in defying the odds led
to searches for supporting evidence. At times, their medical knowledge
abetted these physicians in dismissing risks. For example, Jacob read PET
scans, and consequently was able to dispute a radiologist's perception of
a lesion. Though Jacob's interpretation may have been accurate, he illustrated a broader pattern of challenging other physicians' unfavorable
prognostications.

> The radiologist said, "There's an abnormality here." But I know
> a little more about PET scans than most people, and realized I had a
> muscle strain in the same place. *So I was able to explain it away.*

The possibility of multiple interpretations of data can lead these doctors
to dismiss problems, at times too readily or prematurely.

Others merely fantasized about defying the odds. Yet these wishes can have other effects, prompting more aggressive self-treatment. Dan, the oncologist with chest metastases, said, "I think, 'Let's do everything,' since I fantasize about being free of this: taking another dose of radio-iodine, and having the scan come back negative." Dan sought to support this desire to be cured, and make it come true.

> I have the thought that I can be cured 100 percent, which may or may not be reasonable. It's a belief—lots of people support me in that. That's why I am so aggressive: *the way you cure this is to be aggressive.*

Dan had been very assertive throughout his life, and his cancer had now metastasized to his bone—making it terminal, and further fueling his proactivity.

In sum, inherent tendencies toward optimism and pessimism are prevalent, but subject to change. These doctors either accepted or denied objective data to varying degrees. Similarly, physicians may have intrinsic therapeutic styles of nihilism or aggressiveness toward patients. It is not clear whether these, too, change over a physician's lifetime, and if so, how and to what degree. Presumably they do. Moreover, depending on their conditions, these doctors may be therapeutic nihilists with patients, but more aggressive with their own care. These physicians may treat themselves and others very differently.

"Good Denial?"

These ill physicians came to reassess the roles in their lives of overconfidence, denial, and belief in "defying the odds"—whether these attitudes helped or hindered, and how. Though originally employed by psychoanalysts to refer to an unconscious psychological defense mechanism, the term "denial" has clearly permeated popular psychology and culture.

On the one hand, these doctors argued that certain minimization was beneficial. Jessica recognized her use of this defense, but tried to see it as advantageous: "A lot of my thought processes are a form of denial—but *good* denial." Similarly, Walter felt that such minimization aided him in continuing on in his life. "I can have normalcy reassert itself: I'm not really a cancer patient. It's very positive, because I get on with my life."

But how does one know the difference between such "good" and "bad" denial? Indeed, many rationalized that their denial was *purely* beneficial. Tom, whose lover died of AIDS, argued that "positive" denial was in fact healthy:

> Denial can be very dangerous if you do unhealthy things. But it's healthy to use "positive denial" and not get stuck in bad places. "Negative denial" is making believe something's not true, so that you can do things that aren't good for you. If I was in denial and didn't go to the doctor, that would be silly. But not fretting for three days before the labs come back, and not losing sleep because my count's jumped, is positive. I use "positive denial" to say "Not today." That's healthy.

Here, Tom suggested a continuum between "positive" and "negative" denial, with multiple pants in between.

But self-judgments about the two extremes may be hard to make, and not always accurate. Denial can, after all, foster procrastination and impede essential activities. Deborah acknowledged, "Maybe I should plan to die." But she avoided doing so, since she felt she would then become too depressed:

> Maybe I should keep the fact that I might die as a given in my immediate future. But I don't. If I do, I would be very distraught. I want to write a will, which I haven't done.

Deborah delayed, not completing projects or a will—wanting to keep her hope alive.

> I have uncompleted projects that I should complete—relationships that need to be clarified, writing projects I don't want to do, open family issues. I'm procrastinating, completely resisting doing anything about them.

Deborah questioned how hard she should keep pushing and fighting, and wrestling with these demands, or resigning herself to their incompleteness. Sadly, six months after this interview, she died, with many of these projects unaccomplished.

Feelings about an illness can conflict. One can outwardly appear to accept one's illness in many ways, but still inwardly be terrified. Jessica added, "I never dealt with the fact that I had a serious, life-threatening illness. The face I presented to the world was 'I'm fine, coming to work.'

I never dealt with 'I'm vomiting. My hair is falling out.' " Her external self-portrayal reflected, in part, her ambivalence. She maintained "a permanent core—a fear of dying, sadness—somewhere," but did not integrate these fears and disappointments with the rest of her daily life.

Views may differ as to whether a particular individual's denial is good or bad. As we shall see, one's minimization can potentially be both good *and* bad—helpful in certain ways, but harmful in others.

Influencing the Odds Through Magic

Despite their scientific training, many of these ill doctors indulged more overtly and explicitly in superstitious or magical thinking, believing they could alter their fate—occasionally indulging in even more dangerous forms of denial. As suggested earlier, doctors often believed they were invulnerable to disease. Pseudoscience could bolster their sense that they were inherently lucky or invulnerable.

Magical thinking arose concerning not only prognoses but also the etiologies or causes of disease. Jim, the drug company researcher, was usually very scientific, but was superstitious about the cause of his lymphoma: a fortune cookie may have precipitated it.

> I was cleaning out my night table, and came across a fortune from a Chinese restaurant fortune cookie. I had thrown it in there shortly before I got sick. It read, "You will soon be crossing the great waters," which I now understand is an expression for passing into the next world. I had assumed it meant: you're going to be taking some *big trip*. I tore it into little pieces, and thought: I'm through with this now! This has been sitting next to my head for two years, and now I'm getting rid of it, and feeling better because I'm getting rid of it. *Here is the source of what's happening to me.* This has been causing my lymphoma! I shouldn't have kept it.

Others drew on folk beliefs and old wives' tales. Anne found herself thinking about cultural beliefs with which she had grown up in rural Switzerland: that if you eat a piece of fruit on the first day of spring, it will bring you good luck for the year. Since her diagnosis, she has made a point of eating a fresh plum each year on that day. As a scientist, she realized that this act probably would not help her. But she proceeded, given the low cost of doing it, and the onslaught of her cancer.

The Weighing of Risks

Even those who accepted the statistics had to decide *how to weigh or value these risks*. How important were various less-than-lethal side effects, compared to potential benefits? As patients, they often now balanced risk and benefit data differently than they had as physicians. They also acquired increased awareness of how physicians and patients *differed* in evaluating risks and benefits. Physicians may recognize the possibility of a particular side effect, but *weigh* that risk differently than the patient would. As mentioned earlier, Suzanne, who was on lithium, lamented that her colleagues did not sufficiently value adverse effects such as weight gain and its implications (e.g., having difficulty finding a partner). Likewise, Pascal, the Lebanese internist, spoke of how identification with patients led him now not to "blow off mild symptoms."

In short, these physicians based many decisions on irrational, subjective factors and emotional states. Statistical data about risks and benefits served as a kind of Rorschach test that recipients viewed and interpreted in a variety of subjective ways. Previous experiences, attitudes, and perspectives shaped these doctors' approaches toward data in treating patients and themselves. Indeed, other research has shown that the physician's "practice style," not the patient's prognosis, affects the number of tests doctors order in ICUs (13).

Relatedly, patients, and to a lesser degree, physicians, did not fully understand the meanings of numbers alone, and consequently wanted qualitative verbal interpretations of data (e.g., "good" or "bad"). However, studies have demonstrated that numerical presentations of data are more effective than verbal ones, and less subject to individual variation. Nonetheless, neither quantitative nor qualitative data were always easy to obtain.

Consequently, in presenting statistics to patients, doctors need to be highly aware of these emotional and interpersonal factors. This need has several implications for education and care. For example, the Internet may never fully replace human contact in providing data, since only through face-to-face contact can a physician read and respond to nonverbal, as well as verbal, emotional cues. Medical education also can better sensitize trainees to how and to what extent patients perceive and weigh risks and benefits differently than do providers.

Voodoo and Herbs: Judging Complementary and Alternative Medicines

Complementary and alternative medicine (CAM) threw into bold relief many of these complexities and conflicts concerning assessments of medical information, and had particular implications. Every year, Americans spend as much as $47 billion on CAM (14), and most use CAM in some way (14, 15, 16). In recent years, CAM has received increased attention in the medical literature, with researchers arguing both pro and con. Ill physicians now had to face the possibilities of using these non-Western treatments for themselves. Many remained wary, evaluating claims scientifically, while others became more appreciative of the possible benefits—often despite their own prior biomedical education and long-instilled caution.

Biases Against CAM

Despite claims of benefits from CAM, and the threats from their own illness, a few physicians nevertheless maintained long-standing biases toward Western medicine. Brian, who had hepatitis C, said:

> I'm not averse to alternative treatments. A friend says, "You can't believe in Western medicine alone." But my epistemological approach to data is very scientific. With the one medication, I had a 30 percent chance to clear this disease. I didn't make it, but I took the chance. What are the numbers with milk thistle? I have no idea. Will it help? It could. Can it do any harm? Probably not. So I'll take it. But I'm not going to give up one for the other, unless there's compelling evidence. Indian medicine and meditation might be effective, but you have to really believe in it. I don't know if I'm going to spend that much time learning it to believe in it.

As Brian indicated, he conducted a complex risk-benefit analysis of using CAM, thinking through arguments for and against. He also felt a patient had to *believe* in it—suggesting that it operated in part through a placebo effect.

Doctors can harbor strong biases against CAM, but not recognize them. In contrast, lay patients may perceive and resent this prejudice, and hold it against physicians, seeing conflicts of interest. Jeff, the adolescent specialist, said that his support group mistrusted doctors who were thought to "conspire" against CAM.

> I hear from ten guys who aren't in medicine what it's really like from their perspective: the mistrust. They feel like there's a conspiracy by physicians and pharmaceutical companies against alternative medicine: doctors and drug companies are in cahoots.

Yet physician wariness of CAM may stem simply from its being unproven. Medical education teaches skepticism and rigorous questioning of claims of treatment efficiency. Hence, when seeing media reports concerning treatment, physicians may be cautious. Stuart said, "I don't get stampeded by the popular media or the alternative medicine community. I can read between the lines."

"Faith" in CAM

Nevertheless, as patients, some of these physicians reversed their attitudes and became more favorably inclined toward non-Western treatments. Despite being trained to view alternative approaches with suspicion, several ill doctors began to use such modalities themselves. Charles even conducted underground studies on alternative therapies for his HIV.

> My bubble's been popped as far as thinking that Western medicine is the only approach. In medical school, I was only taught about acupuncture. Yet in my mind, it works, and is finally being approved. Still, it was "voodoo," "ridiculous."

At times, these doctors changed their views seemingly despite themselves. Many came to reassess the value of approaches that had not been scientifically "proven" to work. They recognized more that studies were limited, in part because of obstacles to giving patients appropriate randomized placebo controls. Scott, the internist with the infected foot, was surprised that a treatment ended up working, since he felt his physician was "doing voodoo."

> The skin graft doctor was doing all kinds of unproven stuff: "We don't really know, but we'll try it." He put this therapeutic boot on me. I said, "I looked this thing up, there's absolutely no science on it." He goes, "Yup." But it helped. He said, "Look how well you're doing with this thing on, and there's absolutely no science

behind it: no randomized, controlled clinical trial." It's hard to randomize putting somebody into a cast.

To their surprise, even many who were reluctant to pursue CAM found that it could help. Walter, the politically active internist, said:

Somebody said, "Go see this Chinese herbalist." So I went. It all felt strange, and he wrote out a prescription for Chinese herbs. I went back every two months. When my doctor worked me up, my blood counts came back normal! He was quite convinced that it wasn't going to happen. It may have happened on its own. But maybe the Chinese herbs really did something.

Often, appreciation of CAM and of spirituality increased together, linked. Tom, whose lover died of AIDS, became more open to both these entities. Though drawn to Eastern philosophy beforehand, his affinities now grew. ("Sometimes Western medicine's wrong or stupid. We don't fucking know. We make believe we know, have answers.") Tom reported having lost "*faith*" in Western medicine, intimating the degree to which such matters are, at least partly, those of nonscientific *belief*.

If nothing else, some felt CAM deserved more of a place in medicine because of its potential placebo effect. As Herb, the neonatologist with an MI, said the odds of it working may be small, but not nil.

When my father had metastatic prostate disease, he went to a woman in long white robes up on a stage. The probability that that's going to help anyone is extremely small—but isn't zero. We've got nothing else to do, why not do that? I've always thought the placebo effect was extremely powerful. Your thoughts influence your body, change the way you are. Without explanation, certain physical things can happen. You could probably influence the blood supply and wiring of your heart.

As Herb also inferred, the potential risks of CAM appeared small, and the benefits, huge.

Judgment Calls

Still, even if open to CAM, individuals faced practical questions, unable to try all the CAM options available and reputed to be effective. Patients had to evaluate and compare. As Walter concluded, "I have friends who will try anything. I draw my own limits: 'This is what I'm willing to try, and why.' I just don't have the time and energy to do *everything* you can do."

Though lumped together as a single category, CAM appeared not to be monolithic, but a broad, diverse label that covered treatments with varying degrees of supportive or suggestive evidence. Among nonscientific approaches, these doctors tried to establish criteria for evaluating CAM claims. Charles, the HIV-infected underground researcher, developed several gauges.

> There is a lot of baloney out there. I can separate better than a
> layman what was real from unreal, legitimate from illegitimate. It
> had to meet three criteria: have some scientific or clinical experi-
> ence behind it, be relatively nontoxic, and be available. If it met all
> three of those, there was a good possibility I would try it.

Overall, two critical factors interacted here to affect openness to CAM: the risk involved in the modality and the availability of Western treatment options.

Jacob pursued what he saw as "Jewish" alternative healing, and denigrated other CAM. "The only nonproven stuff that we are allowed to do is Jewish stuff. We do it because the Jewish tradition says it. I consider the other stuff idol worship."

Still, in the end, CAM decisions frequently necessitated difficult judgments. As Nancy said, "It was kind of *a call*" (i.e., not a fact).

Critics may see these beliefs in CAM and spirituality as unscientific, but these doctors wrestled with these issues, varying in skepticism and faith, and generally leaning strongly one way or the other. No doubt, readers of these pages will be split, too, as to the legitimacy of these unproven beliefs. Indeed, conflicts between science and religion, and reason and emotion, have occupied Plato, Pascal, Voltaire, Diderot, and countless others for centuries. In their beliefs, these sick doctors fell across a wide spectrum, reflecting in part the tensions they faced in their roles as physicians and as patients.

In all, patienthood challenged these doctors' assumptions about medical knowledge, and compelled them to reflect on and alter their perspectives. They confronted uncertainties in both their personal and their professional lives. They felt they knew how to interpret statistics, and did not get hung up on the possibility of unlikely side effects. Yet medical knowledge had drawbacks: knowing about "the things the doctor doesn't say" and possible medical errors. Knowledge could serve denial, too.

These ill doctors assessed their own diagnoses differently than those of their patients. Many became more critical of the medical literature, seeing it as falling short, referring only to group means, not addressing individual patients' needs, and even "lying." Many were stunned to receive only "the cold, hard facts" from their physicians.

They varied in how they weighed medical information: whether they accepted or believed they would defy the odds, were pessimists or optimists, engaged in "good" or "bad" denial, and became more open to complementary and alternative medicine. Regarding CAM, some of these doctors had faith, while others remained biased or faced difficult judgment calls.

Medical professionalization shaped these views. Trainees, lacking years of experience and accumulated examples of treatments, often approached risks and benefits differently than did more senior colleagues, overreacting to traumatic cases. Consequently, medical education aims to develop intuition about complex data. Yet how, exactly, does this training instill such acumen? Various adages help, such as "common things happen commonly" and "beware of 'zebras.'" Medical school also inculcates the notion of "theoretical" risks that are extremely low but still exist, and hence, technically, not theoretical. Conversely, "medical student disease" can be seen as resulting from insufficient development of such intuition among trainees.

These doctor-patients revealed, too, the extent to which emotions molded perceptions of risks, and vice versa. Risks fueled anxiety and depression that can in turn influence other decisions, and even disease processes themselves. Ergo, feedback loops exist, as risk perceptions and emotions affect each other. Even anticipation of these emotions can alter interpretations of risks.

Individuals ranged, too, in the degree to which they sought statistics, from avoidance to active pursuit. Presentations of information varied as well. Physicians-of-record often assumed that these ill doctors knew or wanted only the "brute" facts. And even these ill doctors found it hard to challenge their providers' presentations of information. Patients may abet, not correct, their physicians' assumptions, suggesting a degree of collusion. However, such interactions concerning the framing of statistics, including desires not to challenge physicians' expectations of patients, have been under-investigated.

Individuals vary in the precise point at which too much information overwhelms and confuses them. Even among these physicians, capacities and interest in handling numerous, at times conflicting, variables ranged widely. What doctors did not say played a role here as well. Providers' relative emphases revealed styles and biases—as aggressive "overdoers" or minimalists.

Though heuristics and biases that physicians should avoid have been identified, countervailing pressures increase the use of these subjective factors. Even these doctor-patients often used, relied on, and wanted verbal, rather than numerical, presentations of data.

The fact that these doctor-patients were surprised by the importance of these issues is itself surprising, highlighting how much professional socialization impedes awareness of these issues. These physicians' use of statistics reflected a vocabulary, a thought process of probabilistic reasoning, and a set of attitudes—about the knowability and predictability of medical outcomes—instilled in them through their training, both cognitively and emotionally. These uses of statistics suggest underlying attitudes about how uncertain future events may, in fact, be predicted. The fact that patients seek meaning in statistics (e.g., "Do I have to worry or not?") pressures providers, and no doubt fosters the continued use of qualitative verbal expressions, despite their limitations. Such desires for certitude may also contribute to physicians ordering increasing numbers of tests and procedures.

Providers, patients, and their families should be as aware as possible of these areas. To patients and their families, doctors must carefully explain statistics and assess understandings of these complicated calculations. Providers need to realize, far more than presently, how much their views and approaches toward statistics can vary from patients'.

8

"Being 'Strong'"

Workaholism, Burnout, and Coping

Inevitably, as their illness progressed, many of these doctors had to consider the possibility of giving up their work, either partially or fully, which forced them to evaluate the many meanings of their careers. For these physicians, work provided structure, gratification, and income, all of which illness now threatened. These doctors revealed how deeply ingrained professionalism remained. They struggled with problems that all physicians—and professionals in other fields—will one day face.

Workaholism: The Meanings of Work

Work had taken on enormously important personal significance for these doctors. Many spontaneously described themselves as "workaholics" for a variety of reasons, and with both good and bad effects. On the one hand, workaholism resulted from dedication to the profession and to the practice of medicine. Yet it provided, too, benefits in their personal lives, permitting them to avoid issues such as forming or maintaining relationships, or confronting their own diagnoses. Magical beliefs about work also often molded views of jobs, both before and after diagnosis.

External factors promoted workaholism: implicitly, the profession of medicine itself expected such dedication. Kurt explained, "I feared that if I stopped, I would be left behind.... You could spend every waking moment reading, and still not know it all."

These doctors saw the profession as demanding, and rewarding, such conscientiousness. In fact, medicine may preselect for individuals who value such commitment. Jessica, the pediatrician with cancer, said she was "the sort of person who never calls in sick"—indeed, a dedicated and compulsive type. She didn't want her life disrupted because of her illness, but consequently received suboptimal care. From this trait, she derived pride, self-esteem, and structure. Single, her life focused on her work.

Workaholism resulted from financial motives as well. Some physicians tried to treat more patients, so that if they were forced to go on disability, their income would be higher. Steven, the suburban endocrinologist, confessed:

> I need to see as many patients as possible, in case I get sick. The more income you make, the more disability you get. Patients want me now. If I get sick, they won't.

Poor self-esteem perpetuated workaholism, too. Kurt, the internist with HIV who had spiraled downward after using crack, had previously tried to compensate for his past by earning professional kudos.

> I was gay, and never felt good enough in anything I did: athletics, pretty girlfriends. I could only get affirmation by academic achievements. I wanted it to go on.

Indeed, many of these physicians were heavily influenced by how others saw them.

Workaholism resulted as well from other psychological motives, such as past traumas. Despite his illness, Frank, the surgeon who had an MI in the OR, continued to work long days. A refugee, his current ambition arose in part from his precarious history. "When I was younger, for me to work fourteen to eighteen hours a day was not unusual. It's not that unusual even now."

By comparison, other rewards paled. Only work—not materialism or conspicuous consumption—bolstered Neil's self-esteem. "If I worked really hard, people would love me. I bought a Jaguar convertible, and did very materialistic things, but they did not make me happy."

Workaholism also justified spending less time with others in one's personal life. David, the psychiatrist with HIV, said, "If I am working all the time, then I have an excuse for not having a social life." Stuart added about friends:

> They'd let you tell them anything, and they'd believe it. But then I came to realize that it *was* important to remember birthdays, stay in touch with friends....

Socially awkward physicians could hide behind a professional cloak, and interact with others as "doctors"—rather than merely as "human beings."

Physicians who used their profession to avoid intimate responsibilities had an excuse that could not be readily challenged. Eleanor said about her husband:

> It made it really easy for him to avoid dealing with interpersonal relationships. It sounds so socially acceptable: "I have to see my patients." What's the response? "Let them drop dead"? It left me with a very strange sense of where I figured in his hierarchy.

Workaholism Post-diagnosis

Illness can either increase or decrease ambition and drive. On the one hand, several of these doctors went to extraordinary lengths to continue to work and remain responsible, even after getting sick. Jim, the drug company researcher with leukemia, bought a cell phone only when he was admitted to the hospital. There, he also hooked up his laptop.

> I never had a cell phone before, so I arranged to get one at that point, because I was going into the hospital. I gave everybody the number so that they could reach me if they couldn't get me on the hospital phone. I brought in my computer and had it hooked up to the phone.

As a result of illness, some worked harder, feeling more committed and deriving maximal meaning from their professional endeavors. Indeed, some felt more committed *because* they were ill. They worked harder now because they identified more with their patients. If they were healthier, several of these doctors thought they might opt for easier practices. Stuart said:

> I might have been more willing to walk away from my practice, or say, "I can do this in the suburbs." Life would be easier. I could be caring for healthier people.

Stuart's perception of other practices may have partly been fantasy, but nonetheless reflected his sense of commitment.

Post-diagnosis, keeping busy helped doctors avoid thinking about their illness. Deborah, the psychiatrist with metastatic breast cancer, said that maintaining her interests, friends, and family permitted her to think less about her disease, and hence sustained her mentally. She knew busyness constituted a form of denial, yet persisted. She spoke haltingly, indicating the degree to which these issues remained hard to discuss.

> My coping is by denial. That's what keeps me alive. I don't really think about it. It's why I don't get depressed. Basically, I work a lot. I'm a workaholic. I get stressed not over the fact that I'm sick, but that I have too many things to do.

Workaholism resulted from "magical thinking" as well. David, a psychiatrist, was aware of his use of this mode of coping, but continued nonetheless:

> It's basically the "myth of productivity." If I can't be sick, then I won't be. If I am very busy, and being sick would be a *tremendous* inconvenience—it just won't happen.

Workaholism can reflect, too, a form of *bargaining*. Neil observed:

> I know I was bargaining—if I took on this and that, see how healthy I am? I will prove to the world that I can do all of this, and be Superdoc. . . . *If I'm really, really good, and help more people, and take on more, and never say no, then I won't get sick. I won't die.* The bargaining was with God or a higher being: if I work really hard . . . You won't let me die.

Neil expressed a folk belief that spirituality can directly improve health. He also felt that his bargaining was effective medically: "Being so active has been very good for my immune system."

Yet ironically, such intensive commitment, while providing personal meaning, can impair health through stress and fatigue. Hard work could precipitate illness through exhaustion. A vicious cycle can ensue. Neil said:

> It's a Catch-22: the harder you work, the more patients get referred to you, the more people want you, the better you feel about yourself. But I'm seeing patients on my day off, which isn't healthy. It's very tough to balance.

Workaholism can also impede one's health by decreasing the quality and quantity of care these doctors accessed for themselves. Jessica, the pediatrician with cancer, said:

> I had my treatment at the local hospital where I work. Who would go there for cancer treatment? I wouldn't; it's not a good hospital.

But I didn't want to disrupt my life. I wanted to be able to go across the street to get treatment. So I went to an oncologist whom I didn't really respect—who was not very smart. I arranged my treatment for Friday afternoons, so that I could miss the minimal amount of work, puke over the weekend, and feel better on Monday to go back to work. I couldn't write or walk up stairs. But it was important to me to keep working. If I had treatment at a better hospital, I probably would've had to give up a whole day. It's craziness, but worked for me. It was therapeutic, kept me sane, and protected me from being depressed.

Jessica's decision to receive treatment at a hospital of lesser quality stemmed in part from masochism and low self-esteem. Her determination served her well professionally and in some ways psychologically, but threatened to exact high health costs. She suggests how she sharply separated her illness and work identity.

On the other hand, illness led some to work *less*. Disease prompted a few doctors to become less obsessive and guilty about their jobs. Their surprise at the benefits of this change illuminated the extent of their prior beliefs. Bradley, for example, was treated for depression after his MI, and subsequently altered his values:

I've become more relaxed. I can get up and walk home, and leave a mess here—much more than I used to. My capacity to absorb unfinished business has been much better. I do not feel guilty about it. In the past, my Protestant work ethic didn't let me leave loose ends.

Only illness compelled Bradley to change.

These alterations in demeanor can reflect deeper shifts in personality and behavior, and reassessments of priorities and values. Such alterations may become visible only when physicians confront such intense stress. Frank, the surgeon whose MI occurred in the OR, reported that after his illness, his personality changed.

I was very quick-tempered and temperamental, and didn't hold back. If I felt angry, I screamed. Once in a while, I was almost irrational—too angry, considering the event. The yearly resident show imitates me in the OR, as quick-tempered, furious—rage reactions. But I used to pull that more. That's how I got an MI: I got furious in an emergency situation. I pushed a patient into the OR myself. Since then, it's much more controlled. Instead of getting into a real fight, if I see this coming, I will walk away, and come back and discuss it when I feel better. I also take a beta-blocker. It takes the edge off—as a placebo or not, it doesn't matter. I recognized that a temper was unhealthy, and I modified it.

Frank still strove to balance his commitment against his reprioritized values. He didn't want to "die with my professional boots on," but nevertheless continued to work hard.

Still, many doctors wrestled with questions of how much, exactly, to decrease their dedication, when to do so, and how to decide. Brian, the internist with hepatitis C, lowered his zeal due not his illness per se, but to the fact that he was passed over for a promotion as a result of his diagnosis.

For all the work and time I put in the institution, I wasn't chosen as director—rewarded. It made me step back and say, I'm not going to kill myself for stuff that's basically temporary. I put my heart into work, but if I don't get it done, it's not going to get done. I'll do it tomorrow. I'll leave at five or six instead of eight.

Brian cut his hours to a small, but still significant, extent.

Burnout

The workaholism and intense dedication elicited by the profession also reduced balance in these doctors' lives, facilitating burnout—especially when they were ill. Even before becoming sick, many physicians grappled with burnout. Frequently these feelings now increased. Illness prompted sadness and frustration. These doctors then had to figure out how to cope, and generally felt they had to choose between acting strong (as doctors) and emotional (as patients).

The profession offered an ostensible benefit in enabling members to avoid personal social commitments, but a self-reinforcing cycle could then ensue. Stuart, now teaching at the university, observed about colleagues, "They get too emotionally involved with patients, not allowing themselves enough free time to enjoy other things. Some doctors don't have a life." Little variation in one's job, and frustrations with patients, can further contribute to this frustration (e.g., "giving the same spiel to every patient, and they don't listen"). Ironically, some felt that an advantage of managed care was to lessen such dangerously high commitment.

Burnout resulted, too, from physicians feeling unappreciated and not thanked enough. Anger can ensue. Stuart continued:

Physicians who get furious at patients are saying, "No one is saying thank you enough." Good compassionate docs want something
more. Some of them translated it into money: "They're not pay-
ing me enough" or "They're cutting into my fees." I realized that
when I got angry and resentful, in part I just wasn't hearing: patients were saying "Thank you," often in a heartfelt way. But I
expected some translation that I didn't hear.

In fighting patients' disease, helplessness, rather than cures, contributed to this frustration.

Should Doctors Not Cry? Coping

These physicians found it hard to access or use external supports that commonly aided their lay patients. Rather, they felt they had to avoid burdening others. Revealingly, having been trained to be "unemotional" when confronting disease, several feared that weeping would be "weak." "I wasn't sure if I was supposed to cry or not," Deborah said about her reaction to bad test results that she received one day while at work. "I didn't cry. When I got to the clinic, I broke down." Professional norms mitigated against displays of emotionality.

Similarly, in describing the pain of her struggle and secrecy, Suzanne faltered, barely able to articulate the complex loss and shame she felt. She broke into tears, though she had never allowed herself to weep with col-leagues. "I've never cried in front of anybody in my program, but I'm always a little bit ready to."

These physicians felt that their own doctors reinforced this norm of not expressing emotion. At times, physicians-of-record ignored patients' emotional distress, or handled it poorly. For example, Nancy, the en-docrinologist with metastatic cancer, commented about her oncologist, "She immediately tried to medicate away my distress" with anxiolytic medications. Yet Nancy wanted to confront and discuss her terror of dying.

As a defense against distressing aspects of their disease, many physi-cians engaged in intellectualization. For example, Bradley, the internist who was treated for depression after his MI, decided to consult a neu-ropsychologist to test for any new, ongoing cognitive deficits.

A psychometric workup was my defense against "losing it." I'd
be the last one to know it. That was as intellectual an approach
as I could come up with: recognizing the possibility that I was
slipping, and wanting to be defended against that. I didn't tell
anybody.

Bradley relied on medical tests to diagnose potential problems that, if
present, might have been due more to ongoing depression than to neurological disease. But as a physician, he valued objective tests.

Support from Families

These physicians often found it difficult to avail themselves of family
supports that assist many patients. Frequently, these doctors resisted the
aid their families offered. Many family members thought these professionals knew best how to handle the illness, a reflection in part of these
physicians' own attitudes. As a result, certain family members became
less supportive than they might otherwise have been. Many ill doctors
also sought to protect their families from the difficulties of the disease,
though at times that motivation bordered on rationalization. Other doctors had trouble recognizing that their illness caused their loved ones
anguish and stress. Though a few doctors derived some support from significant others, even then, tensions frequently arose, given differences in
medical expertise between physicians and lay family members.

Several physicians had health professional spouses or children, which
helped in accessing care and making sense of the experience of illness, yet
could pose problems of autonomy and hierarchy. Eleanor said about her
physician-husband:

He'd say, "I don't know how I'd do this without you"—in terms
of logistics and managing his pain meds. I had a lot more power
than a spouse usually would because, as a health professional
myself, I could stop staff dead in their tracks.

Eleanor's assertiveness may have bordered on entitlement, but succeeded.
She added:

The resident said, "We never sedate patients coming out of
a coma." So I went and found the head of the MICU, and said,
"Listen, buddy, this is the situation…" Then they sedated him.

At one point, she also told the doctor, "We need a central line!" Her use of the first person plural here underlines the degree to which spouses can indeed become bonded by the disease, seeing themselves as *together* requesting and receiving care.

Yet doctors often "outranked" their familial support systems, making treatment more difficult. Physicians could pull rank with family members concerning diagnoses, treatment, and prevention. Eleanor added about her husband and daughters:

> Being a physician, "he was 'the expert.' " A lot of patients have denial, but if you're a physician, it gets reinforced. The assumption is: you know what you're doing. It allows you to play both ends against the middle—you can understand the consequences of your behavior while you're busy denying that there are any consequences to not modifying your behavior.

Other physicians concurred with Eleanor's assessment of difficulties in treating sick colleagues. Stuart had cared for several doctor-patients, and further illustrated this problem. "Their caretakers at home were always being browbeaten by the patients saying, 'I know what I'm doing. Don't listen to what the doctor said.' "

Support Groups

These physician-patients found it hard not only to draw on family support, but also to participate in support groups. Generally, these groups contained nonphysicians, and many doctors did not join because of not wanting to have to disclose their illness. Rumors about an ill physician could spread. Awkwardness arose, too, from being "the physician" in the room, and being asked medical questions. Suzanne said, "I went to a group, but was the most functional person there. They asked me tons of questions. It just got to be a pain in the ass." As a result of these obstacles, these physicians had fewer resources to rely on.

In a few cities, formal or informal support groups of physicians began at different points, particularly for HIV. Yet, for a variety of reasons, physicians frequently avoided even these entities. Consequently, over time, these groups waned. Charles, the underground researcher, attended a group of HIV-positive doctors, but eventually, they all died. "It was very small, and didn't last very long. . . ." Jerry, the surgeon-lawyer, attended one such support group, but heard too much negativity and complaining. "Two people whining for two hours. I felt, 'This isn't good for me...or where I want to be.'"

The Medical Expertise Retention Program of the Gay and Lesbian Medical Association has helped many HIV-infected physicians, but the fact that it is run by a gay and lesbian organization deterred some heterosexual doctors.

For physicians from other countries, cultural differences can prove to be obstacles, too, in accessing psychosocial support. Mathilde and her husband were both born in South America. She said, "We belong to another culture and don't believe in support groups." Indeed, the notion of individuals opening up freely to one another in a support group may be somewhat peculiarly American.

Others with HIV also recommended a "buddy system," a national meeting, an anonymous 800 number, or a Web site. Jennifer said:

> Some kind of a network, so people could hook up with at least one other person...for prophylactic treatment and for occupational needle sticks—to provide information, give support.

These mechanisms have yet to be established. However, for many, logistics and confidentiality might pose problems with these approaches as well. Still, these strategies may hold promise, and should be considered by local and national professional organizations.

Self-medication and Self-destruction

Several physicians resorted to various kinds of psychological self-medication—from anti-depressants such as Prozac, to drug and alcohol use, and, in a few cases, even abuse. In the latter cases, downhill spirals could ensue. Kurt lost his job at a large group practice due not to his HIV, but to his lateness and absenteeism because of drug use. Once infected, he resorted to drugs, which furthered his decompensation.

A few doctors, trained to believe they could "control" disease, now could not cope, and medicated these conflicts, or contemplated or attempted to wrest ultimate control over their fatal disease through suicide. These approaches varied from suicidal thoughts to near-fatal actions. Dan, with chest mets, who had been very assertive throughout his life, said:

I have thought, "Is it worth going on? Let me take all these pills, and it will all be over." That's passed: I said, "This is stupid. You have a life ahead of yourself." But I have enough pills to kill an army. I'm not sure why I'm stockpiling them.

Dan reasoned against suicide, but kept the lethal pill supply, wanting to maintain the ability to determine his fate if he decided to.

Shattered by the experience of becoming ill, two doctors, both with HIV, in fact tried to end their lives. Roger, a surgeon, attempted suicide when his diagnosis and sexuality threatened to become public.

With one HIV test, everything came crashing down: my sexuality, and choice of job. I was so ashamed and horrified, I didn't tell anybody. On my birthday, my friends took me out to dinner. No one knew. The only way out was to kill myself. I took some meds from the OR, and went up to the roof, which was closed after midnight, and took all the meds. Several minutes later, two kids came up. I was so embarrassed, I wanted to make it look like an accident. I woke up in the ER.

Roger conveyed disconnectedness between his work as a doctor and the rest of his life, using a dissociated tone. Alex said, "I've always believed in taking control over one's destiny." He, too, tried to overdose, illustrating how hard it can be to reconcile radically disparate parts of oneself—one's illness and one's coherent life as a healer. Some felt they could not otherwise integrate these conflicting roles.

Coping by Setting Limits

Yet other doctors sought and found healthy means to reduce burnout and psychological distress by setting limits in various ways. In essence, they altered their conceptions of physicianhood itself, and doctored less than they had before. Concomitantly, many tried to revitalize their personal lives outside of work. Such efforts sought to counter the workaholism and lack of balance that had contributed to burnout in the first place. Some physicians restricted the size of their clinical practice or the length of their career. Stan, an internist, reflected, "I used to say, 'How can I retire at fifty?' I'm forty-three, so: 'sprint to the finish line and be done.' Now, I say, 'Thank God we're not taking new patients.'"

Diversification of practices countered work stresses. Neil, the neurologist, broadened his patient pool, "doing a headache clinic to diversify, do something easier, and see immediate results."

Other physicians adopted more fixed, regular hours. Mark, interviewed in a diner, said, "I chose a job that was not overly demanding: 9:00 to 4:30, five days a week. No call."

Yet such changes and reprioritizations were not always easy to achieve and maintain. Jacob appreciated life more, and was more relaxed, and less bored by his family, but still had limited interests outside of his work.

> I focus a little bit more on the family and kids. I was pretty
> bored by the stuff the family did. . . . But now, if the family is doing
> anything together, I want to do it. I take an interest in what the
> kids do.

Deriving Strength from Patients

In struggling to cope, these physicians also compared themselves to, and learned from, their patients. Clinical experience provided doctors with helpful models in confronting disease and death. These ill doctors had observed lay patients finding hope and sources of meaning, even in the face of adversity.

Seeing patients worse off than oneself can make one grateful for one's own relative health. When seeing such patients, Roxanne, for instance, appreciated her health status more. "I started to become grateful for whatever I have. I was dealt a pretty good set of cards—treatment is available, and if the disease comes back, I could get the treatment again." Indeed, she had flown to the West Coast for an experimental trial. Many patients she saw had fewer advantages. These ill physicians sometimes found that their own difficulties were put into perspective by patients' problems.

Patients' courage and fortitude could inspire these doctors. Many observed patients, even children, endure in the face of larger challenges. As a result of treating others, Jeff, the adolescent specialist, now found the will to go on. "I've seen little kids deal with this stuff, and it gives me more strength."

These doctors often came to appreciate that in comparison, they had at least heretofore enjoyed extended good health. Many thought of patients who had more to endure. Nancy, with metastatic cancer, said:

I've seen patients suffer much worse than I have. A patient with cystic fibrosis had lung transplants, was not going to get another one, and knew he was going to die—never able to marry or have a life. *At least I've had a life and a child!* When I compare myself to people like that, it's hard to feel so bad.

In short, workaholism and potential burnout posed problems to physicians before they became ill themselves, but even more so afterward. Overidentification with patients, and feeling unappreciated, and overwhelmed by the physical, professional, and psychological tolls of their disease and that of their patients could aggravate feelings of burden. Such frustration can ensue particularly after being diagnosed, and continuing to treat patients with one's same or similar symptoms or disease.

Many sick physicians found it hard to counter feelings of burnout and seek psychological support, sensing that physicians had to "be strong." But some managed to set limits on their type of practice, its hours, and the demands it posed on their outside life. Others changed their attitudes or were inspired by patients who persevered. A third group tried to self-medicate with antidepressants, drugs, or alcohol, and even contemplated or attempted suicide.

Ironically, professionalism emerged here as a potential double-edged sword—selecting for, demanding, and rewarding high levels of dedication. This intense dedication also generated workaholism and lack of balance in one's life. The profession enabled one to avoid "having a life," which permitted longer work hours. The field demanded intense commitment to help patients, but precipitated burnout. Thus, these physicians continually had to titrate their commitments appropriately. Their narratives highlighted unique characteristics of physicians: the ways their authority can interfere with accessing appropriate care, and reduce both family members' ability to help, and potential comfort from support groups. As described below, for some doctors, the only solution was to leave the field altogether.

9

"Once a Doctor, Always a Doctor?"

Retirement

"Should I still put the 'Doctor' in front of my name or not?" Stuart, who retired to teach, asked me. "Is a doctor always a doctor?" What if he or she retires, or no longer sees patients? Does his or her identity then change, and if so, how? Not surprisingly, the possibility of retirement and disability posed these dilemmas. Many of these doctors were not sure when and how to alter or reduce their professional schedules. Inevitably, despite efforts to cope, some contemplated and/or chose retirement, and then had to decide if they were still in fact "physicians."

Whether to Retire: Diagnosis as Pink Slip?

These physician-patients confronted tough questions of whether, when, and how to give up their careers. Retiring completely would mean losing the multiple functions that work had served in their lives. Larger moral questions arose, too, of to what degree physicians *should* sacrifice aspects of their lives for those of their patients. How did they view and navigate these options, and decide what to do?

Against Retirement

As mentioned above, the potential or actual loss of one's career can be deeply traumatic. Scott, the internist with the infected foot, broke into tears as he contemplated having to abandon his work. He could barely verbalize his psychic trauma.

I've been having a miraculous recovery, but it's incredibly painful.
I've been out of work since. . . . Six months before this happened,
I got a new lab here, which burnt down. I'm a new researcher, and
it's a new collaboration. . . .

Repeatedly, Scott stopped, unable to complete his sentences, as he tried
to articulate the waning of his hopes and opportunities.

Quitting work could pose additional difficulties—for example, forcing
one to disclose fully to family, friends, coworkers, employers, patients,
and others that one has a serious disease and may die. Jeff, the adolescent
specialist, for example, would now have to disclose to others that he had
AIDS, not another diagnosis. As described earlier, disclosure posed added
difficulties because it forced one to confront the disease more. These issues arose with many diagnoses, not just HIV.

Retirement was hard, too, when physicians had established strong
bonds with patients that could be mutually difficult to dissolve. When
Steven, the suburban endocrinologist, moved to another city, many patients shed tears.

They said, "How can you do this to us?" I'm not ready to go
through that again. I know some of them will cry, and I will, too.

For both sides, breaking the physician-patient bond felt like a betrayal.

Doctors wondered, too, whether they had a *moral obligation* to work.
The profession may implicitly pressure members *not* to retire as soon as
possible. Albert, the sixty-two-year-old doctor who had an MI on the
highway, commented that people had told him he was "not old enough"
to leave work.

These strong motivations to work, and difficulties of making the decision to leave the field, led some simply to avoid the choice. Consequently,
at times physicians continued to practice *too* long, and their work suffered. Stuart said:

How does one take an infected doctor aside and say, "It looks
like you didn't make rounds on Sunday. You shouldn't be doing that." If someone was so tired that they couldn't keep doing all
the tasks, or returning phone calls, and you knew why, you'd have
to tell him, "I don't think I want you covering my patients anymore." It usually didn't come as a shock to them. But there were
some tough conversations. They rationalized that they didn't
know what to do to shut the practice down. They wouldn't get

around to it; money was an issue. But really, they just weren't prepared to make the decision.

Indeed, some physicians literally worked until they dropped, postponing or never retiring—even when fatigue may have impaired their judgment.

Reasons for Retirement

Illness led other physicians to retire promptly—most importantly, because of deterioration of health and physical function. For some physicians, retirement became paramount once further practice could endanger their health. Risk to a doctor's health is understood to be part of the profession (e.g., when treating infectious disease or epidemics, or soldiers in combat). But these physicians now had to decide where, exactly, to draw the line—at what point they should cease to endanger their own health. Ordinarily, physicians' sense of their own invulnerability helped shield them from fully recognizing or confronting this issue. But illness now confronted them with this question anew.

A variety of personal factors entered into understandings of how much sacrifice and risk to accept. Dilemmas arose regarding the exact degree to which physicians should—if at all—sacrifice their own well-being for that of their patients. For example, Dan, who had chest metastases, came to accept, in retrospect, that his research had probably induced his cancer.

I did research using radioactive markers, injecting them into patients—never thinking that I should have a thyroid scan, or take potassium-iodine. My disease was probably due to the iodine from the isotopes.

As mentioned earlier, immunocompromised physicians faced a variety of infectious threats. Many with HIV debated retiring when they risked exposing themselves to opportunistic infections such as TB. Several worried about exposure, but continued to work—often because of wanting to keep their diagnosis secret. Some retired or transitioned to other work. Eventually, Jennifer stopped clinical work due to the dangers of exposure to TB, and growing time commitments to speaking engagements about HIV. She was still able to consult and participate in other activities.

Our clinic had an enormous amount of TB—any public hospital does—and was starting to see drug-resistant cases. A new patient came in with active TB, and coughed over everybody. Six of my coworkers converted their TB skin tests, and patients in the waiting room got infected. My husband said, "This is enough. The last thing you need is to get TB!" I continued consulting and lecturing. I have thought about going back into practice because I miss it. But my physician said, "You really can't go back there"—because of the TB.

Jennifer saw a continuum of risk, and drew a line, initially accepting some danger, but not too much.

Even if one is not immunocompromised, infectious risks may be widespread. For example, physicians and trainees have acquired hepatitis B from patients. Where he trained as a surgeon, Jerry said:

During the five-year residency, a *third* of the residents acquired hepatitis B from intraoperative needle sticks. I worked in a major trauma center, so we would do thirty- or forty-pint blood cases a night on bleeding cirrhotics and a lot of esophogeal variceal bleeds. I had hepatitis B, and was out for three months.

Fears of dementia prompted retirement, too. Loss of cognitive capacity, or fear of such loss, marked particular milestones. Generally, these physicians thought they should and would stop work if and when they began to demonstrate cognitive decline. But such a point was hard to gauge. Charles, the underground researcher with HIV, said, "It scares me if I walk into a room and forget why. I have to give myself a little lecture: I used to do that. But when I'm down, these fears close in." As mentioned earlier, as a defense, Stuart and others asked colleagues to observe them for any such mental slippage.

Retirement also resulted from concerns about how patients might react if they learned of their physician's illness. With an infectious disease, *guilt* over continuing to work without disclosing one's illness to patients could prompt retirement. Those with HIV all quickly restricted their practices or range of procedures to ensure they were in no danger of exposing any patients to the virus.

Trainees confronted particularly difficult questions of whether, given their illness, even to continue in the profession. As a resident, Pascal wondered, "Why should I go through with residency, and put myself through all that?"

Going "Cold Turkey": When to Retire

Dilemmas arose not only about *whether*, but also *when* and *how*, to retire or decrease their work—whether to give up their role abruptly or ease out of it more slowly, over time. Dangers could result from quitting work either too early or too late. Finding the appropriate time was hard.

On the one hand, diagnosis could mean *instant* retirement. For Mathilde's husband, one piece of paper was "both his death sentence and his pink slip.... One day, you are told you have an illness, you are going to die, and at the same moment you are unemployed."

A lack of preparation could exacerbate grief. Juan left work abruptly. He felt he was going "cold turkey," and grieved.

When physicians abandoned their practices suddenly, colleagues and patients were usually unprepared, and found themselves having to react quickly. Stuart said:

> Two docs in our on-call group just abandoned their patients. A letter went out to us and their patients. But how do patients get their medical records? What do they do? It was very chaotic and unprofessional. These two docs reached a point where they just threw up their hands, and said, "I've got to get out right away."

Though delaying retirement could lead to problems, so could retirement that was *too early*. Some HIV-infected physicians quit practice early and later regretted doing so. Others thought of retiring and going on disability, but in retrospect were glad they hadn't—observing others who did so and then became bored. Dilemmas arose in finding the "right time," though none may exist.

When the Doctor Is Sicker Than the Patient

Doctors who found they were more ill than their patients faced poignant questions of retirement. These physicians felt they had to be healthier—that if their patients were healthier, the physician had de facto passed a certain boundary between the roles of doctor and patient. It was then hard to integrate the roles of patient and healer, and to continue to treat patients without potentially compromising the care provided. At that point, physicians felt they should permit themselves to surrender the stoic mantle of the healer, and be healed. Doctors had not only to treat patients, but also to

be healthy relative to them. Physicianhood thus existed relative to patienthood, falling on the same continuum. When he was not feeling well, Paul
tried to focus patients on *their* problems. He realized that it was probably
not best for him to work then, but he often did so anyway.

> If I'm not feeling good, it's really difficult to listen to other peo-
> ple not feeling well. Sometimes patients can tell. Other times, I
> have to say, "I'm really not feeling good this morning, so we need
> to focus on what we need to do today." It's much easier to do
> that than to try to skirt the issue. Since my practice has only two
> doctors, *I work certain times when it's not best.*

As noted earlier, severely sick patients can cause added stress, reminding ill physicians of themselves. Doctors became frustrated when they
were worse off than patients who nevertheless complained. When their
problems grew worse than their patients', others then quit their practice
altogether. They envied patients' milder conditions. Jeff, the adolescent
specialist, remarked:

> With parents' nagging concerns—a parent saying, "My daughter
> doesn't eat vegetables. Talk to her" or "My son flunked a test,
> and he usually makes B's. Talk to him!"—I felt, "If you only knew
> what I have to deal with—peripheral neuropathy and fatigue." Life
> is too short!

Frustration also arose when a doctor treated a patient who was healthier, but nonetheless on disability. David, the psychiatrist, said:

> I've seen people on disability, and their numbers are better than
> mine, and they have not been that sick. I think: "I'm working fifty
> hours. You're on disability: What are you complaining about? You
> have no idea what trouble is."

At these times, ill physicians had to monitor and screen their frustrations.
Such health disparities could also prompt a physician to disclose his or
her diagnosis.

Whether to Return to Work

Several retired physicians, particularly some with HIV, felt better on
new medications, and debated whether to return to work. But returning to one's previous field, after being away from it for several years,

could require retraining, which could prove daunting if not utterly prohibitive.

Others feared they would no longer be able to obtain malpractice insurance. Simon, the radiologist with HIV who refused to be audiotaped, felt he wouldn't be able to get malpractice insurance because of his illness. Consequently, he felt he lost his profession ("My status. Everything"), and thus his self-esteem and "usefulness."

Some who left their clinical practices and missed work still dreamed of eventually returning. Jerry, the surgeon who went to law school, literally dreamed of being back in the OR. However, he suggested apprehension and ambivalence as well.

> I dream I'm back at work in these bizarre situations: not knowing what surgery I'm supposed to be doing. Or I'll be naked in the OR, unaware of what's going on.

Reinventing Oneself

Short of stopping work entirely, medicine provided key benefits through wide professional fluidity. Many physicians altered their mix or type of activities within the field. Options included taking on more administration or research and fewer clinical responsibilities, working part-time, teaching, or consulting—transitioning into other roles. Even before the onset of illness, many physicians had combined different professional activities. John, the public health official, said:

> I've had three careers: as a student for twelve years post-college; then as a health services researcher/administrator/clinician/teacher; then doing public health. Maybe it's time for a fourth.

Once they had become ill, other physicians changed their activities within the field for the first time, reassessing and reprioritizing their personal and professional values. Generally, many felt that research work would stress them less than clinical care. Many valued their remaining time more, and didn't want to work as hard.

Yet such fluidity was not universal. Midway through their education, trainees, in particular, faced difficulties in altering their professional lives. Once entered, medicine was hard to transition out of entirely.

Still, diagnoses received before the completion of training could shape initial choices of field and job. Trainees often assessed which fields posed the least physical or psychological risk to them. Suzanne, the psychiatrist, said:

> If I didn't have bipolar disorder, I would be in ophthalmology now.
> I had everything going for me—looks, athleticism, good personality, nice family, smarts. And then *boom*, in college, I started having
> problems. It slowed me down.

Switching into another field could necessitate additional training. Some physicians thus tried to scale back work to part-time, but doing so was difficult. Medicine forced full-time commitment—long hours of following up on patient details. Roxanne felt she couldn't work less because of professional demands.

> There's always so much to do—charts to dictate, papers and grants
> to write. If I don't do it, it won't get done. The more I do, I still
> don't catch up. I'm always anxious. Sometimes I just shift the piles
> of paper around. But if I get rid of these piles, there will be more.

Patients were often sick enough to require quick and maximal attention. Given calls and emergencies, it was hard to "transition out" of medicine, and practice only part-time. Stuart commented, "You could cut the number of patients, but not stop the number of phone calls. . . . There wasn't enough money to hire another doc." Plans to reduce the amount of work proved elusive, too, since medicine took on a life of its own. Stuart continued:

> Every time I came back from vacations, I said I would contain the
> time. But within a week, the stuff we had planned had failed. I
> thought it was just the nature of the practice, of patients' demands,
> and of the illness. But some of it was just obsessive-compulsive.

Again, the profession selected for, and rewarded, such drive.

Working only part-time diminished the amount of disability insurance one would eventually receive, which had to be weighed against other, competing desires and goals. These physician-patients thus encountered quandaries, balancing work gratification, retirement, and health.

Volunteerism

Even after formally retiring from paid employment, many doctors endeavored to continue to use their medical skills and knowledge by *vo-*

lunteering their services. Even if no longer practicing, they tried to remain in the field in some way.

Yet here, too, dilemmas arose. Albert, who had an MI on the highway, redefined himself, but yearned to be involved in additional activities (e.g., grants and teaching fellows) as well. Charles, with HIV, went so far as to begin to investigate new drugs on his own.

I'm doing a study . . . underground, without a permit, without FDA approval, using my friend's office. I go outside of conventional trials, use unapproved drugs, and take risks to treat myself and others. I could get sued.

At one point, Charles and activist colleagues even treated patients in a motel.

We secretly rented a wing of a motel, and brought in six patients with adjoining rooms, and kept them there for two days with anesthesiologists, four doctors, and seven nurses. The motel didn't know what was going on. We knew it was potentially dangerous. I started IVs, checked them, and hoped to God nobody crashed.

This new work as a medical researcher and activist supplied much-needed purpose in Charles's life. He did not know if he could ever return to private practice now.

Charles altered his attitudes not only about work, but also about broader political commitments.

I now see myself as part researcher, part crusader. There's nothing like coming down with a fatal illness to make you decide where your loyalties and interests lie, to make you reexamine why I was a knee-jerk Republican.

Still, such transition to volunteerism remained hard, as it provided meaning, but not status. Charles insinuated to others that he was working more than he was.

I had to wrestle with the idea that "I'm not working now." I feel I'm not part of society because other people go to routine jobs nine to five, and my work is very sporadic and totally self-motivated. There'll be weeks that I do practically nothing. At times, I imply to other people that I work more than I do, because I feel shame about not working.

Charles still felt peripheral because of both external realities and internal uncertainties and doubts. "I'm fringe, not associated with a major university." His new identity as a "researcher" buffered his self-esteem, and was particularly important, since he felt his role as a physician had vanished. But he felt he had less prestige and respect than if he were a "full doctor."

Who Am I Versus What I Do? Retirement and Identity

Many questioned whether they still were physicians if they no longer saw patients. They were forced to examine whether and how much of being a physician was either an identity or an activity.

Concretely, they disagreed even as to whether to call themselves "doctors" when no longer seeing patients. Some shifted their identity to encompass only the parts of the role that they maintained. For example, Nancy, who had brain metastases, now saw herself as "a researcher" more than "a physician," drawing a fine, but to her, meaningful distinction. She explained: "I think of myself as 'kind of an academic'—not really 'a physician' anymore—because I've given up my patients. I've stopped viewing myself as a doctor, really."

Here, being a doctor required *doctoring*—specifically, treating patients. Similarly, Herb, the neonatologist with an MI, taught part-time, and no longer saw patients. As a result, he felt like an educator. "I feel I'm still a teacher and a resource."

Others still attempted to cling to their identities as physicians, resisting retirement and seeking to maintain the trappings and symbols of continued practice. Though he would never work again, Eleanor's husband insisted on renewing his license, because, he said, "It's so much a part of *who I am*."

Conversely, others felt that their professional identity was ingrained to such a profound degree that they would *always* be doctors, even if not practicing. Their profession was deeply instilled. Juan said:

Once I got an MD, I got it for life. Somebody said, "Since you're not a physician anymore...." I'm not in practice, *but I'll always be a physician*. I'll always be Puerto Rican....*I feel more like a "retired physician"*—I can pick and choose what I want to do. I have been put in an obstacle course and have jumped all the obstacles—

medical school and residency—being up sixty-eight hours in a row. I have it under my belt. Nobody's going to take it away from me. I don't think of things the same way as the general public. I've had too much exposure to illness and death.

Juan qualified his position as a physician, but remained one: for him, being a "retired physician" was still an identity, a role.

The notion that physicianhood constituted a deeply ingrained identity supports the concept that despite the onslaught of managed care, medicine still involves "professionalism," rather than being merely a job. Physicians clung to this role of the doctor, fixed and well-established due to professional socialization.

Yet debates still arose since identity entered numerous daily social interactions in real and symbolic ways—from reserving a restaurant table to introducing oneself to strangers. Ill physicians debated whether they were still entitled to use the title "doctor" when no longer fully functioning in that role. Analogously, as medical students, they had often wondered about being called "doctor" as they began to assume some, but not all, aspects of the role. Retirement forced Stuart, for example, to change radically his sense of self, leaving him puzzled.

Adding "Doctor" in front of my name means there's more to explain as to why I'm sitting here at four in the afternoon: "What kind of doctor are you?" It just opens up questions that I'm not prepared to answer. It's hard to say, "I'm retired." They look at me (I'm forty-five) and go, "That's curious." I use a tone of voice that keeps them at arm's length.

Tone of voice, as well as words themselves, conveys information about his identity. Stuart's communication told listeners how to respond to him; the form of permissible discourse.

These individuals had to navigate the widening gap between their changed social definition and self-definition. Stuart added:

Now, when I get blood drawn at the lab, I'm just myself. I don't use the title "Doctor." Some of the techs remember me, and some don't. I don't . . . walk through the back entrance. I go to the pharmacy and pick up the prescription, rather than giving my title and blustering my way through. I might be fifth in line. If I used the title "Doctor," they wouldn't be as brusque with me. They might even pull me out of line and put me forward. For twenty years, I

was "Dr. G...." While I wouldn't make a reservation in a restaurant under "Dr. G...," much of my life was my professional
life, and people knew who I was. *I was that persona.* Now, most
people who come into contact with me in supermarkets have no
idea who I am. Now, *the part that's a doctor is very small and
contained.* I'm teaching, volunteering. With students, when I introduce myself as "Doctor," rather than just giving my first and last
name, I get totally different reactions. A title means so much to
students. Everybody has one. When I don't use the title, I get
treated like shit. I might just be the librarian. Very quickly after
making that mistake and getting pushed around by first-year medical students, I found I had to pull rank. To them, the pecking order
is very important. So there, I still use "Doctor."

In different social contexts, Stuart felt he had to legitimate his use of
the title, and adjusted his moniker—not using it in the lab or pharmacy,
but doing so at the medical school. He wanted neither special attention nor disrespect, but his altered view of himself collided with others'
views of him. These physicians encountered predicaments of how much
information or explanation they needed to provide in different social and
professional situations, and what the norms and expectations for truth-
telling are: the "wholeness," quantity, and quality of information provided. Misinformation (saying that he was "on sabbatical," rather than
"retired.") in turn created problems, particularly when the initial year
finished.

They could relate to sabbatical. But as the year is ending, students
have come up to me, asking for summer electives: "Are you in a
practice? Do you still see patients?" I'm still searching for a phrase
that makes sense.

Stuart did not want to disclose his illness, and preferred to continue to be
known as a "good teacher" rather than as merely a patient.

Ironically, outsiders perceived these decisions of what to call oneself
very differently. Stuart's decision to forgo the title of "doctor" impressed
some people by what they perceived to be his humility.

Neighbors have said, "You did some community organizing, and
didn't use the MD!" One man thought it was the most modest
thing he'd ever heard: "It's nice that you're a doc and can just be
yourself when you're talking to neighbors."

In sum, illness forced many physicians to struggle with the deepest meanings of their careers in their lives. Many described themselves as "workaholics," due to high job satisfaction, demands of doctoring, boosts to self-esteem, prior psychic traumas, degree of illness, or magical thinking—beliefs that work would somehow immunize them against illness. Such magical thinking persisted side by side with scientific attitudes. Disease could augment, rather than reduce, these doctors' motivation and ambition.

Against this backdrop of workaholism, these physicians had to contemplate reducing or ending their careers, whether as a result of disease, feared or real dementia, or the prospect of having to disclose their disease to others. They faced disturbing questions of when and how to retire, and debated pros and cons. They retired at different points, from too early to too late. Many continued to seek ways to use their skills, or longed to do so, but that goal often proved elusive. Ordinarily, patients' views of doctors and doctors' perceptions of themselves reinforced one another. But for these physicians, that was no longer the case.

These struggles highlighted the importance of doctoring in these physicians' lives—how they integrated their professional identities into their most profound senses of self and their lives; and how and why they encountered difficulties in surrendering that role. These phenomena raise fundamental existential questions: to what degree one is what one does, and what one is when no longer practicing one's profession. In the current age of increasing corporatization and outsourcing, many individuals must reinterpret and reconstruct their identities in the world, and face problems in doing so. Recently, identity has been examined through the lens of "identity politics" based on broad ethnic, religious, or cultural groupings—such as being Islamic, Christian, black, or gay. Yet here, identity based on work, education, and profession also shaped views of self, others, and the world—and outsiders' perceptions. Self-conceptions can fluidly shift, molded by a range of internal and external factors. For each individual here, some aspects of the self changed while others remained the same. Identity thus can be not only political, but also professional.

Concretely, more attention to these issues, and clearer guidelines and professional opportunities available for potential retirees—how they can continue to use their vital skills and find meaning—can assist countless individuals in medicine and other fields.

10

"Touched by the Light"

Spiritual Beliefs and Their Obstacles

Ill physicians now came to appreciate, as never before, the importance of spirituality. Past studies have been divided as to whether and how physicians resembled, or differed from, patients in spiritual beliefs and practices. Early studies found that patients were more religious and spiritual than physicians as a whole, but more recent investigations suggest more commonalities (1). Still, comparisons remain difficult. Possible differences are significant because patients often wish to talk about religion with their physicians, but hesitate, sensing that physicians are not interested or too busy (2). Doctors' spiritual beliefs may also influence their clinical decisions. For example, among physicians, Catholics and Jews have been less willing than Protestants to withdraw life support (3). Doctors who are more sensitive to spiritual concerns may discuss these issues more readily with patients.

Confrontations with their own mortality forced many of these ill physicians to grapple with fundamental existential and spiritual questions in new ways. They revealed continua of different forms and contents of beliefs, illuminating how illness and the acknowledgment of mortality can spark spiritual journeys and quests that unfold in complex stages. In the *Oxford English Dictionary*, "spirit," from the Latin *spiritus* (meaning "breathing"), is defined as "The immaterial part of a corporal being...the soul" (4). "Religion," from the Latin *religio* (meaning "obligation" or "bond" in late Latin), came to mean "a state of life bound by religious vows...of belonging to a religious order" (5).

Forms of Spirituality

Being Spiritual to Start With

Some physicians felt spiritual or religious before their diagnoses. Roxanne, the gastroenterologist with cancer, said religion had always been important to her. In fact, when on call, she would ask a clergyman to pray for her. "I'd go to a priest and say, 'Father, I'm on call,' and he would bless me. I'd say, 'God, help me not to make a decision when I don't know what to do.' "

Nevertheless, though religious or spiritual to start with, doctors often increased the significance of spirituality in their lives, changing priorities or developing a greater sense of appreciation. After becoming sick, many developed or expanded spiritual activities in their lives, adding further dimensions.

Others returned to spiritual beliefs from which they had meandered away over time. Brian, the pediatrician with hepatitis, suggested the extent to which the experience of spirituality can exist in a series of gradations traversed forward or back. Though trained as a Jesuit, he had become less religious, until his illness inspired him to recultivate, and return to, his previous beliefs and practices.

> I was in medical school, training to do missionary work. So I
> am religious in a sense, but I am not pious. I consider myself
> spiritually-oriented in that I try to be quiet, and listen to my-
> self. The illness actually brought me back to that. Not that I had
> drifted from it, but I had become less attentive. . . . I didn't re-
> serve special, quiet time for myself.

Other physicians did not return to a particular tradition, but as result of illness, increased their appreciation of life and nature more generally. Kurt, the internist with HIV, said:

> I've been more reflective, and learned to appreciate things—the
> ocean, the sky—to take time for people. Not just important peo-
> ple, but anybody. It's made me a lot happier.

Spirituality Despite Oneself

Occasionally, physicians became more spiritual without inviting it, almost despite themselves. For example, Walter, when critically ill with lymphoma, had what he considered a spiritual experience. But, long influenced by Karl Marx, he did not know how to process and integrate it into his agnostic inclinations. He struggled with conflicting feelings about faith—wanting to believe in an afterlife in order to acquire a sense of comfort, but unable to accept this concept fully.

> I certainly don't have any relationship to any kind of deism or God. At some points when I've been really sick, I remember thinking, "It would be really good to be able to find some serenity in really believing that there was an all-powerful figure who was going to look after me during, as well as after, death." But I could never quite bring myself to do that. Human beings can share something with each other—through touch or caring. I'm not sure where that falls in any spirituality range.

Walter indicated, too, how a degree of ambiguity and ineffability pervaded these domains.

Despite his uncertainties, when acutely ill, Walter nevertheless felt himself drawing on a strength that came from *outside himself*.

> One really strange story that probably was a result of delirium: I had already been in septic shock, and was going downhill. For a couple of days, I had a very strong sensation that (1) I was strongly rooted in the ground...I had almost a tree root from my back through the bed, into the ground, and that it was rooting me, and giving me strength. And (2) I was getting strength from outside myself. I was quite surprised. I didn't know how to process it. There was nothing I could do about it, but it was a strong sensation. It lasted a couple of days, and never came back. I was not delirious. Sounds like some of my more psychotic patients: I felt like there were vibrations coming from outside...and they did good things inside me.

Though at first Walter joked that the experience was probably due to "delirium," he later emphatically said that he had *not* been delirious. This contradiction reflected his embarrassment at what others might consider "irrational," a phenomenon that he was unable to process fully, and that had no place in his existing system of beliefs. This conflict reflected broader controversies, spanning centuries, concerning the seeming irrationality of spiritual notions and, ultimately, of the existence of God.

Being Spiritual, but Not Thinking of Oneself as Such

Some who felt they were not spiritual nevertheless engaged in what others might regard as spiritual practices. In so doing, several doctors further distinguished between their own and others' views of themselves. David, the psychiatrist with HIV, said others would probably describe him as spiritual, though he did not think of himself as such. He followed rituals but felt he lacked "true faith," perceiving himself as, if anything, "religious, but not spiritual." Similarly, Charles, the underground researcher, felt the need to simplify his material life, and thought this urge perhaps stemmed from a desire to be humble and "atone" for his sins:

> I had a beautiful house, and suddenly felt I had to get rid of it. In retrospect, I probably did it to atone for my sins: I needed to strip myself of this symbol of that kind of life, and live much more simply and more humbly.

Both implicitly and explicitly, Charles invoked spiritual concepts, but did not see himself as spiritual or religious.

Wanting, but Being Unable, to Believe

Like Walter, who desired serenity through faith, but was unable to reconcile himself fully to a belief in God, some ill physician wanted to believe, but found it difficult to do so. A few tried to seek or attain "more spirituality"—having some faith, but wishing for "more"—again suggesting the existence of varying *degrees* of spirituality, and the extent to which acquisition of faith is not entirely or necessarily self-willed.

Several physicians wished they felt a connection with a faith, in order to draw support from it, but battled with doubt about the nature of beliefs and adherents who rely on these. Steven, the suburban endocrinologist with HIV, wanted to be more spiritual, desiring a stronger sense of faith to help him cope with his illness, but his skepticism lingered.

> I wish I were more spiritual. I'm open to the idea—at least I think I am. It makes a big difference in most people's lives.... Those who do have some kind of centering around a spiritual belief seem to do better. As a kid, I used to pray a lot because you're supposed to. Even to this day, I find myself praying—that this blood result will be good, that You're going to let this be good news—without

planning it or thinking about it consciously. Once in a while, I'll pray at night. . . . I don't know why I don't do it more often; perhaps I should. I would do better if I had it in my life *more*. I just have this darn skeptical. . . . On the one hand, I want and need it; on the other, I feel it's what weak, simple people rely on: a crutch.

As he spoke, Steven searched, and at times stumbled to articulate his thoughts on this elusive subject.

Others, too, struggled to grasp the discrepancy between their desire for comfort through faith, and their more limited beliefs. Mark, the internist interviewed in the diner, explained, "Faith is a good thing for people that have it." Yet he expressed uncertainty in self-assessing his faith, saying, "I don't think I really have it *too much*. Sometimes I wish I had it, because it gives some people a certain high." He resolved these tensions by deprecating the solace that faith might provide. "I don't think it's a *real* high. I don't really believe in it. It's like being hypnotized. I think some people, if they really believe in it, maybe can really be hypnotized."

Scientific training can foster such skepticism, and hinder desires to be more religious. Charles, the internist and underground researcher, perceived a contradiction between his beliefs in science and the ethereal, seemingly irrational qualities of religion and spirituality.

I'm looking for a spiritual component, but I tend to be kind of an agnostic. I wish I weren't. It would be comforting. But I have such a scientific bent, and organized religion, and most people out there who believe that, with their crystals . . . it's such a turnoff. It's difficult for me to open up to it. I'm trying to be open to that. . . . It just seems like it's just a more successful way to live. *But I don't know what to do about it.*

Charles saw benefits of moral behavior—feeling good and living successfully—yet these didn't overcome his doubt. He struggled back and forth to make sense of his need for, but wariness of, beliefs, and his uncertainty about how to proceed.

Continuing to Doubt

Religious doubts could persist more strongly and prevail throughout an illness, without change. Frank, who had his first MI in the OR, remained an atheist. He "reconsidered," but had not yet altered, his beliefs.

Of those physician-patients who said that they wanted to believe but could not, some appeared to be depressed. Here, questions arose as to which came first: the depression or the inability to believe. Specifically, depression may thwart beliefs in something beyond oneself; and failure to find such a belief may contribute to depression. For example, though she had metastatic breast cancer, Anne, the Swiss internist, continued to work, feeling driven, estranged from her family, and "not knowing what else to do" with her life. She, too, wanted to believe in a higher entity, but found it difficult to do so while simultaneously feeling depressed.

Other physician-patients were jaded by religion, perceiving hypocrisy among organized traditions and some adherents. These physicians either held nonspecific spiritual beliefs, while maintaining "ideals" concerning human conduct, or became atheists or agnostics. Jessica, the pediatrician with cancer, explained, "What negative feelings I have aren't toward religion, but some of the practitioners—which is a little different. I enjoy some of the ceremonial aspects." While not wholly irreligious, she also quipped, "Religion hasn't given me much."

Unpleasant or off-putting personal interactions with the church prompted others, especially gay physicians, to avoid organized religion—even to their possible detriment.

Also, bad interactions with the church could lead to fluctuations in one's religious beliefs over time. Peter, the student, joked that he was "religious only when it's convenient." Yet he then described a critical point in his life, in which he established a helpful and meaningful relationship with his religious tradition:

> I actually needed to see a priest. I expected the worst, but he was great and actually got me to go back to religion. He said, "In the old school of Catholicism, you have fire and brimstone. You'll burn in hell. But we're not here ... to judge. We're here to help you get through whatever you need to get through." I'm religious personally, but don't do anything with the community.

Peter distinguished personal beliefs from interaction with a broader religious community. Though wary of organized religion because of particular followers, some physicians nonetheless occasionally derived benefit from it.

"Playing the Game": Ritual Without Acknowledging Belief

At times, ill physicians who did not consider themselves religious or spiritual either before or after their illness nevertheless took part in rituals and ceremonies. For example, Deborah differentiated between Jewish religion and culture. Raised Hasidic, she thought of herself as "very Jewish...inside," but not spiritual. While she was hospitalized, many of the Hasidim (i.e., members of a Jewish Orthodox community) visited her, prayed, and at her bedside performed rituals in which she joined.

> I can't say I'm spiritual...I'm very Jewish—but *inside*. I come from a Hasidic family, and in the hospital, people visited me, and prayed, and gave me the book of healing, and read for me, and brought me food. So when I was there...*I let them play the game, and I joined in*. When I came home, the only thing that changed was that I light the candles on Friday night, if I'm not on chemo. But I don't go to synagogue or do anything more than before....
> [T]hese people...asked me if I would do that one thing for them when I came out of the hospital. I said, "Ok, if I come out alive, I will definitely light the candles." It's the most basic, feminine Jewish thing to do.

Returning this "favor" implied respect, and a cultural connection to rituals surrounding Judaism, even if Deborah did not acknowledge any explicit religious beliefs.

From time to time, Deborah had attempted to find a relationship with a religious tradition, but concluded she was not inclined toward spirituality.

> Maybe I should read everything by the Dalai Lama. A friend sent me a book. I read two pages, and...can't finish the book. *Maybe I wasn't touched by the light*. Some people say they have spiritual experiences. I haven't had that. *I'm very down-to-earth*.

Deborah went on to describe how she respected religion and was not antagonistic, but did not feel that it "spoke to her" in a way to which she could relate. She felt that her personality—feisty, down-to-earth, pragmatic—was antithetical to certain aspects of spirituality.

Yet connections with spirituality existed at both intellectual and other personal levels. She continued:

> It's not nonsense. People get a lot of support from being spirit-
> ual. In the hospital, a lady next to me was Christian. . . . I said,
> "That's very nice she's religious, but *it doesn't talk to me*." Once in
> a while when the Hasidim came, yes, I believed in God because
> they were there and supporting the . . . notion of God. But to say
> that I get up in the morning and do the rituals—no, I don't.

Still, ceremony, even without complete faith, can provide meaning. Debo-rah didn't practice Judaism, but felt connected to the people who prayed for her, and was grateful for the kindness they offered her through prayer. In fact, after her hospitalization, she lit candles at home. She added, "My spiritualism is really through my painting. I'm not religious, but I'm a very traditional, culturally-oriented Jew." She made fine, nuanced but key gra-dations of belief and practice. Spiritual connection can be to a tradition and culture.

Contents of Belief

Some physicians felt strong relationships with the particular religions in which they had been raised (e.g., Christianity and Judaism). Yet others invoked a wide range of philosophies and approaches, or combinations of these. For example, Roger, the suicidal surgeon with HIV, became happier and more energetic as a result of a broad, if amalgamated, spir-itual transformation.

> I've done a lot of reading: the Koran, Hindu literature, Mary Baker
> Eddy, Christian Science, and Bible stuff. I found the old parable
> of the elephant helpful: one man feels his leg, one his trunk, etc.
> They've all got a little piece of what's up there.

Roger's new beliefs, though an ensemble of traditions, aided him.

Others struggled, and in the end found comfort in their own unique and particular understandings of, and desires for, greater faith. Mark, the internist interviewed in the diner, said:

> . . . my mom may be a guardian angel for me, if it's possible to do
> that. I was the most important thing in the world to her. If
> you're allowed to have a wish after you're gone, that would be it.

I don't know that I literally believe that that's possible. But I *play with the idea*. I don't know what happens after you die. But if you get to go to somewhere nice, then I'm going to go there and be with my mom again. If I do nothing more than go into nothingness and history, then that's where mom went, too. I find comfort in that.

Though not strictly structured or sanctioned by a tradition or community, such nonspecific beliefs can offer solace.

Openness to a wide range of religious traditions mirrored that of many patients. Jacob, who wore a yarmulke, emanated a certain religious integrity that prompted even non-Jewish patients to ask him to pray for them: "Patients regard me as a little bit special because of the yarmulke."

Nonspecific and vague beliefs persisted, particularly concerning the existence and nature of an afterlife. Though wary of organized religion, Bill, the Southern radiologist with HIV, "grew up Methodist" and felt that life or "energy" somehow "goes on" in an afterlife, though he had not formulated these thoughts further. "I believe in something bigger there...I want there to be an afterlife...I don't know what....It's not necessarily heaven and hell."

Awareness of the continuity of nature and its ability to renew itself inspired awe, and provided a model on which to pattern spiritual beliefs. The processes of nature could represent something greater. Nancy, with metastatic cancer, marveled:

A process is moving forward in some way—some mysterious force. I don't know what it is...if a nuclear bomb wiped out all human beings, there'd still be some little cockroach...and after eons of time...there'd be a whole new population of things. Some things we don't understand.

Nancy found spirituality in biology and science, integrating her beliefs and medical training. Through her hobby of gardening, she increasingly saw the world of nature as exemplifying the transience of life. "The tree or shrub that I love this year, next year is already too big. Things are always changing, nothing stays the same."

Others defined spirituality, or its manifestations, very broadly to include their work as physicians. Scientific principles of medicine could embody spiritual ideals. John, the public health official, viewed his medical endeavors as a way of doing God's work, dedicating himself to people and ultimate goals.

I think of myself as a very religious person, inwardly, deeply. But my religion is around philosophical, mathematical, scientific concepts. I am religious in the deepest sense of the term. I care about people... will fight for principles.... But I don't go to any church.

Helping patients gave doctors a sense of purpose and gratification, further impelling some ill physicians to continue to practice medicine, even as they became sicker and developed metastatic disease.

Spirituality as Involved in Health Events

Beliefs arose, too, that faith and prayer might affect the disease process itself. Though spirituality might promote positive thinking, and hence abet healing and coping, some believed that prayer itself could alter physiology through divine intervention. Roxanne recounted, "Everyone sent me prayer cards and Mass cards. I was in everyone's prayers. It must have worked: I had more energy, which never diminished." Once she was sick, she even made a religious pilgrimage to Lourdes, which she felt gave her additional strength.

Some believed in such physiological effects, but noted colleagues' potential antagonism toward these ideas. For example, Bradley, who became depressed after his MI, came to believe in the power of prayer to treat disease.

A physician-friend was extremely interested in the power of prayer. He would just sit with patients. Some doctors wouldn't send him patients anymore.... [But] you certainly can call on things that you might not be able to describe that make people feel better.

A few actively sought to invoke these physiological effects of spirituality by performing activities that might further these processes. Jacob disclosed his diagnosis to people in order to get them to pray for him. He believed their efforts worked.

I called up five people I consider very holy. They follow Jewish law, without fanfare or publicity. I figure they've got God on their side. I know it helped, because knowing they were doing it, I was functioning better... I believe prayer works. That's part of Jewish belief: you can change the way the world is going.

Jacob said his wife felt they had the power to alter his fate because he was diagnosed between the Jewish High Holidays.

> In the week between Rosh Hashanah and Yom Kippur, one's actions can shape one's fate for the year. This diagnosis was at a very opportune time, instead of if it happened a week after Yom Kippur. We thought we had the power to change the process of fate. I said, "Thank God it's before Yom Kippur."

At times, physicians saw medical events as religious "signs" from God: evidence of divine involvement on earth in illness, and thereby in human affairs. For example, Jacob interpreted as such evidence the fact that his yarmulke covered his surgical scar.

> The lesion would have cosmetically wrecked anybody: it's all a skin graft. But I wear a yarmulke anyway. The margins happen to fit in a way that the skin graft doesn't show. I took that as sort of a *religious reassurance* that whatever I was doing...I should keep doing.

Describing Spirituality

Clearly, religion and spirituality were often intangible and difficult to describe, since these concepts inherently lie beyond words, tied to the mysterious, and ranging in form and content. These doctors did not always understand their spirituality, or know with what to compare it. Spiritual feelings are often innately inchoate; language may simply be unable to convey these states. Hence, terms such as "really," "literally," and "sort of" attempted to qualify and convey beliefs or doubts.

Moreover, discussing spirituality was often taboo. Individuals might strongly disagree about it and fear being perceived as irrational, and thus vulnerable. Eleanor reported that even with her, her physician-husband could not reveal his innermost fears and spiritual concerns.

> ...after he died, I found a book of Japanese death poems that he owned. There was a bookmark. So there must have been some spiritual dimension that he needed to address. But we never discussed it openly. I really don't know if he became more religious or spiritual.

Stunningly, Eleanor's lack of knowledge about her husband's beliefs underlined how *private* spiritual beliefs can be, and how much people are afraid or unwilling to discuss them.

Issues surfaced, too, as to whether and how physicians and trainees could be more sensitive to spiritual issues. Some physicians felt that many colleagues were antipathetic toward religion, and that as a result, spirituality could not be taught. Roxanne said, "You can't teach it. *Spirituality is a gift.* Either you feel it or you don't. How come people don't have the feeling? I don't know. I give it all to God."

Yet physicians can nonetheless increase their sensitivity to the importance of these realms in many patients' lives, even if they do not share these beliefs.

In all, spirituality aided many of these physicians in confronting serious illness, through a wide variety of forms and contents of beliefs and practices. Heightened awareness of these issues can potentially strengthen the relationships between doctors and patients, improving their experiences as they each grapple with disease. Some physicians, who felt a connection to spirituality before their own illness, became more spiritual post-diagnosis, or found that their spiritual inclinations and understandings evolved over time. Many doctors followed traditional religions or mixed and matched beliefs.

Surprisingly, other physicians who saw the benefits of spirituality for their patients, and wanted to become more spiritual themselves, nonetheless had difficulty finding spiritual meaning. Key questions arose as to who is "touched by the light" and why, and why others are not. The reasons appeared to be manifold. Depression may provoke religious doubt and, conversely, religious doubt may prompt or aggravate depression. In other ways, too, spirituality appeared not to be fully voluntary, but tied to complicated and unclear processes. Some people simply appeared more inclined to believe than others.

Yet in part because spirituality cannot necessarily be willed, questions arose as to the degree to which it can be taught. These issues are important because physicians who are not "spiritually inclined" may find it harder to communicate with patients about spirituality in ways that patients find helpful.

The fact that several of these physicians did not feel themselves to be spiritual, but engaged in activities and held beliefs that an outside observer might perceive as spiritual, underscored the difficulty of assessing or measuring this realm. Several researchers have attempted to assess spirituality quantitatively (6). At best, they can evaluate certain measurable components (e.g., church attendance or frequency of prayer), but individuals vary widely in defining these words, and any one formulation may reflect only particular religious systems. The concepts of religion and spirituality may remain ineffable, and measuring them may not ultimately be as fruitful as many scholars hope. The ways individuals struggle with doubt, and may wish to avoid it, but find themselves unable to do so, are important to understand as well. Some managed to overcome their personal uncertainty, while others did not. In any case, heightened physician awareness and sensitivity concerning these areas can help many patients.

Part III

INTERACTING WITH
THEIR PATIENTS

11

"Us versus Them"

Treating Patients Differently

"I do more for patients now than I used to," Deborah, the psychiatrist with cancer, confessed. The experience of illness changed how most of these physicians treated their patients. Frequently, personal experiences of illness reversed years of professional medical training. In facing the darkness of their own disease, these doctors often came to treat patients and to teach trainees better. Nonetheless, "enlightenment" did not always occur. Treating those under their care more humanely was not always easy or successful. Psychological, social, and economic barriers could hamper doctors' improving the care they offered. Other physicians veered too far in this new direction—doing too much for patients, raising questions of how much of an advocate or friend to be. As providers, they often found it hard to arrive at the appropriate balance between being too concerned or too detached. They wrestled to achieve what the sociologist Renée Fox terms "detached concern" (1)—to be simultaneously concerned and, in order to be objective, somewhat detached. Over time, they struggled with this balance, seeking equilibrium—sometimes voyaging too far one way or the other, becoming too close or too removed, and then having to adjust, based on their perceptions of patients' responses.

"We're All in This Together": Reducing the Hierarchy

The experience of being ill inspired many physicians to strive to reduce the barriers between themselves and their patients. Often, doctors now reassessed the doctor-patient relationship, seeing it less as "us versus them" and more as "we're all in this together." Yet these reactions underscored the differential that existed beforehand and presumably would have continued if these doctors had not gotten sick themselves.

At times, new camaraderie ensued. Lou, who had an award on his office wall, now felt with patients: "We're bonded because we're both in the same club: both patients."

They could share not only physiological processes, but psychosocial effects of disease as well. Such identification commonly grew, particularly if these doctors were treating patients with whom they shared a diagnosis. Tom looked differently at patients who had either of his problems: alcoholism and HIV.

> Being an alcoholic, I see alcoholic patients differently. Being HIV-positive, I've had much more engagement with patients' experiences with mortality, discrimination, and difficult decisions of whether to take drugs.

Suzanne, the psychiatrist with bipolar disorder, added:

> It's the same way as talking to an alcoholic who is now a drug and alcohol counselor: they have a comfort level. But most of *them* admit it and say, "I'm a recovering alcoholic."

Even ill physicians who felt they were highly sensitive to patients' experiences to begin with often changed significantly. Most "sensitive" doctors now felt that they had become more empathetic, even if in subtle ways, and more aware of patients' perspectives. Attitudes changed not only toward patients, but also staff. Bradley, the internist who had a heart attack, said that previously, he hadn't considered retiring or helping younger colleagues advance in their careers. Now, he listened more and accepted giving up control.

> My illness affected how I operate my lab. I had eighteen people working here, and I considered myself immortal. I'd never even *considered* the reality of retiring. I have a very devoted, excellent, younger (fifty-five years old) associate, who has been working with me for thirty-one years. He's not a physician, and I had difficulty accepting what he wished to do as being right. Post-illness, I have been more accepting of other viewpoints, leading to my willingness to retire. It no longer bothers me not to be in control. But I did not arrive at these points of view through some intellectual process.

In their multiple roles, both professionally and personally, disease could be an equalizer, but involved unconscious and subjective factors.

Reductions in hierarchy could have several advantages, promoting both less distancing from physicians and passivity from patients. The power differential reflected antagonism that physicians might feel toward patients, and could occlude necessary discussions. For example, Scott, the physician with the foot infection, and several others reflected on the long-standing traditional medical hierarchy, in defining "a good patient" as "one that doesn't bother you." Others defined a "good patient" as one who adhered to medications, and was respectful. Nancy added: one that "did not try to second-guess." "Doctors really deserve courtesy, too—patients not abusing the phone, or calling at weird hours when they can phone during the right hours—not being a pain." The realization that these definitions of a "good patient" prevailed, amazed physicians. Harry, the internist and war refugee with heart disease, was astonished when the nurses told him, "You were such a wonderful patient: you never needed us." The fact that he was liked because of this passivity astounded and disappointed him. This concept of a "good patient" appeared to exist as a clear category in the minds of both doctors and nurses.

This hierarchy between doctors and patients can also be perpetuated by patients' reticence, at times reinforced by cultural and educational differences. Patients felt disempowered, unable to "stand up" to a doctor (even when to do so may have been in their interests) because they felt they were *"patients, not equals."*

Maintaining a Hierarchy

Yet even once they were diagnosed, some doctors continued to separate themselves from patients, maintaining rigid hierarchy and relational power. Hegemony can serve certain beneficial ends, but it creates problems as well. Despite knowledge of its limitations and potential coerciveness, this hierarchy persisted, whether through direct efforts or by default.

Many consciously relied on this power to achieve what they saw as positive ends. For example, their authority could serve to encourage a patient to eschew unhealthy behaviors and engage in healthy activities. Patients might very much want—and need—to feel that doctors were stronger and healthier. Physicians possessed an aura. Stuart said:

Patients needed to believe that their docs were absolutely im-movable allies. Some of it's also an illusion the doctors project. Patients tend to buy into it, too: that physicians' judgments are authoritarian and infallible.

The need for doctors to be stable and constant manifested itself in various ways. Patients assumed that doctors would always "be there." Yet physicians could become ill or die. Paul, who lost a job offer, re-flected on this problem, since his own physician—who was also a friend—had recently perished. Paul felt she was not "supposed" to die: not expected to, and somehow cosmically not *allowed* to. He wept:

> She really was the friend that wasn't *supposed* to die. She had said she would take care of me. There was a huge comfort in that—it wasn't a question or an imposition. So it was totally unfair. Her funeral was huge. Patients talked about how difficult it was: their caregiver dying while *they* still lived.

When the doctor became sicker than the patient, an implicit border was transgressed—in the minds of patients as well as of physicians. Moreover, Paul felt as if his physician were magically immune from death. Thus, in some ways, a physician's death may resemble that of a *parent*, a protector from harm.

To Bolster Magic

In conjunction with their authority, physicians often possessed an "aura," implying a magical or superhuman element. Some of these doctors ex-plicitly observed and commented on this power, surprised by its strength. The placebo effect has been amply documented; and the psychiatrist Jerome Frank (2) has written about the importance of health profes-sionals as "healers" who help persuade patients to adopt healthy patterns of behavior. But do physicians see themselves as having an implicit placebo effect? Talcott Parsons suggested that doctors have a "bias to-ward optimism." Given the uncertainty of many treatments, physicians wish to bolster their confidence, which manifests itself as bias that treatments will work. The physicians here elaborated on how this hoped-for magic can aid patients. Harry, the internist and war refugee with heart disease, for example, found that patients believed that "as long as you took care of us, we were never going to die."

When I retired, I had seventeen letters that said that I was a traitor for leaving them. We have magic. I only realized that, in a comprehended fashion, when I was a patient. Waiting for the doctor to show up and say a few little common words—the faith.

On one level, intellectually, Harry knew this fact beforehand, but grasped it—fully, experientially—only now. This gap illustrated the degree to which book and experiential knowledge can vary. He suggested, too, why waiting for the physician instilled frustration: these longed-for properties themselves were delayed.

Still, this magic remains difficult to understand. Harry struggled to find analogies, seeking other examples.

We transform expectations into magic. It's nothing new: you expect your mother to perform it. I wait for my mail: it's going to transform my life. I'm astounded by how eagerly I look at my mail. I know it's going to be rubbish. But there's some fragment of magic there.

These desires are linked with and can engender a placebo effect. Indeed, physicians' power may have ancient and mythic sources. Harry continued:

A solid figure with unlimited power is going to help you. Whether doctors can or cannot, we're there, and a little authoritative— knowing more. One magnifies the object of one's dependency in order to feel more secure. We have healing powers. Everybody has discovered this: faith healers, quacks, native tribes with their quasi-religious figures dancing around the fire.... As long as she was taking care of me, I knew I wasn't going to die. Because of cheerfulness and positive attitude, people do better.

Though numerous popular jokes deride doctors for "acting like God," here, patients themselves often feel that doctors are like God, possessing special knowledge and powers. Illness can in fact promulgate a search for such special abilities.

But medical training does not explicitly teach or discuss such powers. Harry added, "Doctors are not aware of the extent of this. Maybe they know, but don't talk about it." Yet he sensed that self-awareness of this potency could be beneficial, "to help physicians understand themselves."

Still, such awareness may yield mixed results. Even Harry wavered, pointing out, "If we became totally aware, we'd have bigger heads."

Yet in doctor-patient relationships, this differential in roles, and disease vulnerability had critical implications, as it corresponded to, if not legitimated, a differential in power. Another physician, for example, sensed that patients needed him to be "stronger" than they were.

A lot of time what you're really dealing with—especially with death and dying—is "Yes, I'll be here longer than you will be. I'm stronger than you are. You can lean on me."

Physicians' power can therefore aid patients.

Doctors' powers arose in part from beliefs that they were *healthier* than their patients. Though feeling more aligned with patients than before, Suzanne said, "I still think: *I'm* the all-powerful resident who knows everything, and *these* are mental patients."

Differences in function further this power differential. Physicians perform duties that patients cannot. Doctors not only possess technical knowledge, but they also address emotional and psychological issues, and alleviate uncertainty. Harry spoke of doctors' anxiolytic properties: Physicians had to tolerate worry. Yet he was surprised at the importance of this function.

Nobody told me in medical school, but the toleration of anxiety is our stock in trade. You spend a great deal of your time dealing with others' anxiety. You can't get angry at the patient. You have to be aware of what you feel, and remain calm: sit and let people be anxious, and not be impatient or annoyed by their irrationality and nonsense.

Medically, this anxiety-reducing function of the doctor-patient hierarchy is critical. Anxious patients do not do as well.

Doctors can also use this hegemony to make patients feel valued. Walter, the political activist with lymphoma, saw other psychological benefits to physicians' use of their status.

When patients from poor communities have a doctor with status look them in the eye, and talk to them with respect, as another human being, it gives them a sense of their own humanity—that they ... matter. Particularly when you're sick, that's incredibly important. I go out of my way to *listen to people's hearts*. Every physical, I examine people. It fulfills their vision of being taken care of. If you lay hands on people, they feel you are thorough, and cared enough to do that.

Hence, the doctor-patient hierarchy can be employed to good ends.

But physicians had to decide when and to what degree to exercise this authority. Some used it only sparingly. Others grappled with decisions of when, how, and to what degree to invoke it. Brian, who had hepatitis, drew on this power differential exclusively when patients endangered themselves or others. "The only times the hierarchy becomes important is when patients are refusing treatment that I think is beneficial—or if they're abusing someone." He relied on it only when the potential harms to the patient or others outweighed those to the doctor-patient bond.

These ill physicians thus revealed two related kinds of power. The magical aura and status of doctors, as described here, arose from, and contributed to, healing. This status granted doctors permission to enter dangerous spaces and flout social strictures, probing strangers' nakedness, urine, feces, and blood.

As conveyed earlier, a second, relational kind of power between authority figures and dependent patients grew from, and relied on, this first kind of power, but could also take on a life of its own. Doctors modulated, and used or misused, this second, authority-based power to enhance healing. But patients differed in how much they needed or wanted this relational authority; and its outcomes varied from arrogance to hope.

Hierarchy as Helping Doctors

Hegemony resulted, too, from motives that benefited doctors more directly than patients. Limited time and energy led even the best-intentioned doctors to erect barriers between patients and themselves. Occasionally, physicians found themselves impatient, and rushing or coercing patients. Even Walter, despite his deep egalitarianism, sometimes found himself pressuring adolescent patients, blocking communication through his vocabulary, and hence implicitly coercing them: "I can talk patients into things if I want to—use words they don't understand, and are probably too embarrassed to ask about—if I'm feeling rushed." Despite his liberal, if not leftist, political views, Walter felt that at certain points, the doctor-patient relationship needed to be hierarchical, not equal. Hence, the balance in this relationship was based not simply on *political* views, but also on interpersonal medical ones imbued with special magical properties.

Emotional distance offered by hierarchy can assist doctors, too, in distancing themselves, as a defense in coping with losses and deaths of patients.

Conversely, closeness and hazy boundaries between patients and friends could exact psychic costs. Juan, who had HIV, was friendly with some patients, but later that closeness made it harder for him to treat them. He felt emotionally attached and, as a result, was more affected.

> At times, I felt *calloused from death*—I'm used to it. But with two patients who invited me to dinner—we weren't close, but considered each other to be friends besides doctor-patient—it was almost as if one of my close friends was passing.

To a certain extent, training as a physician numbs one to patients' suffering and death. Juan went on to describe this dullness of feeling, which often manifested itself as a delay in, and muting of, reactions. For instance, he was not upset by one patient's illness until after the patient's death. Only much later did he feel grief.

> There's a lag time. A patient passed, and it didn't hit me for three days. Then it hit me, but not as hard or intense as I thought it would. That's *numbing*—it's *anesthetized*. Once, I had a small surgical procedure on my toe, and they numbed part of it. In spite of the anesthesia, I felt part of it. But most of it hit me after the anesthesia wore off. This patient not being there anymore, his next scheduled appointment was removed from the books. I missed him, thought about him, reminisced about what we had gone through.

Over time, such grief can compel doctors to distance themselves further from patients. With patients, doctors had to titrate closeness versus separation.

Physicians' reactions to colleagues' deaths also further illuminated this chasm between dealing with death and loss professionally versus personally. Ronald, the suburban radiologist, said, "If a patient dies, I feel bad; but if it's a colleague, it's more upsetting."

Doctors appeared to handle death by separating themselves from the patient, not by having magically inured or inoculated themselves against death in general. Rather, they hardened themselves against a patient's demise by seeing the patient as one of "them," not one of "us." Stuart said, "Here's the doctor and there's the patient, and you have to choose your side, and *we* choose to be doctors, so we'll never be patients." As a consequence, it was tougher when disease occurred in oneself or a colleague. In that case, the strong defenses developed against loss of a patient through death did not work. Stuart's comment that doctors will "never be patients" further underscores the fragile illusion here.

Avoiding the Risks of Overidentification

As noted in the beginning of this chapter, physicians who sought to equalize the roles of doctor and patient risked *going too far in the opposite direction*—blurring roles and boundaries too much. Doctors could over-identify or become overinvolved with those in their care. They were not always clear on *how* close or social to be with patients, and had to gauge what were, and should be, the boundaries between the two sides. In small towns, this potential for sociability and hazy boundaries led a few doctors to seek treatment elsewhere.

Particular problems arose in treating friends. Nonetheless, a few physicians ended up doing so. Occasionally, friends became patients, or vice versa. Mark, the HIV-infected internist interviewed in the diner, said:

Generally, they're friends first. I'm flattered they have that much confidence in me. I figure in general I'll take better care of them than anybody else would, because I really care.

Doctors felt threatened, too, seeing patients *younger* than themselves dying. Only at such a point did Walter, for example, feel vulnerable himself. "When your patients who have serious illness or are dying are your own age or less, you feel that it could happen to you, too. I can't separate out those threats." He implied here, as well as earlier, that he had resisted and denied his own mortality.

Boundaries can also muddle for physicians who share diagnoses with their patients. These doctors tried not to think about the fact that ill patients could be them. Yet such efforts at avoidance did not always succeed. Paul said:

I think all the time, "God, that patient could be me." You don't let yourself get there. If you get too close, you're going to fry. I'm sure there's huge denial there.

Dangers lurked, but as Paul realized, attempts to avoid such identification could border on maladaptive defenses with added psychic costs. Doctors risked overidentifying with patients because of sharing not just medical diagnoses, but also other psychological or personal characteristics. For example, David, the psychiatrist with HIV, strained to guard against overidentifying with patients who had his "issues," psychologically.

Doctors' Problems with Blurred Boundaries

Firmer boundaries may make medicine more straightforward to practice, but were not always easy to maintain. At times, doctors socialized with patients, problematizing professional-client relationships. Patients could then take advantage of the friendship. Patient-friends may call at hours that are appropriate for friendships, but not for professional relationships. Stuart described the situation thus:

> Sometimes the friendship gets abused. Somebody calls on a Sunday at 7 A.M. and has a question. I'll ask them, "Why are you doing this?" They have a reason that I don't think is very good. So I say, "...If you behave like a patient, you will get good care....Please come to my office." Once in a while I'd say, "Don't do that again...."

Talcott Parsons described roles of doctors and patients in the abstract (3, 4); when these boundaries eroded, unexpected tensions could arise. The doctors here struggled to decide how to respond—whether as providers (with respect) or as friends (with anger).

Physicians faced questions of exactly how close to be with patients—for example, what to do if they saw a patient in a social context engaging in unhealthy behavior: eating poorly, smoking, drinking, or using drugs. Physicians could later broach these topics in the office with the patient. As a result, at times patients opted not to consult doctors they knew.

Particular dilemmas about diffuse boundaries arose when doctors had to decide whether and how often to give out their home phone numbers. Some physicians provided these to patients, while others refused, or did so only very selectively. Juan and many of his patients had HIV. He said:

> I gave my home phone number or pager number to a lot of patients I identified with and felt needed me. So people paged me in the middle of movies, or sex. It was hard to keep the boundaries clear. I thought that if I was in their situation, I would want my doctor to be that available. So it was hard to say, "This is unreasonable." The boundaries got very blurred....A lot of times if somebody

gave me just the littlest guilt or shame about not being there, I would be there extra. But doing that took more and more time . . . impinging on my personal life. . . .

Within the complex intricacies of daily practice, doctors gave out their outside numbers for other motives as well (e.g., to entice patients in various ways). Kurt, the internist with HIV, handed out his home phone number in order to be seen as "the best doctor" in his group practice. Other doctors in his group then resented him.

> The only way I could be a better doctor was to make myself available at odd times. In the beginning, I got off when patients switched from their doctor to me. I would spend a lot of time with them, give them hugs, pat them on the back. The senior docs liked to take a lot of vacations; I would see their patients while they were gone. But one doc yelled at me . . . three of his patients saw me and wanted to see me again.

Kurt paid a price, too, for his weakened boundaries. Patients, once his, would then continue to demand his time, which he found difficult to supply. He subsequently tried to reduce the amount of time he allotted to patients, or became resentful.

Patients could also seek, but then reject help, frustrating physicians. Uncooperative patients, including those with drug abuse or borderline personality disorder, received particular rebuke for requesting, but then refusing, assistance. Antagonism can ensue as part of what psychoanalysts term countertransference (i.e., a physician's feelings toward a patient).

Fuzzy distinctions between doctor and patient could interfere, too, with treatment decisions. For example, several HIV-infected physicians reported knowing HIV-infected doctors who would "not let their AIDS patients die, and kept them alive too long," when patients' families or lovers thought it was time to "pull the plug" and not continue heroic measures to prolong the patient's life. Having been infected with HIV by a needle stick, Jennifer found that her illness made it more difficult for her to care for patients, because she feared she would suffer from their same devastating symptoms.

> I had no professional objectivity! I couldn't handle it, and was making bad decisions. I would say, "Don't ask me. Just pull the plug." It was tough to see the disease all the time, knowing so much about it. Outpatients were easier. A lot were very

motivating—they lived positively with their disease. But it was hard to watch very painful deaths, people losing their dignity, becoming demented, their bodies falling apart. . . . I can take anything, but don't let me lose my mind! Anytime I would forget something, I would freak out.

The prospect of dementia terrorized her and others.

Physicians who felt they became too close and "a little soft on the boundaries," posed dilemmas about balancing opposing approaches, and defining the "softness" or "hardness" of boundaries. Jennifer indicated how knotty maintenance of appropriate professional distance can be.

I'm sure patients thought, "Why is she so hung up about a feeding tube and total parenteral nutrition through a central line?" I would say, "You need to consider these things." *I probably went too far in the other direction*, giving patients much more information than they wanted. Some staff said, "Do you think you *really* need to be talking about this?" I'd say, "Yes, this is very important." I may have been hung up on stuff because of where I was *personally*. I felt I needed to meet all of my patients' needs, because no one was listening to *me* when *I* would go to *my* doctor.

When physicians overidentified with patients, assisted suicide raised particularly troubling personal and professional issues. Several of these physicians encountered difficulties concerning this issue, or tried to establish and maintain clear protocols for themselves concerning these controversial acts.

Establishing Styles of Doctoring: Distance Versus Warmth

To deal with these conflicting pros and cons of hierarchy, ill doctors also established general practice styles: models and boundaries with which they felt most comfortable. These physicians described a range of such styles with regard to how close or distant to be with patients overall. In addition to styles of nihilism versus aggressiveness described earlier in the context of choosing doctors, this spectrum of distance versus warmth constituted another key dimension of physicians' approaches.

Styles of closeness could profoundly shape a physician's practice. For example, Jessica, the pediatrician with cancer, chose to join a group that had a style similar to hers in terms of being "warm and fuzzy" with patients.

> At job interviews, I was very much impressed with the vibes I got.
> At one interview, I didn't get a good vibe, so I chose another job.
> I wanted to work with a female colleague I knew and respected; we
> have very similar practice styles because we trained together.

Jessica's group practice inculcated new members into its approach, suggesting how doctors may choose practice settings through processes of mutual selection. "We trained a resident in our clinic for four years, so we indoctrinated her in our style. And she found it attractive, because she wanted to come work with us. *She selected us and we selected her.*"

Styles can also evolve to fit the characteristics of patient populations. Jessica added:

> Most of the staff and patients are Latino. Latinos are very warm,
> demonstrative and friendly. People bring food, and respect me for
> being warm and fuzzy. My approach enhances my stature with
> patients.

Others tried to balance *with each individual patient* the benefits of a hierarchy versus the desire for equalization. Hence, physicians may adjust their styles to meet the needs and challenges of particular patients. Over time, physicians dynamically equilibrated of their closeness with patients. These styles resulted from inherent character traits, and implicit rather than explicit teaching.

Gradients of Shared Decision-making

Physicians reassessed and often altered not only the boundaries of their relationships with patients, but also their specific approaches to decision-making, adopting a spectrum of models from traditional "doctor knows best" to more equal "sharing." Doctors modified traditional stances in various ways—from patients essentially making decisions alone, without strong physician input, to engaging in mutual processes of negotiation.

Many patients wanted not to share decision-making completely, but to re-equilibrate the relationship, and have the physician simply *explain decisions better*. Harry, for example, said:

In the past, the authoritarian physician could do what he or she thought was best for the patient. Maybe it *was* best for some given percent of patients a high percent of the time. Patients probably weren't totally happy, unless they liked authoritarian physicians. Other patients wanted more "say," and understanding: not be as much "say" as "understanding."

Though some patients wanted decisions made for them, or sought only explanations, at the far other extreme some doctors now saw patients as full equals with whom to make *joint decisions*. With his patients, Juan, for example, sought as much balance as possible.

> My role is as an advocate, a teacher, so that they can understand the "medicalese"—the concept behind the drugs—and make their best decisions. I now tell patients, "I'm not going to tell you what to do. I'm just going to give you the information so you can make the best decision." Patients said that that approach was different from what they got elsewhere, and that was why they were coming to see me.

Patients thus selected or rejected Juan based on his stance toward them. Other patients preferred more direction and "answers." Ronald, the suburban radiologist, reported that after he gave patients information for them to make decisions, *a third* would ask him, "What would *you* do if you were me, doc?"

> Sometimes I'm just talking over their heads, even though I'm trying not to use big words. One of the hardest things we try to explain is why, with unresectable lung cancer, I wouldn't cut it out anyway. Patients say, "Why don't I just undergo surgery?" It's difficult for them to understand: It's not going to influence their survival.

The many inherent ambiguities in medicine were difficult to convey because of high degrees of uncertainty, invasiveness of treatments, patients' potential understandings, and personal communication preferences.

Physicians' nondirective approaches could even offend and confuse patients. Sally, who brought her laptop to the ICU, explained, "When I laid out some options, one family said, 'Doc, don't *you* know what to do? You want *us* to decide?' I tried to explain my rationale to them. It was far from what they expected from a doctor!"

Other physicians came to take a different approach to decision-making by presenting more choices: not necessarily sharing decision-making, but making it more transparent and giving patients more leeway. Even Dan, with chest metastases, who had always been very assertive, now became *"less dictatorial."* "I'm offering my patients more choices: 'We can do A, B, C, or D—I think we ought to do A, but if you want to do B or C, we'll do that.' "

Here, too, doctors tried to adapt their styles to meet their perceptions of individual patients' desires. Suzanne, the psychiatrist with bipolar disorder, said:

> I'll sense what patients need. If they need me to just take control and be the authority, I'll do that. If *they* need to be the one making choices, I'll do *that.*

Yet determining patient preferences can be intricate. Patients may or may not concur with their physicians' assessments of how "authoritarian" to be, and may change over time.

In sum, their experiences as patients led many of these physicians to try to establish an appropriate balance of "detached concern," varying from upholding a traditional hierarchy between doctors and patients on the one hand, to becoming more "equal" with patients on the other. At times, this hierarchy—encompassing properties of aura and magic—turned out to be a powerful tool, sought by patients. *These doctors themselves possessed a "placebo effect"* that could help patients ameliorate anxiety and uncertainty. Yet medical training rarely, if ever, explicitly taught or discussed such "magic." This hierarchy could grow, too, from physician callousness and antagonism, separating doctors and patients, and widening due to competing demands on physicians' time. This power, reflecting both magic and relational authority, could take on a range of forms. Many physicians now felt closer to patients, but still struggled to avoid overidentification and to gauge *how* close to be, adopting different styles over time. In grappling with these boundaries, they followed different models of decision-making, from "the doctor knows best" to the doctor merely providing options and letting patients decide by themselves.

Medical information emerged, then, not as a monolithic or static entity, but rather as something exchanged in variable, dynamic contexts of doctor-patient relationships, in which decision-making played key roles. Physicians adopted different roles, depending on a variety of factors, including physician and patient preferences. Mutual self-selection may occur, too, as both physicians and patients sought members of the opposite group who exhibited preferred patterns of communication.

Again, surprisingly, many of these doctors only now, as patients, became fully aware of the importance of these phenomena in their day-to-day interactions—underscoring the need to make their colleagues and patients more aware of these issues.

12

Improving Education

Can Empathy Be Taught?

Does a doctor have to get sick in order to become more sensitive? The physicians here posed critical questions of how to improve sensitivity in the profession: whether trainees and other providers can be taught to be more empathetic, and if so, how. Clearly, formidable internal and external obstacles exist to improve patient care, including implicit stigma: the fact that physicians often see patients as somehow "less than." To bolster themselves and conquer disease, many doctors distanced themselves from, and identified less with, patients. Yet overall, these physicians changed their practices in ways ranging from small to large. Recently, questions of how to make doctors better have received attention (1). But the doctors here suggest additional ways, and their intimate stories offer insights that made even "good" physicians better. They came to reassess and alter their relationships with patients: approaches to tests and diagnoses, treatment problems, poor adherence, nonmedical aspects of care, and communication about end-of-life and other taboo topics. Though potentially, illness could merely embitter and frustrate a doctor, that was overall not the case here. Indeed, many now wanted to take on, as a mission or legacy, improving the training of future providers. Through their pain, these doctors hoped to enlighten and inspire others.

Nonetheless, some joked that ideally, medical students should be hospitalized and forced to sleep in patient rooms, to experience the disruptions, inconveniences, powerlessness, and humiliations that patients routinely encounter. Eleanor described how such an experience, with its loss of power over one's very body and life, and its confrontation with the unknown, could transform trainees.

They should be admitted through the ER—have people bustling back and forth, nobody saying what's going on, why they are doing particular evaluations, what anybody is thinking, what the differential diagnosis may be, how long it's going to take—leave them with all that uncertainty.

In its ability to make physicians appreciate fully what it is like to be a patient, patienthood was seen as unique. Ernie, who had Huntington's disease, thought that *only* the process of becoming ill would make medical students more empathetic.

If you're not personally affected, it's *impossible* to imagine what it's really like. I'm not sure what would make students more empathetic. Maybe you *have to* go through it yourself.

Potentially, health care professionals can be taught to see more clearly that they have only one point of view, and that it is just one of many, differs from that of patients, and can be restrictive. Humans evolved such that each person generally sees through just one main vantage point, his or her own. Unfortunately, that creates problems. Novelists and filmmakers know and illustrate these limitations. Faulkner's *The Sound and the Fury* and Kurosawa's *Rashoman* each depict one event from differing individuals' perspectives. Perhaps only narratives can reveal another person's point of view—the experience of literally being inside another skull, seeing the world through his or her eyes. Otherwise, we usually rarely realize the constrictions on our perspectives. To each of us, our views seem coherent, and correct. The doctors here can impel others to become more aware of the extent to which physicians' ways of seeing infact differ from those of patients, and are ultimately bounded.

These doctors illuminate, too, how and why book and experiential learning differ. As patients, these doctors learned much that they had not fully realized before. Not until now did they truly see and learn what it was like to be in the opposite role. *Illness taught them what books failed to.* Thus, these doctors limned the divide between intellectual and experiential knowledge, and the extent to which experience involves emotions and deeper layers of self. The discrepancies can be vast. Yet awareness of this gap can help bridge it.

To heighten these sensitivities, several physicians thought that medical school can more effectively teach specific skills in ways other than by hospitalizing all students. Much of doctor-patient relationships and communication was best instilled not explicitly through lectures, but *implicitly* through role-modeling. Jessica, the pediatrician with cancer, tried to instruct students and residents informally, by example:

> ...almost by osmosis. They observe me. I try to get across...the way I relate to patients and parents. It's just very informal. That's part of pediatrics. But I am *especially* informal.

These approaches get communicated subtlely, indirectly.

Some doctors attempted to achieve educational goals by other means, similarly trying to draw on student emotions. But, given the medical profession's prevailing "macho" culture, they were not always successful. One ill physician described how on rounds once a medical student had said bluntly to a patient, "You have cancer." The chief of medicine then turned to the student and said, "You, get out of this room! You are hereby kicked out of this medical school. And I will make sure you never get into another medical school in this country." Crushed and confused, the medical student slowly stumbled out of the room. At the last possible moment, the chief said, "Come back. I just wanted to make you aware of what it's like to be given a death sentence." Such a pedagogical approach may foster sensitivity, but not reduce the hierarchy in medicine between doctors and patients, or instill humanity.

Not surprisingly, some questioned or viewed skeptically the ability to teach compassion to medical students. Others concluded that such training might have unclear efficacy, but was still worthwhile. Jerry, the surgeon-lawyer with HIV, said:

> I go back and forth: students are either going to have that sensitivity and treat patients in a kind and decent way or not. Every year, I spoke to the third-year students about being an HIV-positive physician and being gay. I thought at times that it was good, but at other times that that was something you can't train. It's still good to teach them...but I wonder if it does any good.

Cynicism lingered about the ability of education to make students more empathetic. Albert, who had an MI on the highway, said:

> Med school applicants want to work in soup kitchens all their life, and practice urban-missionary medicine. But many physicians won't get out of bed at night to see a patient. So, I'm a cynic. My partners...are compassionate, caring. I don't know how well you

can evaluate that. I say to medical students, "In terms of your interaction with people, you're going to be where you already are. Do you treat people nicely? Then that's going to be the way you practice medicine. If you're not, we can't change that.

Albert raised several issues here: whether students can shift; how such alteration can be evaluated, if at all; and the degree to which trainees differ in underlying compassion for others.

Still, for the most part, illness opened these physicians' eyes. Every medical student probably won't be required to stay in a hospital bed, tied to an IV for a few nights. But the next best thing, I think, is to have trainees increase their awareness of these issues through narratives such as those here.

Reconnecting with Patients: Improving the Process of Care

Despite these questions about teaching empathy, ill physicians offered several specific, explicit ways to improve patient-doctor communication. The experience of being patients themselves led many to treat their patients differently, using a variety of techniques. They made suggestions, large and small, offering advice that can benefit both doctors and lay patients. I do not mean to reduce the richness of their narratives to a few quick, pat phrases, but several of their recommendations can be readily and widely adopted.

Communicating Better: Providing More Time and Attention

In response to becoming sick, these providers not only reassessed their relationships and decision-making processes with patients, but often managed to provide *more time* for interactions with their patients as well. To do so, they had to confront and navigate a series of obstacles, and did not always succeed as much as they had hoped.

Some felt motivated by their own doctors taking extra time with them. When Roxanne, the gastroenterologist with cancer, now took a history, she reflected on her own physician's generosity.

What surprised me most is being inspired by my doctor. He's very patient. He never felt threatened by my getting a second opinion. He took a detailed history and was never rushed...when I'm getting a history, I think about that.

Unfortunately, countervailing pressures compelled many doctors to feel too hurried to obtain full histories. In fact, colleagues denigrated such efforts to take extra time. Roxanne continued:

Patients have told me that I'm the only doctor who listened to them. I'll ask fellows a question about a patient, and they'll have to go back and ask. Patients come here because they've seen other physicians, and have inches of papers of blood work and X-rays that I don't look at. But get a detailed history, and the patient will tell you their diagnosis. They'll say, "I get pain that comes after I eat," and diagnose their ulcer. Other doctors have not had the time. Everything is driven by efficiency now. If a fellow is slow, it's seen as bad, even if it's because he's taking more time with patients.

Consequently, as a result of these pressures, as antidotes some physicians developed special approaches or mechanisms for giving more time to patients—often revisiting and speaking to them at other times than while on rounds. Deborah, the psychiatrist with cancer, said:

A nurse told me, "You have a special way of talking to patients. You come back—you don't just leave them, or not show up. You listen." I didn't want to say, "It's because I am a patient, what do you expect?" I really feel compassion. *I can't explain it.* Sometimes I check on patients when the other interns aren't here, because I think patients talk to me much more honestly than with a whole group.

As Deborah said, doctors often talked with patients only on group rounds, which can discourage thorough or optimal communication. Yet she indicated, too, that she can't wholly describe the difference she now felt—the heightened empathy. No doubt, this interaction involved emotional, not just intellectual, connections, and can be subtle and nonverbal.

Many physicians now *offered more information* to their patients. These doctors may explicitly share their uncertainties more, or check if patients have additional questions. As a result of being a patient, Roger, the HIV-infected surgeon who became suicidal, divulged more than before his clinical reasoning to those he treated.

I'm much more likely to explain why I'm doing things. Other physicians make decisions, but don't say what they're thinking about to patients. . . . I give . . . my rationale, doubts: "Basically, this is a crapshoot. We don't know what we're dealing with here. We'll take our best shot." A lot of doctors rush out, but I just *psychologically fold my hands and listen.*

Though sensitive and compulsive in the past, many of these physicians now found room to follow up with details even more.

Others tried to communicate better by providing information not only about the content of decisions, but also the *process* of clinical care—what to *expect* from treatment and its course. Tom, whose lover died of AIDS, wanted to give patients "a road map" to guide expectations. "With managed care, it's even worse, because you have to wend your way through the system. I say, 'Don't expect this doctor to really be a human being, just expect them to cut out your gallbladder.'" Brian, the pediatrician with hepatitis, also became more proactive with patients.

I've always been good at explaining, but I'm more vigilant now than before, in talking about side effects and what to expect. I say, "An hour before you get this, the nurse ought to be giving you a pill. Make sure you get it." You can do that with some, but not all, patients.

These suggestions—to be proactive and explicit—can benefit other physicians and their patients as well.

Ill doctors came to realize the importance of both verbal and *nonverbal* interactions as well, and the range of such interchanges. For instance, rubbing a patient's back can help alleviate an existential sense of aloneness and isolation. Walter, the political activist, said:

Giving a back rub was so incredibly important to me. It was profoundly human—an act of caring. Even with painkillers, there's suffering and pain. Those back rubs were...somebody affirm[ing] that I mattered.

Yet, as mentioned in the previous chapter, such heightened sensitivity toward patients was not always easy. Competing pressures and demands can overwhelm. For instance, occasionally, in part for personal reasons (e.g., if she had a long day), even Jessica, who had a "warm and fuzzy" style, still paid little heed to certain patient complaints.

If I am not in a really good mood, I've blown off patients' complaints. I'll listen, but sometimes when every organ system causes pain, I can get a little dismissive.

Although they would like to provide ideal care, many factors can stymie these doctors' best intentions. In the end, physicians were only human.

In the current, ever-changing health care system, professionalism itself
is in crisis. Many concluded that doctors were often less conscientious,
and that medical education needed to embrace professionalism and a
sense of responsibility more. As Nancy, the endocrinologist with cancer,
observed, "We should teach not just humanism, kindness, and empathy;
but how to behave professionally."

Reduced supervision by overworked attendings can further lower
standards. Nancy complained of physicians becoming "lax." For example, she felt that chief residents no longer reviewed patients' charts to
check for errors or suggest improvements far less. She added:

> There are all kinds of abdication of responsibilities. Residents are
> technically not supposed to do things, but it's sort of ok, and ev-
> erybody gets used to this loosey-goosey kind of moral responsi-
> bility. A nice chief resident had been doing little procedures for
> attendings on the side, unsupervised. He wasn't supposed to. But
> the department had kind of set a tradition. He got caught. I'm sure
> he thought: they have been doing it for years. It's all sort of lack-
> adaisical. It's probably necessary in a hospital, to avoid losing
> money while taking care of poor patients. A strength of our pro-
> gram is that you are very autonomous.

Nancy herself was ambivalent about the pros and cons of such independence as a trainee, citing both advantages to students and costs to
patients, and highlighting the conflicting pressures teaching hospitals
confront.

Some of these doctors urged trainees to collect detailed histories despite increased pressures to do otherwise. However, given the shortened
amount of time physicians have with patients, trainees often resisted
gathering such "ideal," full medical backgrounds. Harry said, "I taught
students to do an hour and a half initial history. They said, 'What are we
going to do with *that?*'" Students perceived that such attention was no
longer the norm. Stuart remarked:

> I told students how to take a history and a sexual history. They
> turned to me as if I were speaking Greek: "We've been in primary
> care offices. *Nobody does this.*"

Concrete Practice Behaviors

Since extra attention was not always easy to provide, these doctors described several other concrete behaviors to be more sensitive to patients—even small ways to be available and accessible. A doctor sitting down in a patient's room, rather than remaining standing, proved important. Similarly, Harry, the internist and war refugee with heart disease, wrote chart notes in patients' hospital rooms rather than at the nursing station.

> I learned something useful from one doctor. He was busy and wonderful—considerate, insightful—and used to take the chart into the patient's room, and sit there writing his notes, rather than sitting out by the nurse's station. That gave him an extra four minutes. While he was writing, he might ask questions. I've tried to incorporate that. So simple. The doctors' station for writing notes is a refuge.

Likewise, Harry mentioned, regarding acknowledgment of the indignities of patienthood, that such interchanges don't "have to be very long: five to ten minutes . . . some sign of awareness of the helplessness, dependency." A physician simply saying to patients, "I'm sorry about keeping you waiting," can diffuse potential patient frustration.

Many tried to transmit their insights to trainees, urging more openness with patients. Brian, the pediatrician with hepatitis, felt that his experience as a patient made him more likely to ensure that his trainees asked if patients and their families had any questions.

> I am more attentive to making sure that medical students and residents sit down and talk with parents to really understand parents' concerns. I've always done that, but I'm *a little bit more attentive* now, asking them, *"Anything* you don't understand?"

Additional practices arose, too, that allowed more time with patients. Roxanne, the gastroenterologist, chose a university-based practice to give her longer periods with patients than private practice would permit, even though her salary was consequently less. Given that she sought thoroughness, in private practice she would see fewer patients and "starve."

Improving Content: Specific Areas of Increased Sensitivity

As a result of experiences with their own providers, these doctor-patients often became more sensitive not only to the *form* of interactions, but also to several specific *content* areas.

"Routine" for W*hom?* Increased Sensitivity to Medical Tests

Frequently, these physician-patients altered their understandings of the meanings of diagnostic tests. They came to realize that every test, even if they considered it "routine," was critically important to the patient undergoing it. Jennifer, the internist infected with HIV from a needle stick, commented:

> Here we doctors are, sitting with a piece of paper. We tell them the
> result, and want them out of our office for the next patient,
> without really going through the emotions of what that one result,
> what that specific one, means.

Seen from patients' perspectives, tests were no longer merely ritual or rote, but traumatic and defining, with profound implications.

Waiting for Test Results

As a result, several physicians now tried to provide patients with test results more swiftly. Jacob, the radiologist with cancer, for instance, was more likely to interrupt what he was doing to give patients their results.

> I always try and run out to them to tell them the results of their
> scan. . . . But now, I'll interrupt *anything* I'm doing to tell them the
> results. In the past, I would get them the results as quickly as
> possible, but if I was talking to someone else, I wouldn't get up.
> Now I pretty much drop everything, or call the tech: "Go and tell
> the patient everything is ok." I prefer to do it myself. When pa-
> tients say, "It's nice you did that," I say, "I've been there, and know
> what it feels like."

Yet again, competing pressures can hamper physicians' ability to respond as fully and immediately as they would like. Daily challenges ensue.

Increased Sensitivity to Symptoms

Ill physicians may now be able to diagnose symptoms better in others, having confronted these symptoms themselves. Certain symptoms (e.g., pain, nausea, insomnia, anxiety, and depression) constitute inherently ineffable subjective states, and are difficult to quantify objectively or convey verbally. Those who have experienced them acquire a distinct, though not unalloyed, advantage. Psychiatric symptoms pose particular problems, as ill physicians may run the risk of overdiagnosing them. For example, Suzanne now overestimated bipolar disorder because she sometimes overidentified, though "I try to really notice that."

Yet one's own experience of illness can increase awareness of the difficulties of diagnosing subtle evidence or absence of disease symptoms in others. For instance, Suzanne could detect individuals who tried to deceive doctors, claiming to have psychiatric disorders in order to obtain secondary gains.

> I am good at smelling out if a patient is really psychotic or malingering. When someone comes to the ER, I can really tell if they're lying. Either I really know what it's like to be mentally ill, and can tell that they're just not; or I am really good at identifying if somebody is manic versus on cocaine. One guy said he was just a mess, an emotional wreck. But then he went to sign something, and was ok: got the pen and pulled it together, no problem. If somebody says they're hearing voices or are really paranoid, or seeing things, you just watch where their eyes go, listen to the way they talk.... You get a hunch. A lot has to do with relatedness. When you're sick, you're "off." There is a sort of "offness" about you. Three times, patients were going to kill me when I told them they couldn't get admitted. I knew they were bullshitting me. They'd get up and say, "You fucking bitch, I wasn't going to kill anybody, but I just wanted to...." We have a park nearby, and they do crack, then come in here for a good night's sleep.

Suzanne also now better distinguished between early mania and anxiety. She used a metaphor of *smelling* diagnoses to suggest how her awareness increased of the subtle, and indescribable aspects of determining diagnoses, involving additional vaguer, and more nuanced kinds of information than many doctors use.

Given that part of the problem communicating about certain symptoms, particularly psychiatric ones, is their inexpressible nature, individuals who have experienced these symptoms have sometimes found ways of conveying them from which other practitioners can learn. Her experiences led Suzanne to establish quick rapport:

> I just say, "Does it feel like there's a dark cloud in front of you, and it's hard to put one foot in front of the other? You can't get where you want because there's this hump you can't get over?" That's what depression feels like. Patients' eyes light up: "That's exactly what it feels like. How did you know?" They feel so comforted that somebody understands. We feel very connected—three sentences into our conversation.

Patients feel gratified when physicians not only empathize but, more specifically, "clarify or summarize" such states. Suzanne continued, about panic attacks:

> I say to patients: You're somewhere and feel you just need to get out, immediately. It doesn't matter what you're doing, you just need to get to a safe place. Patients say, "Yeah, that's exactly what it feels like." Or "You feel like you're going to die. There's this load on your chest. All of a sudden it feels like you're wearing a tight turtleneck." They say, "Oh my God, that's exactly it." Or when people get antsy and can't sleep, I'll say, "Does that anxiety sometimes get to the point where it's more like agitation, like people start to really bother you?" They say, "Yeah!"

Suzanne's realizations illustrated the degree to which physicians otherwise have difficulty communicating and connecting with patients about these disturbing but inchoate symptoms.

Physicians also drew on their own experiences of illness to teach patients quick ways to stymie symptoms. For example, based on his own history, John, the public health official with HIV, taught patients tricks to recognize and treat early herpes symptoms.

> Since I've had a lot of herpes myself, I tell people how to recognize it: that the first thing you get is tingling. I said, "Keep acyclovir in your medicine cabinet. As soon as you feel that tingling, pop eight capsules, and see if you can abort it!"

Yet diagnoses informed by personal experiences may conflict with more conventional diagnostic assessments arrived at by other clinicians. Suzanne described how her "hunch" that one patient's symptoms resulted from bipolar disorder collided with a professor's view that drug abuse was the cause.

> I was convinced a patient was hypomanic to manic. I just knew it. I could just feel it—his whole story. He vehemently denied any drug use, and seemed honest. The attending said, "What's this guy on?," totally discrediting the fact that the kid could be hypomanic or manic. The attending was prejudiced....I said, "I bet you that there are no drugs involved with this." So we did a urine toxin screen.

The next week, she phoned me to report that the tox screen turned out to be negative.

Such heightened attunement to subtle diagnostic signs highlighted what other clinicians may miss. Suzanne explained about this patient:

> For me, all these buzz words went off: ADHD [attention deficit hyperactivity disorder] as a child. I was diagnosed with ADHD as a kid. My psychiatrist said, "It was probably because you were prodromal. That's what it looks like as a kid."...When I was hypomanic, everywhere I went and everything I did was an event. Every interaction was this big to-do. In every single state or country this patient went to, there were security problems. This or that would happen. That happens when you're hypomanic: you get into "situations." Every day my life was one mishap after the next. I'd always bump into things, and had bruises all over. He did, too.

Less Hard on Patients: Increased Sensitivity to Poor Adherence

As a result of having been patients themselves, many of these physicians approached treatment problems differently, especially concerning poor adherence, often becoming "less hard" on those under their care. Their own battles with side effects led many to be much more sensitive to adherence problems. For example, Paul, the internist who lost a job offer, said:

> When someone talks about missing doses, I try to pinpoint what's happening. For me, it's easy on workdays, but not on weekends.

Other times, [patients] just get sick of the schedule.... Or they're feeling sick, so they don't want to take a pill that makes them sicker. Trying to ferret it out makes it easier.

The arduousness of sticking to a schedule often startled these doctors, who then became more sympathetic with patients' struggles. Steven, the suburban endocrinologist with HIV who had considered trying a diabetic diet, but ultimately did not because of the burden, now understood even better and more clearly patients who had trouble adhering to treatments other than those he himself took. For example, he had more understanding for a diabetic woman who had been checking her glucose too frequently.

I give patients more slack. This morning was the first time I saw patients after...taking medication myself. I saw a diabetic woman who had delivered an infant and was still taking six to eight shots of insulin a day. During pregnancy, that's ok. After that, it's unreasonable. She was checking blood sugar eight to ten times a day. Her husband checked her blood sugars at night while she was sleeping! She thought maybe she shouldn't be on this schedule the rest of her life. I said, "*For sure* you can't!" Some endocrinologists wouldn't say that.... Previously, I would have said, "You have to do this."

Again, it took one's own illness to realize how to approach such patients more effectively. Steven reframed patients' adherence failures as well.

Now, I acknowledge very small steps—if patients don't do 100 percent of what they're supposed to, but just a little bit. In the old days, instead of saying, "You've really made some improvements," I'd say, "You need to work a lot harder."

These doctors also became less likely to lecture patients about other poor health behaviors. Steven said, "I have a better understanding of what they're going through. For folks with diabetes to successfully treat their disease, they have to make major lifestyle changes. I'm seeing how hard that is for *me*!" These physicians thus became less judgmental, and more aware of disease management outside the clinician's office. Previously, medical training and the functional separation between doctors and patients had impeded these recognitions.

These physicians also mentioned specific methods of promoting *preventive* health care. For instance, Sally urged doctors to consider "well-child preventive care" for adults: "getting on an exercise program, worrying about your bones if you're on steroids....Doctors weren't thinking about it."

"I've Become Like a Social Worker": Nonmedical Aspects of Care

Ill doctors became more sensitive to *nonmedical aspects of care* as well. Many came to address more regularly and thoroughly questions of whether patients could afford medications, and had transportation home, and adequate home care. Ronald, the suburban radiologist, said, "I've become like a social worker"—highlighting the degree to which physicians ordinarily saw such duties as outside their role. Many of these physicians had overlooked nonmedical aspects of patients' lives (e.g., applying to Social Security for disability benefits), and now extended the scope of their responsibilities.

Some ill physicians now addressed more than before *psychotherapeutic issues* (e.g., having patients develop and work toward "life goals"). Deborah, the psychiatrist with breast cancer, came to make sure patients had aspirations for themselves and future plans. In doing so, she felt she deviated from traditional doctoring. As a result of her own illness, she urged patients more regarding not only establishing, but also achieving, personal goals.

> Previously, I'd help them do this and that, but now *I push them.*
> Sometimes I think I'm crazy about it. Before, I would have said,
> "Do whatever you want." But now people come back and tell me
> what they've done. Somehow, my system works.

The narrowness of the biomedical model, and competing time pressures, inhibit physicians from ordinarily addressing such issues with their patients. Yet patients may benefit from physician interest in treating the "whole" person in these ways. Appropriate training in these approaches would clearly be helpful. In these ways, physician hierarchy could further be used to good ends.

Physician Assistants have more time than physicians, and could provide services for which the latter have inadequate time. Patient advocates could help, too. Sally, the internist with cancer, suggested that tertiary care doctors in particular hire more nurse practitioners "to do the things other than fighting the fires."

Protecting Privacy and Confidentiality

These physicians often spoke more to their patients about threats to medical privacy, and took extra measures to protect patients' confidentiality. A few physicians now went so far as to inform patients that privacy no longer existed: that despite policies to protect privacy, leaks could occur. ("It's illegal, but the *reality* is that at work, the employment person might sit across from the benefits person, and the information might get passed.")

Doctors also took extra measures to protect patients' privacy. These threats were particularly high for celebrity and VIP patients. In such cases, Harry said, "You have to give the chart to the secretary and say, 'Nobody is to look at this but me.'"

To protect confidentiality, at times doctors even engaged in or encouraged deceit. For example, increasingly, schools and camps ask for medical information that may not be necessary. Given these growing invasions, to protect confidentiality, Jessica felt that professionalism necessitated a degree of duplicity. She said:

> A mother was agitated because her daughter was recently diagnosed with epilepsy—petit mal seizures, not the kind where someone falls on the floor and shakes. The girl just stares into space. The teacher wants to tell the class, so they won't be scared if the girl falls and shakes. I got angry. Schools and a lot of people are very inappropriately interested in other people's health problems. *There's no confidentiality.* Schools are always asking for information they don't need and that has no impact on the kid. Why does the school need to know if there is a family history of high blood pressure? Even things that are against the law: they'll ask about drug use, violence, or sexuality. A lot of times, I tell parents, "Don't tell the school," or I leave it off forms.

Talking About Taboos

These physicians saw the need to educate medical students and physicians more about taboo areas. Yet improving communication between physicians and their patients about such stigmatized topics posed challenges. Nonetheless, several ill doctors now developed methods for talking about these areas better. Specific techniques can assist in desensitizing students to these topics. For example, Jerry, the surgeon-lawyer, saw other ways to improve communication skills concerning sexuality: teaching medical students in history-taking not to ask, "Are you married?" but "Do you have a partner?" In speaking about safer sex with patients, Paul had learned to use blunt, rather than medical, terms to open up conversation ("saying 'fucking,' 'sucking,' and 'going down' instead of using technical words, tends to open things up"). Professional roles can prompt professional language that may suboptimally convey information.

Doctors also used their own failures to talk to their providers about health behaviors, such as unsafe sex, to approach patients more effectively. Jeff, the adolescent specialist with HIV, drew on his experience of how hard it was to follow his own physician's advice concerning nonadherence to safer sex and medications.

> I assume health-negating behavior, and take it from there. Doctors say teenagers lie to them. But teenagers don't. They *can't* tell me the truth because I'm not being effective in getting to it. So it's *my* problem. When I hear false stuff from a teenager, *I've* screwed up; they haven't.

Jeff admitted that he had in fact dissembled to doctors, and hence learned to ask his patients about health behaviors more effectively than he had before.

> I won't ask, "Do you use condoms?" but "Do you use condoms some of the time, never, or all the time?" If they want to say 100 percent of the time, I say, "Absolutely 100 percent of the time? Most people slip up once. When did you? How?" Again they have to say, "No, I've never done that." I assume drug experimentation. The other day, a former patient thanked me: "I couldn't tell you many things, but you would tell me, so then I didn't have to tell you."

Usually, such nonpsychiatrist physicians see these patients first or exclusively, making this ability to gather delicate information crucial.

Giving Bad News: Framing Information

These physicians heightened their sensitivity, too, to how they presented medical information—the contexts in which they used it, and the need to ground it in a realistic sense of patients' experiences. Particularly with poor prognoses, these doctors highlighted the importance of "framing data."

Increasingly, they saw the delivery of such medical information as a "talent," especially since many patients misunderstood and "twisted" what they heard. This task took dedication. Neil, the neurologist, commented:

> Information is good, as long as it's delivered in a way the patient can understand. But many doctors don't have that talent, so it's useless. Some patients take a little information and misunderstand.

As a result, Neil tried to be as careful as possible, "to be gentle when I give bad news."

Many became more sensitive to communication about difficult decisions concerning death and dying, and to addressing these areas in a more sensitive and timely manner. Jennifer said that after her diagnosis, with patients, "I talked a lot more about end-of-life issues and resolving things and being very open and up front about it." She suggested, though, that despite her relative openness about many clinical matters, death and dying remained difficult topics for her.

Even physicians who felt they were sensitive to end-of-life issues to begin with nonetheless changed. Mathilde described the heightened attention she gave to these topics after her husband's death.

> Now, I put myself in my patients' clothes. When I talk to them, I really talk to myself: How would *I* react to what was being said? If people used my words toward *me*, would I consider them too blunt? If I ever had any rough edges, I smoothed them.

Mathilde suggested the aesthetic considerations in such discussions: avoiding either bluntness or "roughness," trying to smooth transitions, and perhaps softening information—or at least its impact.

Many physicians altered how they discussed not only death, but also poor medical outcomes. Following the loss of her husband, Mathilde became even more sympathetic than she had been before toward framing as positively as possible other major changes in patients' lives.

> My husband's illness led me to have even more sympathy than I ever expressed. When I had to tell patients that their kidneys had failed, and that they had to go on dialysis, I would say, "I don't tell you: you have to die. I tell you that you're going to have *another* life. It's different and difficult, but you are going to live." I'd use my husband's example, if they knew him: "I wish his doctor had said the same thing. I'm not saying you're lucky, but within the

illness, you are lucky because you can have a life—at times, completely normal. You can travel, have a transplant...a second chance. My husband did not."

As part of such enhanced empathy, many physicians improved their ability to discuss and make "do not resuscitate" (DNR) orders for patients. Confronting one's own mortality can make it easier to confront that of others. Mark, the internist with HIV whom I interviewed in a diner, reported:

I've dealt with my mortality. A lot of doctors are not good at dealing with code status because they haven't dealt with their own mortality. When somebody becomes demented, it's really easy for me now to draw the line.

Other Aspects of End-of-Life Care

Several of these doctors thought that issues of death and dying were still not taught with enough time, quality, or follow-up. Deborah said:

A lot of hospitals and medical schools address end-of-life, but not enough or well enough. No staff is really dealing with end-of-life, except hospice. Doctors think, "This is never going to happen to me."

This topic requires meaningful, not superficial, attention.

Hospice training was rare. To improve care around the end of life, Deborah felt that every resident, especially in psychiatry, should receive some experience in palliative care:

...to really deal with dying patients, and see how they die....A resident should talk to dying patients about their needs—spiritual, religious. Our hospital has a rabbi, but I've never seen him.

Attitudes toward death and dying need to be changed as well. For example, doctors should not view a patient's *death as a failure*. Eleanor added:

The phrase "there is nothing more we can do for you" ought to be banned. There is a lot more we *can* do for you, even if we can't cure your current physiological problem—talking to patients...as opposed to just doing procedures.

Goals of positive outcomes of treatment need to be redefined. Physicians' refusals to recognize fully that they, too, would one day face these issues in their own lives had psychological and adaptive advantages. This attitude allowed for denial of painful truths about death all around them, but could clearly cause problems, too.

Obstacles to Improving Care

Still, the more sensitive and enlightened practices and attitudes mentioned by these ill doctors were not always easy to follow. *Empathy emerged as a daily challenge.* Entering into the life of the patient, of "the Other," and seeing that in medicine "a person waiting is a person suffering," was hard. Even Roxanne, the gastroenterologist who, when on call, would ask a priest to bless her, occasionally found herself being rushed and preoccupied: "Sometimes I catch myself about to leave the room in a hurry, and ask, 'Do you have any questions?'" Despite their best intentions, physicians could readily slip back into old patterns.

Roxanne tried now to think before speaking insensitively, but doing so was not always easy. "I try and stop a millisecond before blurting out something, but I'm sure I've blurted out stupid things. It requires a lot of self-control. You *always* have to be careful of your comments."

In incorporating lessons from their experiences as patients into their work as physicians, these ill doctors confronted troubling trade-offs. Spending more time with each patient forced them to see fewer patients overall. Jennifer said, "I probably became slow as molasses because I just wanted to make sure that every patient had everything taken care of for them." Finally, unable to reconcile the conflict, she left clinical work entirely to devote herself to patient advocacy.

Some doctors did not feel instinctively communicative all of the time, and hence had to *force themselves* to enter the role of "the caring doctor." Harry described doctors' efforts to be empathetic as "playing" a part.

> Part of what we do is *play-act sincerity*. We are there to be sincere, but some is *playing our roles* as confidante and dispenser of wisdom, security, and hope. I did not ever think of that as part of my persona.

Yet, patients may occasionally have unrealistic expectations or demands for time. Kurt said, "At times, I would spend tons of time with people; and with some, it just never was enough."

Though doctor-patient relationships contain important elements of aura and magic, questions arose of whether at any point, increased awareness of this magic could lessen its effects. It may be important that the mystique of the healer not be entirely removed; but magic can be dangerous and misused. In *The Sorcerer's Apprentice*, failure to appreciate the responsibilities, burdens, and potential danger of one's magical powers easily renders harm (2). Presumably, increased self-consciousness about a physician's own placebo effect would not necessarily dampen it, but is there a point at which it might? Certainly, if it promulgates arrogance or misuse among physicians. But these boundaries were not always clear.

Unfortunately, these issues emerged against the backdrop of growing constraints on resources. A doctor may try his or her best, but patients may remain frustrated or disappointed. At times, consumers may set too high a standard—expecting doctors to have ample compassion and time—while wanting to pay the least possible for care.

Better Systems and Policy

These doctors had critical suggestions for improving policy, yet means of providing feedback to alter the system appeared scant. Nonetheless, even simple, low-tech alterations may be helpful. For example, taboos against physicians criticizing each other could impede improvements in care. Professional hierarchy stymied complaints or efforts of trainees, who were less socialized into medical institutions, and hence generally more open to, and sympathetic with, patient perspectives. Trainees observed problems, but felt powerless to change them. Repeatedly, potential benefits of a national health insurance system became evident. Needs emerged to improve informed consent as well. For example, Jerry felt that current policies and policy debates about how much information to provide to patients in order to obtain informed consent were not sensitive enough to the realities of clinical practice. "Lawyers don't realize that most patients don't want to know all the information. If you try to give it to patients, they'll tune you out."

Jerry and others saw needs for flexibility, and for improvements in education about medical ethics and law.

I had no idea what the whole legal doctrine around informed consent was, yet I was getting consent every day from patients. I was probably doing things ok, but not discussing enough detail.

Several changes were suggested for the *system* of medical practice. Eleanor, for example, said:

Medicine is a business, or would like to be a business, but doesn't play by business rules. I wish more bright businesspeople would go into hospital administration and cure these problems.

Administrative problems, like medical problems, require treatment. And policymakers and administrators would benefit from heeding more the problems with the bureaucracy and the physical plant that these ill doctors voiced.

Simon, the radiologist with HIV who refused audiotaping, saw a need to revamp disability insurance to allow doctors to return to work if they feel better, yet not lose their disability insurance. ("People should not have to leave medicine.")

Current policies also contributed to HIV-infected health care workers facing stigma and discrimination that impaired their lives, work, and care. Arguments have been made that a physician should disclose his or her HIV status to all patients, regardless of the procedures performed. Yet such policies need to be carefully considered since they can hamper the lives of these providers, causing stresses that can threaten the quality of care these physicians deliver to their patients. Policies should ensure the least possible bias against these doctors, and establish adequate safeguards to prevent discrimination. If these physicians can be offered as much support and the least discrimination as possible, they can be of even more assistance to their patients.

Strongly entrenched norms in the profession—that physicians have to "be strong," not "weak" or emotional—contribute to burnout, and hence should be reassessed and altered. Medical training would benefit from explicitly and proactively trying to ameliorate these problems, so that trainees can best prepare for, and remedy, these difficulties. For ill doctors, interventions can be designed using physician-only support groups; helping doctors' family members in aiding ill physicians; providing guidance and consultation on how to establish and maintain appropriate boundaries; identifying and treating mental health symptoms proactively (e.g., overcoming stigma surrounding physician mental illness); and assisting with consideration of, and transition to, other jobs. Local and national medical groups and societies (e.g., the AMA and local medical associations) should be aware of these intricacies, and can play vital roles, but need to tailor programs appropriately. Burnout and resistance to treating it can impair these doctors' abilities to access care.

Future research can probe the effectiveness of the techniques mentioned above as antidotes to burnout, examining their impact on patients' clinical outcomes as well. The profession needs to explore whether and how physicians can reduce workloads, how such changes can be maintained over time, and whether such efforts indeed reduce burnout, and if so, how much.

These doctors suggested other underexplored aspects of doctor-patient relationships and communication for further study: for example, how doctors' and patients' interpersonal dynamics evolve over time, what the costs and benefits of such alteration are, and whether spirituality can ever be better expressed quantitatively, and so, how.

Overall, these physician-patients increased their sensitivity to anxieties, difficulties with adherence, multiple personal meanings of tests, and nonmedical aspects of care. Many ill doctors sought to improve communication with patients, providing more time to address taboo topics such as mental health problems, sexuality, and end-of-life issues. Some arrived at simple mechanisms, such as charting at the bedside. But heightened sensitivity was not always easy. Hence, efforts to humanize and reform medical education must overcome several critical obstacles, from competing pressures on doctors' time, to physicians' instinctive responses to the interpersonal stresses and demands they faced.

Are these doctors setting the standard for communication *too* high? Will they encourage patients to expect too much? As it is, increasingly medical students are opting for residencies in which they don't have to deal with patients (e.g., pathology, where patients are dead; anesthesiology, where patients are unconscious; radiology, where patients themselves aren't seen; or ophthalmology, where doctors deal only with limited parts of patients' bodies).

I do not at all mean to engage in, or encourage, "doctor-bashing"—quite the opposite. The doctors here repeatedly impressed me with remarkable dedication and selflessness. The material presented here is what these doctors candidly said to me. Not presenting these data because they may make doctors "look bad" or heighten patients' expectations too far would be both ethically and scientifically suspect. Still, in the end, despite certain limitations, medicine and its practitioners embodied here extraordinary nobility and idealism in an era when these virtues are increasingly rare.

Some of these doctors wanted more spiritual connection, but felt they could not attain it. The positivistic scientific medical model led some to shun ambiguities, mysteries, and inchoate subjective experiences. Steven said, "I wish I were more spiritual," but he remained skeptical. Increasingly, evidence-based medicine spreads, valuing only the objective, the objectifiable, and the measurable. Medical training itself wounds in ways that can callous and distance doctors from patients, rather than heightening sensitivity and warmth. The threat of disease and death can also overwhelm doctors, who then minimize, avoid, or deny their injury, rather than acknowledge, embrace, and grow from, it.

Yet concurrently, the benefits of these physicians' own experiences with illness are not unalloyed. I do not mean to be a Pollyanna, touting the benefits of disease on medical practice. Clearly, personal illness can affect one in both good and bad ways. Empathy often, but not always, increases. At times, these doctors lost patience with those whose medical problems seemed comparatively minor, but who nevertheless complained, and failed to adhere to effective treatments. Most doctors did not go so far as to rebuke patients as did Nancy (e.g., saying, "You have the ability to make yourself better, and I don't"). But many of these physicians shared her irritation. They realized, too, the limitations of their field—for example, that medical knowledge does not wholly alleviate pain. From side effects such as nausea and weight gain, to pain and discomfort from lumbar punctures, biopsies, and feeding tubes, physicians often underestimated how much they *harmed* their patients. Doctors may tell patients, "Don't worry, this procedure won't hurt," or "will hurt only a little," or "just in the beginning," or "the scar will be nothing," "this is routine." Yet at times, such statements are simply untrue. These physicians are then giving false information.

Hopefully, these narratives will encourage physicians to optimize as much as possible the time they *do* have with their patients. Even if they have only ten minutes with a patient, doctors could often be more sensitive. *Physicians should at least be made more aware of the limitations they confront—from patients' perspectives.* Healers need to realize the impact of their constrained time and resources—how patients at the other end of the stethoscope see their treatments and providers.

13
Conclusions

The Professional Self

"What do you do?"

Perhaps more than almost any other profession, except possibly the priesthood, medicine compels its members to define themselves by their work. Novitiates endure a physically demanding and self-sacrificing apprenticeship, or process of "socialization," that deeply ingrains the values and identity of the field into its members. Consequently, as we have seen, the threat of losing their job can challenge their deepest senses of meaning and self-definition.

Their profession permeated their very beings. Generally, they had integrated their professional selves and identities, and now, when forced to abandon their careers, faced crises. As Juan quipped, "Once a doctor, always a doctor," even if retiring or no longer seeing patients. But they struggled.

These physicians illustrated the complexities, nuances, and subtleties of these roles and identities, revealing varying boundaries and conceptions of professional identity. Physicianhood emerged as potent, even post-retirement. The more they fought disease in patients, the more they were doctors, and vice versa. Even if no longer working, they tended to define themselves as physicians, an identity that appeared to be a complex amalgam of both "doing" and "being." Many needed to be doing something to justify still being a doctor in their minds. "Being" emerged from "doing," but took on attributes and a life of its own.

These providers illuminated tensions between different aspects of themselves—personal versus professional, patient versus physician—and how they bridged these gulfs. Deep conflicts emerged between the social roles they put on, and other aspects of themselves. While sociologists such as Talcott Parsons discussed the "sick role" and other social identities, the delineations between these roles and other aspects of oneself are not always clear. The individuals here put these roles on and off, often each day, in the service of personal needs, whether good or bad (e.g., aggressive self-treatment or denial). In some ways, physicianhood appeared as a role one put on daily at the office and did not always fully integrate into how one behaved.

But doctoring emerged here, too, not merely as a matter of education and academic degrees. Physicianhood did not constitute merely a socially constructed role. Rather, these doctors *internalized* the white coats they wore. Even when they were no longer practicing medicine, this career permanently stamped them. This identity became profoundly embedded, functioning at multiple levels and springing from deep-seated fears and desires that at times operated despite these individuals, shaping their views, experiences, and responses in the world. Not surprisingly, as a result, they generally at first resisted surrendering this position and adopting that of the patient. In diagnosing themselves, they frequently saw themselves as if they were a doctor looking at someone else—until the pain or symptoms overwhelmed them. Only then did some became patients. Over time, the precise boundaries between this role and identity shifted. Frequently, these doctors acted the part, and in doing so, to varying degrees, it became part of them.

Yet these physicians' responses revealed not only similarities, but also differences. We are each unique amalgams of social roles and individual psychological traits and quirks—products of our unique experiences. These individuals had varied personal and family histories, experiences, psyches, self-conceptions, and specializations (e.g., pediatrics versus psychiatry). For instance, Harry, in part because of his experience as a war refugee, believed there was a limit to how much doctors could alter external "other Forces." Deborah, Juan, and Charles grew up in Hasidic, Latino, and white Anglo-Saxon Protestant families, respectively. These backgrounds shaped their responses, too. Variations in personal histories and social and political commitments could influence individual "styles," approaches, and preferences with patients.

Nonetheless, as I have tried to show, as they moved from doctor to patient, clear underlying patterns cut across their experiences. These individuals often transcended, and at times rejected, neat categories. Deborah had dismissed most of her family's religious practices, though now starting to light Sabbath candles; Charles left the Republican Party after developing AIDS. Bradley was the son of an academic physician, and thus more committed than he may have otherwise been to helping those less fortunate. He started out more liberal than Charles, and grew up with a strong sense of social conscience, yet illness changed him, too. His depression prompted him to become more open to younger colleagues' perspectives, and to less biomedical forms of spiritual healing.

Psychological traits also shaped these physicians' responses. Inner sense of self and outward role molded each other. Dan, who had chest mets, had always been very assertive. Now, as a patient, he still "yelled and screamed" and got what he wanted. Juan, a gay Latino, had felt bad about himself growing up, and now clung to the role of physician as a key source of self-esteem, even as his disease worsened.

Illness itself could also modify character traits. Frank became more relaxed about his cancer after his MI in the OR.

Serious disease compelled these men and women to grapple with the most fundamental existential issues. All patients, not just physicians, wrestle with mortality, suffering, and pain. But physicians encounter death and dying daily as part of their job, and thus more than most others. They each developed their own responses to their patients' pain, finding stances or styles with which they felt comfortable, even if at times becoming calloused or distanced.

Through these experiences, holding on to one identity appeared easier than combining two or more. Reinventing or reconstructing oneself takes energy and creativity. Their institutions tended to see these individuals only one way or the other—as functioning doctors or as patients—and could not widen this conceptualization. Institutions wanted doctors to be powerful, unimpaired. They tended to see ill physicians first as still doctors, and then later as "merely" patients. For example, Deborah was told she had to be at rounds at 9 A.M., even if she was receiving radiation therapy. No exceptions would be made. Later, her institution would not even give her back voice mail, appearing to have written her off as dead. Institutions had difficulty seeing these ill doctors as occupying both roles.

In part, as a result, these doctors had trouble integrating these identities, as demonstrated in their puzzlement over what to call themselves when no longer practicing. Importantly, others played vital roles in how one structured and viewed oneself. Disease altered one in one's own eyes, and those of others. Forging identity emerged as a complex and *interactive social process.*

Through these journeys, these doctors became *wounded healers*, providers who themselves have suffered in some way (1). Anthropologically, certain other cultures and psychotherapeutic schemas value this category. Western biomedicine generally does not, but their experiences gave these doctors rare insights and wisdom.

At the same time, though these physicians integrated their profession into their lives to impressive extents, they did not always do so fully, as evidenced by their not taking optimal care of their health. Medical training, while providing strong senses of meaning, gratification, and self-esteem, did not necessarily alter their own health behavior for the better. Clearly, changing behavior, particularly health behavior, is enormously difficult; knowledge, even among medical school graduates, appears insufficient. Conflicting demands and desires—for Big Macs, "drug holidays," and unsafe sex—linger and have to be overcome. In addition, medical school teaches professionalism, but not self-care. Perhaps medical schools should give lectures on caring for one's own health. Still, it is unclear exactly what such a course would teach, and how effective it would be. Despite the adage "Doctor, heal thyself," many failed to do so.

These doctors raised broader questions, too, about professionalism, and how it may differ between diverse fields such as law, nursing, and the clergy. Do lawyers who get sued come to treat clients differently? Surely, lawyers do not always act ethically or legally—and they may view and make decisions about such transgressions in ways that both resemble, and differ from, doctors. A doctor diagnosed with a serious disease must struggle with fundamental crises of selfhood and soul, in ways that sued lawyers, though stressed, probably do not. Self-doctoring also has life and death implications. Compared to other patients I have seen, the force and bluntness with which these doctors often acknowledged their own mortality impressed me. Many were very matter-of-fact about dying—realistic and stoic in the fullest senses of the terms, accepting death as a part of life.

Through these narratives, *power disparities* loomed, about which these physicians provided unique first-hand perspectives. These doctors had, and now often lost, clout over patients and family members, causing stress, and challenges in redefining themselves. As these doctors now reflected back on the position they once had, they revealed key aspects of the scope and impact of their power: how it asserted, protected, and maintained itself. They conveyed its complexity, relativity, and ambiguity. As mentioned, in much of postmodernist and post-Marxist theory

(2), power is, essentially, wholly suspect. These approaches have responded to the fact that institutions (including the medical profession) have tended to be hierarchical, ignoring the relative impact of these power relations on those served (e.g., patients), and reflecting gender and race inequalities. The views of the disempowered are crucially important. Hence, much critical theory serves as a needed corrective. However, its implications could potentially go too far in certain domains.

The doctors here offer nuance to these understandings, suggesting some of these potential limitations, and thus contributing to discussions about these issues. These doctors were parts of larger systems. Physicians held much sway, but their power did not explain everything they did. Even prior to their illness, in some ways they felt weak—unable to change the system. Their level and use of hierarchy may vary, too, depending on several factors, such as specialty. Surgeons may be more likely to "blow off" patients, radiologists and pediatricians, less so. Other factors can shape possible interspecialty differences, including who is attracted to each of these fields in the first place. Hierarchy was entwined, too, with other personal and psychological issues and differences, and entailed costs. Status can impede optimal self-treatment—the profession and its hierarchy can jointly fuel denial.

Indeed, even when seriously ill, doctors often prioritized maintenance of their authority over promotion of their health. The effects of this hierarchy can extend widely in the lives of these individuals and their patients, colleagues, and institutions. Hierarchy can shape interpretations of language in doctor-patient interactions (e.g., definitions of time). The health care system facilitates and promulgates hegemony. Hospitals tolerate few dents in physicians' armor. Hence, questions emerge for further studies of *whether and when power differentials are legitimate and/or beneficial* in society, and how such determinations are to be made.

Patients here often *wanted* doctors to be potent. Hierarchy—intrinsic to the placebo effect, and hence to much of the healing process itself—can be used for good. As opposed to scholars who are wary of all forms of power, needs for professional fortitude arise here to abet the placebo effect and quell anxiety. Certain authors, from Aristotle in *Politics* to Alexander Hamilton in *The Federalist Papers*, have seen power as not all bad, depending on how it is used (3, 4). Removing the placebo effect and discarding its illusion may impede doctoring, making patients less well. These points may be controversial, but they have surfaced here and deserve more systematic inquiry. In all, doctors need to modulate their authority based on patients' needs, but may not always do so optimally.

These physicians frequently had difficulty fully integrating these divergent aspects of their identities, beliefs, and roles. For example, despite their medical education, irrational underlying attitudes persisted, such as fears of being blamed for their disease. Postmodernism suggests, too, a sense of discontinuities, of parts of the self that do not cohere (5). Proust portrayed people as each consisting of separate selves. In *Operation Shylock*, two Philip Roths wander about Jerusalem (6). We each have many selves. Some individuals more than others can live with seeming "negative capability," as Keats described it—"being in uncertainties, Mysteries, doubts without any irritable reaching after fact and reason" (7).

Toleration of ambiguity can vary widely. Many people feel compelled to seek definitiveness and unity. They may even ignore parts of their experience that do not fit into this schema. Yet randomness persists in individuals' lives. These phenomena have not yet fully entered into social science, but can contribute to forming the basis of new understandings of selfhood, professional identity, and mind in future scholarship. Suggestions have been made to build a new psychology of chaos, analogous to work on fractals in physics, probing such discontinuities, inconsistencies, and irregularities at multiple levels of an individual's life (8). The narratives here can perhaps help in considering and developing these approaches, elucidating the ways multiple identities can exist, interrelating and shaping each other. These doctors varied in the degrees to which they either integrated roles or resisted patienthood: in self-prescribing, self-prognosing, colluding with colleagues, and accepting their illness and mortality.

Yet the individuals here intimated, too, what I term a *"will to wholeness."* They strove to achieve a sense of cohesiveness in order to grapple with the experiences they now faced due to illness. They were not wholly successful. At times these disjunctions merely generated puzzlement, insufficient to render change.

Methods and Lives

Methodologically, these narratives can be viewed from diverse perspectives: psychologically, sociologically, anthropologically, historically, or linguistically. A scholar from any one discipline may focus on his or her own viewpoint. Humanists who prioritize the integrity of narratives may value each person's *story* told as a whole; sociologists may seek underlying *social structures*; psychologists may prioritize relevance to *psychological theory*. Yet human lives are messy and complex. Illness threatens not only jobs and power, but all aspects of one's life. Hence, to provide a sense of the whole, I have tried to integrate vantage points from these diverse fields. As such, these doctors shed light on approaches of, and interfaces between, the social sciences, humanities, and sciences. For each individual, a wide range of factors and experiences combined in unique and complex ways that narratives rather than quantitative assessments can limn best.

This analysis can add to psychological theory; for example, though theoretical literature has suggested that individuals either seek (i.e., "monitor") health information or avoid (i.e., "blunt") it (9, 10), here, some "monitors" change, becoming "blunters" at a certain point. At times, ill doctors who had eagerly sought information became too sick or too anxious to do so. Sociologically, as a subtype of the sick role, these physicians suggested that a "dying role" or "death role" may exist. The individual is no longer expected to get well, and others may distance themselves more, at times even starting processes of mourning and grief.

Similarly, though postmodern theory focuses on issues of race, class, and gender, the individuals here are often of the same race, social class, and gender, but still differ widely, suggesting how more nuanced and dynamic views of social construction are vital to understand the nuances of individual lives. Postmodernists and post-Marxists often fail to appreciate such individual variations, arising from psyche and personal history, that are critical in comprehending individual interactions within any one group or, potentially, dyad. These physicians' actions reflected not just hegemony, but other complexities of their lives. They posed questions about other factors that may account for differences between them.

To probe what we know and don't yet know about doctors, patients, and medicine today, and thus to arrive at the next level and generation of questions has been one of the goals here. Future scholarship needs to explore further these intersections of theories and individual lives.

Historically, these physicians' stories both resembled and differed from those of sick doctors in the past. To make sweeping generalizations about possible historical change over the lives of many individuals is hard. But some differences emerged. Since other compiled reports by different doctors, over two decades have passed, and the medical profession has shifted in key ways. For example, as one set of these earlier editors observed, the doctors in these books never mentioned payment or insurance. That has clearly altered. At the least, money serves as an additional hurdle and hassle these doctors now face. Heretofore, many of these physicians underappreciated their patients' struggles with insurance and medical bills.

But, though money has impinged on relationships, professionalism and trust persist. *Doctoring is still not yet merely a job.* Despite more HMOs, managed care, and shortened on-call hours, professionalism is still alive and well. In part, the processes of socialization and training remain arduous and transforming. Doctors continue to work with intense dedication and moral commitment, deriving an enormous sense of meaning. Many love their work with patients, who teach and inspire them in significant ways. Physicians' roles represent not merely desires for, or exercises in, power, but moral commitment. Though some other careers also reflect that, not all do. These doctors touch patients physically, and have unique closeness that transforms them. Many felt they did not have the right to give up the profession, to let people suffer.

These doctors also revealed critical areas that have been less explored in the past concerning how they view hierarchy, time, risks and benefits, their medical selves, spirituality, their own poor health behaviors, and collusion with providers. In the past 20 years, medical consumerism has spread, transforming doctor-patient relations. Yet concomitantly, certain problems voiced in the past persist. Despite improved treatments, mental illness (particularly depression) remains a sources of deep stigma and shame.

More than in past reports, concerns appeared here about confidentiality. Due to electronic medical records and changes in insurance, fears of privacy now loom large. HIV demonstrates how far these concerns can go, illustrating these fears in bold relief.

These narratives have broader implications as well. Their scientific training did not inure these physicians against irrational, nonscientific beliefs and behaviors. The degree to which "magic" and irrationality persisted in the lives of these scientifically trained doctors surprised me. They often perceived medical knowledge as overrated, and magically imbued. *Despite this age of ever-increasing scientific knowledge, magic endures.*

This phenomenon has several ramifications. America as a whole is becoming more spiritual; fundamentalists and conservative Christians have exercised political clout, spurring antagonism toward science among many Republicans. Beliefs in creationism and intelligent design, as opposed to evolution, flourish. The data here suggest that these beliefs cannot be fought simply with science. Rather, *mythologies and magic remain deeply ingrained in human needs and psyche*, and no doubt will always exist and prompt wariness toward science. Science is making inroads, but perhaps will never be able to rule wholly. Critics of the Religious Right may benefit from grasping as fully as possible the complex roles of magic and irrationality in the psyches of even scientifically-trained physicians, to understand the fears and psychological pressures that help fuel these beliefs.

Are Doctors Bad Patients?

Since starting this project, I have often been asked whether doctors make better or worse patients. Many people assume the latter. Yet in the end, I realized that doctors as patients are different—in some ways better, in other ways worse.

This question, though, raises others that are far more important: After all, *what is "a good patient"?* Is it indeed one who "leaves the doctor alone"? If that is the definition, at least in the minds of many health care providers, then numerous implications emerge for patients, families, health care delivery, and educators. Should other models be promulgated, and if so, what? For example, the definition of a good patient could be based in part on health outcomes. Yet, if that were true, "bad patients" might then merely be the ones who get sicker. Are good patients those who are more adherent? That view may reflect attitudes about the primacy of physician authority. Doctors may even communicate this expectation to patients. But patients who disagree with their physician are not necessarily "bad" (especially given how much doctors may disagree among themselves, for example, in aggressiveness or nihilism).

In confronting disease, these doctor-patients both resembled and differed from lay patients. Clearly, they have more medical knowledge than lay patients. The latter may "self-doctor" in certain respects; but only physicians can order their own tests and prescribe medications. Physicians may impair their own care, and be more difficult than lay patients in going "too far" managing their own case. Yet this phenomenon depends on the extent of the physician's illness and expertise. Self-doctoring can foster a minimization of disease, the sense that one can manage one's own problems. Hence, denial can promote self-doctoring and vice versa.

Ill physicians may be "worse" than lay patients in having the power and authority to compel doctors to defer to them in denying problems. Generally, if these ill physicians did not want to get care, no one in their family or social networks could push them.

Moreover, collusion occurred—doctors selected physicians for themselves to accomplish the same ends as self-doctoring, reinforcing resistance to entering the role of patient. But such collusion has received little, if any, attention.

"Good denial" arose, too, as a concept, representing perhaps no more than hope. Yet the demarcation between good and bad denial was not always clear: who determined it, how, and with what accuracy. Talcott Parsons suggested that doctors' functions are to "do everything possible" for their patients. These doctors pursued this standard for themselves, but were often *less able to do so for their patients*, due to financial constraints. This double standard needs to be appreciated more fully, so that if they wish, some patients can be offered choices of "riskier" treatments that doctors might ordinarily seek for themselves, but not for their patients.

These physician-patients found coping hard, and could benefit from enhancements in colleagues' and others' attitudes and available supports. Yet these physicians generally avoided support groups that help many nonphysician patients. Doctors don't want to be seen as "the expert in the group." The presence of a physician member could turn the group into a "let's ask the expert" session. But a network could be created of ill doctors who could offer peer support to each other. This could be done at least in part online, or through periodic meetings. Support groups of HIV-positive doctors, generally initiated earlier in the epidemic ad hoc and informally from the ground up, often functioned for a while, until members became more severely sick or died. Then, these groups tended to fizzle out. Nonetheless, such entities could be effective, particularly as doctors become older, to discuss these issues. Local medical societies could more actively support such groups and networks. Possibilities for such peer support, in part through local and national physician organizations, should be further explored.

Lessons for Patients

In the beginning of this book, I wrote of being depressed. After several weeks, treatment helped me, and these symptoms passed. But I remained profoundly struck by the oddness and "otherness" of that experience. It taught me much that I wanted to understand better, and thought might help others—both patients and providers. The experience radically changed how I saw what I and other physicians did, the wrong assumptions we made each day, and the width of the wall we build separating us from patients. We may sense what the experience of patienthood is like, but don't fully grasp it or its implications.

We try to incorporate what patients say into the terrain of our own worlds and words. In our descriptions of patients in medical charts, after the opening phrase—the patient's chief complaint (the patient's verbatim response to the question, "What brought you here today?")—we revert to medicalese. We need at least to be aware that our accounts and understandings are missing something that, at least according to the testimony of the doctors here, is vital.

These doctors had crucial lessons for lay patients: about how to communicate better with providers, realize that doctors are only human, set realistic expectations and standards, and understand the pressures and difficulties that even doctors face in the medical system. To avoid their own mistakes, many of these physicians wanted to teach other providers and patients. Patients need to be educated further—for example, about the benefits of adopting a *proactive stance*, and how to achieve that approach most effectively. For example, if these sick doctors found it hard to get second opinions, lay patients must face even more difficulty. At the same time, the intricacies of denial—its dangers—as well as the possible need for "good denial" or hope need to be further recognized and explored. The distinction between helpful and hurtful denial can be murky, but such ambiguity may be an inevitable feature of the human condition. Through education and reflection, patients can better understand the complexities of choosing a doctor, appreciating physicians' stylistic biases (e.g., as minimalists versus "overdoers") and tastes (i.e., partly aesthetic judgments). Patients can assess not simply whether doctors have good bedside manner versus technical skill, but also what mix of these traits might be best for a particular medical procedure and patient. Despite magazine lists of "The Best Doctors," the providers here questioned the notion of reputations, and even what the phrase "the best doctor in town" means.

The stories here can assist patients, too, in anticipating and handling more effectively communication problems that arise. Studies on patient outcomes and satisfaction rarely, if ever, assess *dignity*—the loss of which emerged as important here, and needs to be further investigated. These doctors can help patients to better see how to approach statistics, noting how easily these numbers can be misunderstood or misconstrued.

Public health campaigns and professional education can help in teaching and encouraging skills to promote such insights as much as possible. In improving doctor-patient relationships and communication, and the health care system as a whole, knowledge alone is not enough. Attitudes of physicians need to shift as well.

These doctors had vital lessons for professionals and trainees as well—specific ways to be more empathetic with, or sensitive to, patients. Yet obstacles arose as well in caring for patients. These doctors didn't always become saints; they encountered conflicting impulses and frustrations. Day-to-day, optimal empathy was hard to sustain. Nonetheless, their struggles can enlighten many.

Through this project, I have learned much. I was moved by the humanity and enormous generosity of spirit demonstrated by these doctors—their openness about their lives; honesty about their foibles, failures, and limitations; and commitment to medical ideals. Methodologically, combining narratives and integrating stories is hard. Presenting a meaningful whole that both reflects broader underlying themes and social structures (e.g., about medicine, doctoring, doctor-patient relationships, disease and coping) and does justice to these individuals and the coherence of their lives requires a fine balance. Biographies generally examine only one life at a time. Plutarch compared two figures at a time. Modern technology makes it easier to record and document multiple lives. Still, individuals operate as both social and psychological beings, and exploring themes across individuals' lives remains challenging, but I think provides rich rewards, as I have tried to show.

Vividly, I recall these physicians and my conversations with them. They inspired and moved me, and taught me much.

What became of them?

I have incomplete follow-up on several. I have seen David, a fellow psychiatrist, at professional meetings, and he is doing well, still wry. After I interviewed Bradley, we became friendly. He appears healthy, and not at all depressed. He successfully transitioned to half-time work, and is more involved in teaching and medical humanities. At one point, after coming across my name in the newspaper, Jacob called. He and his wife invited me to a Shabbat dinner. I politely declined the invitation. I sensed they wanted to persuade me to become more religious. I was wary, and also felt that my primary role with them was as a researcher. At a party of doctors, I saw Lou. "I have a vested interest in this man's research," he announced proudly to others standing near us. He, too, seems to be doing well. Suzanne has finished her residency, and is proceeding successfully in her career. Walter has started a new, second career as a political activist—seemingly despite himself, surprised at his continued health. "I'll keep it going as long as I can," he says, shrugging in typical modesty. "What else am I going to do?"

But others have fared less well. Nancy died shortly after I interviewed her. Now, at my university, all medical students each year watch a video I made of our interviews in which she shared her insights. Six months after I met Deborah, she phoned and left a voice mail message: "I happen to have a folder of articles about doctors who become patients," she said. "I was wondering if you wanted it. I could send it to you. If you're interested, leave me your address." I called her back immediately and left a message, saying yes. I recalled her comment during our meetings that she felt she was not preparing herself for possible death as she should by tying up loose ends in her life. One week later, I received an envelope containing the articles. No note. Two weeks later, she died.

Sally continued to work and kept her lab operating. I saw her once more, at a reception. She looked thin and frail. "I don't know what else to do," she said. Only at the last moment did she close her lab. When she died, her hospital mourned her death, and scheduled a memorial service in her honor.

A few months ago, when I was leaving for two weeks at a conference and then vacation, Anne called. When I returned to town, I was overwhelmed with work, and unable to phone her back for several days. I left a message, but never heard from her again. I have been afraid to call again.

Yet despite their disparate outcomes, they all left me with countless gifts—legacies and lessons. In their memory, I wish to pass these on, so that others may learn from them, too.

In the end, all of us—including doctors—will one day be patients. We may not want to fully realize or acknowledge that fact—to do so challenges our denial of death. But such realizations can go a long way in narrowing the widening chasms in our lives.

Not all doctors are, or will soon be, patients. But those who have been seriously ill themselves can inspire and teach others. Through their pain, these men and women arrived, often without seeking to, at insights that can potentially benefit us all—whether as providers, patients, family members, or combinations of these. I hope that through their words, each of us may eventually conclude, as did Jennifer: "My eyes were completely opened."

References

Chapter 1: Introduction

1. Jung, CG. *The Practice of Psychotherapy: Essays on the Psychology of the Transference and Other Subjects* (trans. RFC Hull). Princeton, NJ: Princeton University Press, 1966.
2. Klitzman, Robert. *A Year-Long Night: Tales of a Medical Internship.* New York: Viking Press, 1989.
3. Klitzman, Robert. *In a House of Dreams and Glass: Becoming a Psychiatrist.* New York: Simon & Schuster, 1995.
4. Parsons, Talcott. "Illness and the role of the physician: A sociological perspective." *American Journal of Orthopsychiatry* 21 (1951): 452–460.
5. Parsons, Talcott. "Social structure and dynamic process: The case of modern medicine." In Parsons's *The Social System.* New York: Free Press, 1951, pp. 428–479.
6. Foucault, M. *The Birth of the Clinic: An Archaeology of Medical Perception* (trans. AM Sheridan Smith). New York: Vintage Books, 1994.
7. American Bible Society. *Good News Bible,* 2nd ed. 2001.
8. Frankl, V. *Man's Search for Meaning.* New York: Pocket Books, 1997.
9. Lifton, RJ. *The Broken Connection: On Death and Continuity of Life.* New York: Simon and Schuster, 1979.
10. Malinowski, B. *Malinowski and the Work of Myth* (ed. I Strenski). Princeton, NJ: Princeton University Press, 1992.
11. Rosenstock, IM, Strecher, VJ, and Becker, MH. "Social learning theory and the health belief model." *Health Education Quarterly* 15 (1988): 175–183.
12. Prochaska, JO, DiClemente, CC, and Norcross, JC. "In search of how people change: Applications to addictive behaviors." *American Psychologist* 147(9) (1992): 1102–1114.

13. Houlihan, GD. "The evaluation of the 'stages of change' model for use in counselling clients undergoing predictive testing for Huntington's disease." *Journal of Advanced Nursing* 29 (1999): 1137–1143.

14. Hartmann, Heinz. *Essays on Ego Psychology: Selected Problems in Psychoanalytic Theory*. New York: International Universities Press, 1965.

15. Lacan, Jacques. *The Four Fundamental Concepts of Psycho-Analysis* (ed. Jacques-Alain Miller; trans. Alan Sheridan). New York: Norton, 1981.

16. Foucault, M. *The History of Sexuality*, vol. 3, *The Care of the Self* (trans. R Hurley). New York: Vintage Books, 1988.

17. Foucault, M. *The History of Sexuality*, vol. 1, *The Introduction* (trans. R Hurley). New York: Vintage Books, 1990.

18. Foucault, M. *The History of Sexuality*, vol. 2, *The Use of Pleasure* (trans. R Hurley). New York: Vintage Books, 1990.

19. Goffman, Erving. *Stigma: Notes on the Management of Spoiled Identity*. New York: Simon and Schuster, 1963.

20. Bok, S. *Lying: Moral Choice in Public and Private Life*. New York: Vintage, 1999.

21. Kant, I. *Groundwork of the Metaphysics of Morals* (trans. Mary Gregor). New York: Cambridge University Press, 1998.

22. Goffman, E. *The Presentation of Self in Everyday Life*. Garden City, NY: Anchor, 1959.

23. Starfield, B, Wray, C, Hess, K, Gross, R, Birk, PS, and D'Lugoff, BC. "The influence of patient-practitioner agreement on an outcome of care." *American Journal of Public Health* 71(2) (1981): 127–131.

24. Tulsky, JA, Fischer, GS, Rose, MR, and Arnold, RM. "Opening the black box: How do physicians communicate about advance directives?" *Annals of Internal Medicine* 129(6) (1998): 441–449.

25. Suchman, AL, Markakis, K, Beckman, HB, and Frankel, R. "A model of empathic communication in the medical interview." *Journal of the American Medical Association* 277(8) (1997): 678–682.

26. Selwyn, PA. "Prospects for improvement in physicians' communication skills and in prevention of HIV infection." *Lancet* 352(9127) (1998): 506.

27. Laine, C, and Davidoff, F. "Patient-centered medicine: A professional evolution." *Journal of the American Medical Association* 275 (1996): 152–156.

28. Stewart, M. "Effective physician-patient communication and health outcomes: A review." *Canadian Medical Association Journal* 152 (1995): 1423–1433.

29. Roter, DL, Stewart, M, Putnam, SM, Lipkin, M, Stiles,W, and Inui, TS. "Communication patterns of primary care physicians." *Journal of the American Medical Association* 277(4) (1997): 350–356.

30. Ong, LM, de Haes, JC, Hoos, AM, and Lammes, FB. "Doctor-patients communication: A review of the literature." *Social Science & Medicine* 40 (1995): 903–918.

31. Kaplan, S, Greenfield, H, Gandek, B, Rogers, WH, and Ware, JE. "Characteristics of physicians with participatory decision-making styles." *Annals of Internal Medicine* 124 (1996): 497–504

32. Groopman, J. *How Doctors Think*. New York: Houghton Mifflin, 2007.

33. Grant, VJ. "Making room for medical humanities." *Medical Humanities* 28 (2002): 45–48.

34. Meakin, R, and Kirklin, D. "Humanities special studies modules: Making better doctors or just happier ones?" *Medical Humanities* 26 (2000): 49–50.

35. Pellegrino, ED. "Teaching medical ethics: Some persistent questions and some responses." *Academic Medicine* 64 (1989): 701–703.

36. Shapiro, J. "How do physicians teach empathy in the primary care setting?" *Academic Medicine* 77 (2002): 323–328.

37. Burack, JH, Irby, DM, Carline, JD, Root, RK, and Larson, EB. "Teaching compassion and respect: Attending physicians' responses to problematic behaviors." *Journal of General Internal Medicine* 14 (1999): 49–55.

38. Tosteson, DC. "Learning in medicine." *New England Journal of Medicine* 301 (1979): 690–694.

39. Mattern, WD, Weinholtz, D, and Friedman, CP. "The attending physician as teacher." *New England Journal of Medicine* 308 (1983): 1129–1132.

40. Feudtner, C, and Christakis, DA. "Making the rounds: The ethical development of medical students in the context of clinical rotations." *Hastings Center Report* 24 (1994): 6–12.

41. Whitley, TW, Allison, EJ, Gallery, ME, Cockington, R, Gaudry, P, Heyworth, J, and Revicki, DA. "Work-related stress and depression among practicing emergency physicians: An international study." *Annals of Emergency Medicine* 23(5) (1994): 1068–1071.

42. Belfer, B. "Stress and the medical practitioner." *Stress Medicine* 5 (1989): 109–113.

43. Shapiro, ED, Pinsker, H, and Shale, JH. "The mentally ill physician as practitioner." *Journal of the American Medical Association* 232(7) (1975): 725–727.

44. Davis, DA, Thomson, MA, Oxman, AD, and Haynes, RB. "Changing physician performance: A systematic review of the effect of continuing medical education strategies." *Journal of the American Medical Association* 274 (1995): 700–705.

45. Charon, R. "Reading, writing, and doctoring: Literature and medicine." *American Journal of Medical Science* 319 (2000): 285–291.

46. Shapiro, J, Morrison, E, and Boker, J. "Teaching empathy to first year medical students: Evaluation of an elective literature and medicine course." *Educ Health* 17 (2004): 73–84.

47. Hulsman, RL, Ros, WJG, Winnubst, JAM, and Bensing, JM. "Teaching clinically experienced physicians communication skills. A review of evaluation studies." *Medical Education* 33 (1999): 655–668.

48. Sacks, Oliver. *A Leg to Stand On.* New York: Simon and Schuster, 1989.

49. Mullan, Fitzhugh. "Seasons of survival: Reflections of a physician with cancer." *New England Journal of Medicine* 313(4) (1985): 270–273.

50. Heymann, Jody. *Equal Partners.* Boston: Little, Brown, 1995.

51. *The Doctor.* Dir. Randa Haines. Perf. William Hurt, Christine Lahti, Elizabeth Perkins, Mandy Patinkin, and Adam Arkin. 1991. DVD, Buena Vista, 2005.

52. Pinner, Max, and Miller, Benjamin, eds. *When Doctors Are Patients.* New York: Norton, 1952.

53. Mandell, Harvey, and Spiro, Howard, eds. *When Doctors Get Sick.* New York: Plenum, 1987.

54. Stoudemire, Alan, and Rhoads, Marc J. "When the doctor needs a doctor: Special considerations for the physician-patient." *Annals of Internal Medicine* 98 (1983): 654–659.

55. Court, Charles. "British study highlights stigma of sick doctors." *British Medical Journal* 309 (1994): 561–562.

56. Donaldson, Stewart, Graham, John W, and Hansen, William B. "Testing the generalizability of intervening mechanism theories: Understanding the effects of adolescent drug use prevention interventions." *Journal of Behavioral Medicine* 17(2) (1994): 195–216.

57. Chappel, JN. "Physician attitudes towards distressed colleagues." *Western Journal of Medicine* 134(2) (1981): 175–180.

58. Ingelfinger, FJ. "Arrogance." *New England Journal of Medicine* 303(26) (1980): 1507–1511.

59. Fromme, Erik, Hebert, Randy, and Carrese, Joseph. "Self-doctoring: A qualitative study of physicians with cancer." *Journal of Family Practice* 53 (2004): 299–306.

60. Fromme, Erik, and Billings, Andrew. "Care of the dying doctor: On the other end of the stethoscope." *Journal of the American Medical Association* 290 (2003): 2048–2055.

61. O'Connor, PG, and Spickard, A. "Physician impairment by substance abuse." *Medical Clinics of North America* 81(4) (1997): 1037–1052.

62. Christakis, N. *Death Foretold.* Chicago: University of Chicago Press, 1999.

63. Klitzman, R. *Being Positive: The Lives of Men and Women with HIV.* Chicago: Ivan R. Dee, 1997.

64. Klitzman, R. *The Trembling Mountain: A Personal Account of Kuru, Cannibals, and Mad Cow Disease.* New York: Perseus, 1998.

65. Klitzman, R., Thorne, D., Williamson, J., & Marder, K. "The roles of family members, health care workers and others in decision-making processes about genetic testing among individuals at risk for Huntington's Disease." *Genetics in Medicine* 9(6) (2007): 358–371.

66. Klitzman, R., Thorne, D., Williamson, J., Chung, W., & Marder, K. Disclosures of Huntington's Disease risk within families: Patterns of decision-making and implications. *American Journal of Medical Genetics* (in press).

67. Klitzman, R, Thorne, D, Williamson, J, Chun, W, and Marder, K. "Decision-making about reproductive choices among individuals at-risk for Huntington's disease." *Journal of Genetic Counseling,* June 2007.

68. Geertz, Clifford. *Interpretation of Cultures.* New York: Basic Books, 1973.

69. Charon, R. *Narrative Medicine: Honoring the Stories of Illness.* New York: Oxford University Press, 2006.

70. Terkel, S. *Working: People Talk About What They Do All Day and How They Feel About What They Do.* New ed. New York: New Press, 1997.

71. Terkel, S. *Race: How Blacks and Whites Think and Feel About the American Obsession.* New York: Anchor, 1993.

72. Strauss, Anselm, and Corbin, Juliet. *Basics of Qualitative Research: Techniques and Procedures for Developing Grounded Theory.* Newbury Park, CA: Sage, 1990.

Chapter 2: "Magic White Coats"

1. Dewey, John. *The Essential Dewey*, vol. 1 (ed. LA Hickman and TM Alexander). Bloomington: Indiana University Press, 1998.

2. Woods, Sherwyn, Natterson, Joseph, and Silverman, J. "Medical students' disease: Hypochondriasis in medical education." *Journal of Medical Education* 41(8) (1966): 785–790.

3. Moss-Morris, Rona, and Petrie, Keith J. "Redefining medical students' disease to reduce morbidity." *Medical Education* 35(8) (2001): 724–728.

Chapter 3: The Medical Self

1. Aach, RD, Girard, DE, Humphrey, H, McCue, JD, Reuben, DB, Smith, JW, Wallenstein, L, and Ginsburg, J. "Alcohol and other substance abuse and impairment among physicians in residency training." *Annals of Internal Medicine* 116(3) (1992): 245–254.

2. Vegni, E, Mauri, E, and Moja, EA. "Stories from doctors of patients with pain. A qualitative research on the physicians' perspective." *Supportive Care in Cancer* 13(1) (2005): 18–25.

3. Gafni, A, Charles, C, and Whelan, T. "The physician-patient encounter: The physician as a perfect agent for the patient versus the informed treatment decision-making model." *Social Science & Medicine* 47(3) (1998): 355–356.

4. Schneck, SA. "'Doctoring' doctors and their families." *Journal of the American Medical Association* 280(23) (1998): 2039–2042.

5. Althabe, F, Belizan, JM, Villar, J, Alexander, S, Bergel E, Ramos S, Romero, M, Donner, A, Lindmark, G, Langer, A, Farnot, U, Cecatti, JG, Carroli, G, Kestler, E, and the Latin American Caesarean Section Study Group. "Mandatory second opinion to reduce rates of unnecessary caesarean sections in Latin America: A cluster randomised controlled trial." *Lancet* 363(9425) (2004): 1934–1940.

6. DiPiro, PJ, van Sonnenberg, EE, Tumeh, SS, and Ros, PR. "Volume and impact of second-opinion consultations by radiologists at a tertiary care cancer center: data." *Academic Radiology* 9(12) (2002): 1430–1433.

7. Staradub, VL, Messenger, KA, Hao, N, Wiley, EL, and Morrow, M. "Changes in breast cancer therapy because of pathology second opinions." *Annals of Surgical Oncology* 9(10) (2002): 982–987.

8. Newell, S. "The threat of therapeutic nihilism." *Journal of Pediatric Gastroenterology and Nutrition* 29(3) (1999): 237.

9. Bronson, R. "Detection of antisperm antibodies: An argument against therapeutic nihilism." *Human Reproduction* 14(7) (1999): 1671–1673.

Chapter 4: "Screw-ups"

1. Gilligan, Carol. *In a Different Voice: Psychological Theory and Women's Development.* Cambridge, MA: Harvard University Press, 1993.

2. American Medical Association, Women Physicians Congress (WPC). "Table 1, Physicians by gender (excludes students). Available at www.ama-assn.org/ama/pub/category/12912.html. Accessed June 26, 2006.

3. Lacan, Jacques. *The Four Fundamental Concepts of Psycho-Analysis* (ed. Jacques-Alain Miller; trans. Alan Sheridan). New York: Norton, 1981.

4. Braddock, CH, and Snyder, EL. "The doctor will see you shortly: The ethical significance of time for the patient-physician relationship." *Journal of General Internal Medicine* 10 (2005): 1057–1062.

5. Husserl, Edmund. *Phenomenology of Internal Time-consciousness.* Bloomington: Indiana University Press, 1964.

6. Sorokin, Pitirim A. *Sociocultural Causality, Space, Time: A Study of Referential Principles of Sociology and Social Science*. New York: Russell & Russell, 1964.

7. Klitzman, Robert. *The Trembling Mountain: A Personal Account of Kuru, Cannibals, and Mad Cow Disease*. New York: Perseus, 1998.

8. Ballard, DI, and Siebold, DR. "Communication-related organizational structures and work group temporal experiences: The effects of coordination method, technology type, and feedback cycle on members' construals and enactments of time." *Commun Monogr* 71 (2004): 1–27.

9. James, William. *The Principles of Psychology*, vol. 1. New York: Dover, 1950.

10. Light, D. "The sociological calendar: An analytic tool for fieldwork applied to medical and psychiatric training." *American Journal of Sociology* 80 (1975): 1145–1164.

11. Dandoy, S, and Hansen, R. "Tuberculosis care in general hospitals: Arizona's experience." *American Review of Respiratory Disease* 112 (1975): 757–763.

12. Roth, Julius A. "Consistency of rule application to inmates in long-term treatment institutions." *Social Science & Medicine* 20 (1985): 247–252.

13. Zerubavel, Eviator. *Patterns of Time in Hospital Life: A Sociological Perspective*. Chicago: University of Chicago Press, 1979, pp. 113–116.

14. Roth, Julius A. *Timetables: Structuring the Passage of Time in Hospital Treatment and Other Careers*. Indianapolis: Bobbs-Merrill, 1963.

15. Christakis, Nicholas. *Death Foretold*. Chicago: University of Chicago Press, 1999.

16. Francis, AM, Polissar, L, and Lorenz, AB. "Care of patients with colorectal cancer. A comparison of a health maintenance organization and fee-for-service practice." *Med Care* 22 (1984): 418–429.

17. Chin, S, and Harrigill, KM. "Delay in gynecologic surgical treatment: A comparison of patients in managed care and fee-for-service plans." *Obstetrics and Gynecology* 93 (1984): 922–927.

18. Mechanic, D, McAlpine, DD, and Rosenthal M. "Are patients' office visits with physicians getting shorter?" *New England Journal of Medicine* 344 (2001): 198–204.

19. Weeks, WB, and Wallace, AE. "Time and money: A retrospective evaluation of the inputs, outputs, efficiency, and incomes of physicians." *Archives of Internal Medicine* 163 (2003): 944–948.

20. Stafford, R, Saglam, D, Causino, N, Starfield, B, Culpepper, L, Marder, WD, and Blumenthal, D. "Trends in adult visits to primary care physicians in the United States." *Archives of Family Medicine* 8 (1999): 26–32.

21. Bogaty, P, Dumont, S, O'Hara, GE, Boyer, L, Auclair, L, Jobin, J, and Boudreault, JR. "Randomized trial of a noninvasive strategy to reduce

hospital stay for patients with low-risk myocardial infarction." *Journal of the American College of Cardiologists* 37 (2001): 1289–1296.

22. Every, NR, Spertus, J, Fihn, SD, Hlatky, M, Martin, JS, and Weaver, WD. "Length of hospital stay after acute myocardial infarction in the Myocardial Infarction Triage and Intervention (MITI) project registry." *Journal of the American College of Cardiologists* 28 (1996): 287–293.

23. Neutel, CI, Gao, RN, Gaudette, L, and Johansen, H. "Shorter hospital stays for breast cancer." *Health Rep* 16 (2004): 19–31.

24. Shabbir, J, Ridgway, PG, Lynch, K, Er Law, C, Evoy, D, O'Mahony, JB, and Mealy, K. "Administration of analgesia for acute abdominal pain sufferers in the accident and emergency setting." *European Journal of Emergency Medicine* 11 (2004): 309–312.

25. Tait, IS, Ionescu, MV, and Cuschieri A. "Do patients with acute abdominal pain wait unduly long for analgesia?" *Journal of the Royal College of Surgeons of Edinburgh* 44 (1999): 181–184.

26. Goldberg, RJ, Mooradd, M, Gurwitz, JH, Rogers, WJ, French, WJ, Barron, HV, and Gore, JM. "Impact of time to treatment with tissue plasminogen activator on morbidity and mortality following acute myocardial infarction (the second National Registry of Myocardial Infarction)." *American Journal of Cardiology* 82 (1998): 259–264.

27. Feddock, CA, Hoellein, AR, Griffith, CH, Wilson, JF, Bowerman, JL, Becker, NS, and Caudill, TS. "Can physicians improve patient satisfaction with long waiting times?" *Evaluation & the Health Professions* 28 (2005): 40–52.

28. Leddy, KM, Kaldenberg, DO, and Becker, BW. "Timelines in ambulatory care treatment: An examination of patient satisfaction and wait times in medical practices and outpatient test and treatment facilities." *Journal of Ambulatory Care Management* 26 (2): 138–149.

29. Thompson, DA, Yarnold, PR, Williams, DR, and Adams, SL. "Effects of actual waiting time, perceived waiting time, information delivery, and expressive quality on patient satisfaction in the emergency department." *Annals of Emergency Medicine* 28 (1996): 657–665.

30. Thompson, DA, Yarnold, PR, Adams, SL, and Spacone, AB. "How accurate are waiting time perceptions of patients in the emergency department?" *Annals of Emergency Medicine* 28 (1996): 652–656.

31. "Patient," Def. B1b. *The Oxford English Dictionary*, compact ed. 1973.

Chapter 5: "They Treated Me as if I Were Dead"

1. Robert, LM, Chamberland, ME, Cleveland, JL, Marcus, R, Gooch, BF, Srivastava, PU, Culver, DH, Jaffe, HW, Marianos, DW, Panlilio, AL, and

Bell, DM. "Investigations of patients of health care workers infected with HIV. The Centers for Disease Control and Prevention Database." *Annals of Internal Medicine* 122(9) (1995): 653–657.

2. Spielman, B. "Expanding the boundaries of informed consent: Disclosing alcoholism and HIV status to patients." *American Journal of Medicine* 93(2) (1992): 216–218.

3. Grace, E, Cohen, L, and M. Ward. "The public's attitude toward physicians and the card of AIDS patients in the state of Maryland." *Journal of the National Medical Association* 84 (1992): 681–684.

4. Aoun, H. "When a house officer gets AIDS." *New England Journal of Medicine* 321 (1989): 693–696.

5. Aoun, H. "From the eyes of the storm, with the eyes of a physician." *Annals of Internal Medicine* 116 (1992): 335–338.

6. Mitford, Jessica. *The American Way of Death.* New York: Simon & Schuster, 1963.

Chapter 6: "Coming Out" as Patients

1. Gostin, L. "HIV infected physicians and the practice of seriously invasive procedures." *Hastings Center Report* 19 (1989): 32–39.

2. Beach, MC, Roter, D, Larson, S, Levinson, W, Ford, DE, and Frankel, R. "What do physicians tell patients about themselves?" *Journal of General Internal Medicine* 19(9) (2004): 911–916.

3. Frank, E, Breyan, J, and Elon, L. "Physician disclosure of healthy personal behaviors improves credibility and ability to motivate." *Archives of Family Medicine* 9 (2000): 287–291.

4. Tinsley, JA, and Mellman, LA. "Patient reactions to a psychiatrist's pregnancy." *American Journal of Psychiatry* 160 (2003): 27–31.

5. Dilts, S, Clark, C, Harmon, R. "Self-disclosure and the treatment of substance abuse." *Journal of Substance Abuse* 14(1) (1997): 67–70.

6. Goffman, Erving. *The Presentation of Self in Everyday Life.* Garden City, NY: Anchor, 1959.

7. Bok, Sissela. *Secrets: On the Ethics of Concealment and Revelation.* New York: Vintage, 1989.

8. Nicholson, N. "How hardwired is human behavior?" *Harvard Business Review* 76(4) (1998): 134–147.

9. DePaulo, B, Kashy, D, Kirkendol, S, Wyer, MM, and Epstein, JA. "Lying in everyday life." *Journal of Personality and Social Psychology* 70(5) (1996): 979–995.

10. Gostin, L. "HIV infected physicians and the practice of seriously invasive procedures." *Hastings Center Report* 19 (1989): 32–39.

11. Anonymous. LRP Publications. "Court retracts mandate that physicians must disclose HIV." *AIDS Policy & Law* 14(3) (1999): 5.

12. Klitzman, R, and Bayer, R. *Mortal Secrets: Truth and Lies in the Age of AIDS*. Baltimore: Johns Hopkins University Press, 2003.

Chapter 7: Double Lens

1. Fox, Renée. *The Sociology of Medicine*. Englewood Cliffs, NJ: Prentice-Hall, 1989.

2. Seneca. *Letters from a Stoic* (trans. Robin Campbell). New York: Penguin, 1969.

3. Tversky, A, and Kahneman, Daniel. "The framing of decisions and the psychology of choice." *Science* 211 (1981): 453–458.

4. Shiloh, S, and Sagi, M. Effect of framing on the perception of genetic recurrence risks. *American Journal of Medical Genetics* 33 (1989): 130–135.

5. Gigerenzer, G, Todd, PM, and ABC Research Group. *Simple Heuristics That Make Us Smart*. New York: Oxford University Press, 1999.

6. Redelmeier, D, Rozin, P, and Kanheman, Daniel. "Understanding patients' decisions: Cognitive and emotional perspectives." *Journal of the American Medical Association* 270 (1993): 72–76.

7. Wertz, D, Sorenson, J, and Heeren, T. "Clients' interpretation of risks provided in genetic counseling." *American Journal of Human Genetics* 39 (1986): 253–264.

8. Kong, A, Barnett, G, Mosteller, F, and Youtz, C. "How medical professionals evaluate expressions of probability." *New England Journal of Medicine* 315 (1986): 740–744.

9. Grimes, D, and Snively, G. "Patients' understanding of medical risks: Implications for genetic counseling." *Obstet Gynecol* 93 (1999): 910–914.

10. Bergus, GR, Levin, IP, and Elstein, AS. "Presenting risks and benefits to patients: The effect of information order on decision making." *Journal of General Internal Medicine* 17 (2002): 612–617.

11. Woods, Sherwyn, Natterson, Joseph, and Silverman, J. "Medical students' disease: Hypochondriasis in medical education." *Journal of Medical Education* 41 (8) (1966): 785–790.

12. Klitzman, R. "Clinical Neuroethics." In *Neuroethics* (ed. J. Illes). New York: Oxford University Press, 2005, 229–241.

13. Elstein, AS, Christensen, C, Cottrell, J, Polson, A, and Ng, M. "Effects of prognosis, perceived benefit, and decision style on decision making in critical care." *Critical Care Medicine* 27 (1999): 58–65.

14. Eisenberg, DM, Davis, RB, Ettner, SL, Appel, S, Wilkey, Van Rompay, M, and Kessler, RC. "Trends in alternative medicine use in the United States, 1990–1997: Results of a follow-up national survey." *Journal of the American Medical Association* 280 (1998): 1569–1575.
15. Barrett, B. "Complementary alternative medicine: What's it all about?" *Wisconsin Medical Journal* 100 (2001): 20–26.
16. Barnes, P, Powell-Griner, E, McFann, K, and Nahin, R. "Complementary and alternative medicine use among adults: United States, 2002." *CDC Advance Data Report #343.* May 27, 2005. http://nccam.nih.gov/news/report.pdf.

Chapter 10: "Touched by the Light"

1. Daaleman, T, and Frey, B. "Spiritual and religious beliefs and practices of family physicians: A national survey." *Journal of Family Practice* 48 (1999): 98–104.
2. Hebert, RS, Jenckes, M, Ford, D, O'Connor, DR, and Cooper, LA. "Patient perspective on spirituality and the patient-physician relationship." *Journal of General Internal Medicine* 16 (2001): 685–692.
3. Christakis, N, and Asch, D. "Physician characteristics associated with decisions to withdraw life support." *American Journal of Public Health* 85(3) (1995): 367–372.
4. "Spirit," def. 2. *The Oxford English Dictionary*, compact ed. 1973.
5. "Religion," def. 1a. *The Oxford English Dictionary*, compact ed. 1973.
6. Hill, Peter, and Hood, Ralph, eds. *Measures of Religiosity.* Birmingham AL: Religious Education Press, 1999.

Chapter 11: "Us versus Them"

1. Fox, Renée. *The Sociology of Medicine.* Englewood Cliffs, NJ: Prentice-Hall, 1989.
2. Frank, Jerome, and Julia B. Frank. *Persuasion and Healing: A Comparative Study of Psychotherapy*, 3rd ed. Baltimore: Johns Hopkins University Press, 1991.
3. Parsons, Talcott. "Illness and the role of the physician: A sociological perspective." *American Journal of Orthopsychiatry* 21 (1951): 452–460.
4. Parsons, Talcott. "Social structure and dynamic process: The case of modern medicine." In Parsons's *The Social System.* New York: Free Press, 1951, 428–479.

Chapter 12: Improving Education

1. Gawande, Atul. *Better: A Surgeon's Notes on Performance*. New York: Metropolitan Books, 2007.
2. "The Sorcerer's Apprentice" (L'Apprenti Sorcière). Music by Paul Dukas. "Der Zauberlehrling" (poem by Goethe).

Chapter 13: The Professional Self

1. Taussig, Michael T. *The Nervous System*. New York: Routledge, 1992.
2. Morris, D. *Illness and Culture in the Postmodern Age*. Berkeley: University of California Press, 1998.
3. Aristotle. *The Politics*. New York: Penguin Classics, 1981.
4. Madison, J, Hamilton, A, and Jay, J. *The Federalist Papers*. London: Penguin, 1987.
5. Lacan, Jacques. *Four Fundamental Concepts of Psycho-Analysis* (ed. Jacques-Alain Miller; trans. Alan Sheridan). New York: Norton, 1978.
6. Roth, P. *Operation Shylock*. New York: Simon and Schuster, 1993.
7. Keats, J. *Selected Poems and Letters* (ed. D Bush). Boston: Houghton Mifflin, 1959, p. 261.
8. Robertson, R, and Combs, A, eds. *Chaos Theory in Psychology and the Life Sciences*. Mahwah, NJ: Lawrence Erlbaum, 1995.
9. Miller, SM. "Monitoring and blunting: Validation of a questionnaire to assess styles of information seeking under threat." *Journal of Personality and Social Psychology* 52(2) (1987): 345–353.
10. Case, DO, Andrews, JE, Johnson, JD, and Allard SL. "Avoiding versus seeking: The relationship of information seeking to avoidance, blunting, coping, dissonance, and related concepts." *Journal of the Medical Library Association* 93(3) (2005): 353–362.

Index

CPSIA information can be obtained at www.ICGtesting.com
Printed in the USA
LVOW07*1922130913

352419LV00006B/10/P